AF352408

Y OF U.S. ARMY

ISCHEMIA AND NECROSES
OF BONE

ISCHEMIA AND NECROSES OF BONE

by

R. Paul Ficat
Professor of Orthopaedic
and Trauma Surgery

Jacques Arlet
Professor of
Rheumatology

University Paul Sabatier (Toulouse)

Edited and adapted by
David S. Hungerford
Associate Professor of Orthopaedic Surgery
Johns Hopkins University, Baltimore

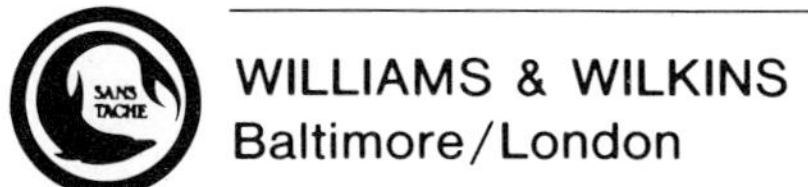

WILLIAMS & WILKINS
Baltimore/London

Copyright ©, 1980
Williams & Wilkins
428 E. Preston Street
Baltimore, Md. 21202, U.S.A.

Copyright ©, Masson, Editeur, Paris, 1977, Ischémie et nécrose osseuses

Made in the United States of America

Library of Congress Cataloging in Publication Data

Ficat, Paul.
    Ischemia and necroses of bone.

    Translation of Ischémie et nécrose osseuses.
    Includes bibliographical references and index.
    1. Bones — Necrosis. 2. Ischemia. 3. Bones —
Blood-vessels — Diseases. I. Arlet, J., joint author.
II. Hungerford, David S. III. Title. [DNLM:
1. Bone and bones — Blood supply. 2. Ischemia.
3. Osteonecrosis. WE225 F444i]
RC931.N43F5213   616.7'1072   80-10110
ISBN 0-683-03199-6

Composed and printed at the
Waverly Press, Inc.
Mt. Royal and Guilford Aves.
Baltimore, Md. 21202, U.S.A.

Dedicated to the memory of Dr. Dallas Phemister whose pioneering work formed the initial stimulus for our involvement in the circulatory disorders of the bone.

FOREWORD

The transition of medicine from art to science, begun as an evolution during the 19th century, has gained revolutionary forces—and unpredictability—during recent decades. The spectacular development of clinical chemistry, clinical physiology, and clinical immunology has forced clinicians into the laboratories and experimental scientists to the bedside. The normal and abnormal function of the thyroid, the heart, the liver, and the kidney can be described in precise numerical terms so that rational therapy can prevent gross destruction of form.

Orthopaedic surgery has participated less in this development than most of the other great clinical specialties. The virtual elimination of classic orthopaedic disease such as tuberculosis, rickets, and polio was an effect of scientific and general social developments with little or no contribution by the surgeon. It is true that orthopaedic surgery has graduated from sequestrated institutions for chronic victims of locomotor disease to become a full partner at the active city and university hospitals. This development, however, is more an effect of wartime experience, the rising toll of motor accidents, and the anatomic perfection of arthroplasties and less of deeper, scientific understanding of disturbed locomotor function. Indeed, chemical and physiologic methods are used in the evaluation of orthopaedic disease, primarily for the elimination of other etiologic factors than fracture, osteoporosis, and osteoarthrosis. As a consequence, the definition and classification of diagnostic groups in orthopaedics are still generally based on descriptions of form rather than measurements of tissue function.

Until quite recently, therefore, we have had to rely on radiographic evidence of gross anatomic abnormality to establish such diagnostic entities as arthrosis, osteomyelitis, osteonecrosis, primary bone tumor, and metastases to bone. By definition, the opportunity to prevent malfunction in most of these conditions has thus been lost already at the time of diagnosis. It is against this background that we must welcome the authors' ideologic conviction that examinations of bone circulation in individual cases have clinical relevance equal to traditional radiographic methods. In this book, they have documented their belief that radiographic criteria of orthopaedic disease can now be revised and augmented with exact preradiographic patterns of disease.

The authors look toward the future. Yet, their main message has a firm historic foundation. Until quite recently, radiographic sclerosis was interpreted as evidence that the bone was dead in osteoarthrosis, osteonecrosis, and pseudarthrosis. In all of these conditions, our therapeutic methods were, therefore, aimed at restoring the blood supply to bone. However, 20 years ago Trueta demonstrated that juxta-articular bone in arthrosis is alive, not dead. In the 1960s, Merle D'Aubigne gave tracer evidence of vitality in osteonecrosis. In the 1970s, it became generally accepted that the sclerotic bone in pseudarthrosis is an effect of frustrated repair processes. Radionuclide scintimetry has now established by non-invasive, clinical techniques that the sclerotic bone is metabolically hyperactive by one or two orders of magnitude. Consequently, our therapeutic approach to arthrosis, osteonecrosis, and pseudarthrosis has improved substantially.

Let no one doubt that it has been a formidable task to synthesize, in monograph form, the experimental and clinical evidence of the pathology of bone necrosis. This is a major work which should be received by the orthopaedic world with a curiosity that will, I hope, match the enthusiasm of the authors. In particular, the authors have presented a complex and puzzling problem in a form, linguistically and logically, which is shockingly new and yet is but another branch on the orthopaedic tree—this work reminds us that it grew first from French soil.

For me it is a great honor to write this foreword. I cannot help but speculate on one of the great driving forces in the international development of science—the subtle differences between national and local schools of thought. French medicine is not the same as Anglo-Saxon medicine. In this context, the names of Leriche and Phemister come to mind as exponents of this difference. Many hold language to be the decisive factor in maintaining the individuality of scientific subculture. I rather feel that general social conditions and educational tradition are more important in this respect.

One may read this book as an expression of the School of Toulouse, international, yes, but also regional, a team-work, yes, but with the provocative flavor of the individuals!

Monday, March 18, 1977
GÖRAN BAUER

EDITOR'S FOREWORD

It is the responsibility of any translator to convey to the new audience the meaning and intent of the authors he translates. A "simple" translation will seldom do. I have heard an Englishman complain about how "awful" an article was in a foreign language publication when such did not seem to be the case. I believe he was reacting to the form in which the ideas were presented, which was "foreign," rather than the content or its scientific worth. One has only to read any French medical journal to see that their style or "form" is much different from the commonly accepted form in English.

This monograph contains much which will appear novel to the English-speaking scientist. Ideas are presented and defended which have not yet been widely circulated in the English language scientific literature. In order to present these ideas in the most "comfortable" form to the English-speaking scientific community, extensive rewriting has been carried out so as not to present the reader with both "foreign" ideas and a "foreign" style.

Paul Ficat and Jacques Ariet have been working together on problems of bone circulation for nearly two decades. This monograph is a synthesis of their experience. In addition to the wide-ranging clinical and laboratory findings in many forms of bone necrosis, which this monograph presents, it also documents their refreshing approach to Orthopaedic problems. Nothing is taken for granted. The operating room becomes a physiology laboratory. Clinical presentation, x-rays, physiological parameters, and histology specimens are compared and interrelated. Hypotheses are constructed and refutation sought. It is an approach which seeks to expand diagnostic possibilities to the point where disease processes can be arrested or reversed. It is a much needed approach today for all aspects of Orthopaedics.

There is much in this monograph to stimulate controversy, but through controversy, criticism, and the construction and refutation of hypotheses, the truth may be approached. The Toulouse school has laid down the challenge.

David S. Hungerford, M.D.
Baltimore, Maryland, 1979

PREFACE

At each step in the diagnostic process of osteoarticular pathology, we are reminded that standard x-ray has significant built-in limitations. Routine x-ray can only give an indirect and late picture of pathological processes. It seems that both orthopaedists and rheumatologists are not sufficiently aware of this fundamental concept which at first may seem somewhat revolutionary but, nonetheless, is true for all pathology except trauma. From this awareness comes the recognition of a need to develop diagnostic techniques which can detect pathological processes prior to their radiologic manifestation. Such methods of exploration ought also to help us to better understand the pathophysiologic processes involved in disease. It is to this task that we have applied ourselves, seeking those parameters which could reveal all aspects of the pathological manifestations of disease and, particulary, the earliest reliable signs. The earliest signs usually involve a vascular component which may stem from the primary circulatory origin of the disease or which may be manifest at some point in the evolution of other aspects of bone pathology. The results of this approach are presented in this manuscript in a general form which we have christened "the functional exploration of bone circulation."

The manuscript is divided into three main sections. In the first section the fundamental anatomical and physiologic substratum of bone circulation are presented. This framework of reference becomes important because there are few reports which place all of the information in one setting, with the exception of the Thesis of Féry[139] and the Proceedings of the First International Symposium on Bone Circulation held in Toulouse in April of 1973. How can we understand the pathology if we are ignorant of normal function? In documenting what is known, what we seek to learn becomes more clearly defined. In spite of the distance of areas of incomplete knowledge, we have attempted to present a hypothesis of circulation based upon an integration of morphology and experimental physiology.

The second section details the methods of exploring bone circulation. The baseline method of exploration of the hemodynamics of bone circulation includes measurement of intrameduallary pressure, intramedullary venography, bone scanning with radioisotopes, and bone and bone marrow biopsies for evaluating the histologic changes. The latter may include synovial tissue and cartilage when indicated. Methods of exploration which will be used more more rarely include selective arteriography, measurement of bone blood flow, oxymetry, and thermometry. Each of these methods will become more developed in the future. Although other methods will undoubtedly be added, the ones available already offer us a wealth of information which has not yet been maximally exploited. The circulatory aspect of many osteoarticular disorders remains poorly understood even though systemic application of these methods would provide a much better understanding of common disorders. Although fragmentary and incomplete reports may detail certain aspects of bone circulation in relationship to pathology, no one has assembled all of the information in a complete way, particularly as it involves the early pathologic processes.

The third part of this manuscript deals with the application of these methods to human pathology, particularly in the realm of ischemia and necrosis of bone. We have drawn on our experience, comprising more than 800 functional explorations and a series of 136 patients totaling more than 181 hips involved with bone necrosis. In these patients the firm diagnosis of necrosis has been established, allowing comparison of the pathophysiologic changes in the evolution of disease. This series of patients is examined through the two aspects of a statistical study and a search for etiologic relationships. This allows us to completely develop the information which we have acquired in over 12 years of investigation.

Although this work more fully develops osteonecrosis of the proximal femur, the functional exploration of bone circulation opens the way for application to other joints including the shoulder, knee, ankle, hand, and foot, as well as the investigation of other diseases including reflex sympathetic dystrophy, arthrosis, Paget's Disease, tumors, etc. This investigation has allowed us to determine the role and responsibility of circulatory disorders in the evolution of other diseases of bone. We have, in this book, attempted to open a new pathway to the evaluation of osteoarticular disorders by demonstrating all of the information which we have been able to extract in its application. We look to others to add to and complement these investigations.

We believe that there are two important paraclinical methods of diagnosis of bone pathology which are complementary. The comparison of information from each, the radiographic examination and the functional exploration of bone, leads to a wealth of information. This approach can significantly change our specialty as we seek to uncover disease in an early, potentially treatable and reversible state, where previously a nihilistic attitude prevailed.

The authors would like to thank the members of the Department of Osteoarticular Pathology at the University Paul Sabatier, particularly those in the Surgical Section. These include Drs. G. Lartigue, C. Ficat, J.-P. Cuzacq, J.-F.Gourdou, and A. Ricci. In addition, we are grateful for the efforts of Professor J.-P. Géral, Professor Agrégé Pujol, Dr. R. Durroux, Mrs. M.-A. Tran, and Mrs. M. Thiéchart.

The editor would like to acknowledge the assistance of the Division of Audiovisual Programs of The Johns Hopkins University School of Medicine in the preparation of the English edition. Mr. Henri Hessels has considerably enhanced the photographic reproductions. Misses Terry Mack and Anne Yao, in overseeing the technical production, have greatly aided the completion of the English edition. The assistance of Dr. Antoni Trias, in providing a literal translation of the French edition, has been invaluable in the preparation of the authors' work in English.

TABLE OF CONTENTS

CHAPTER I

ANATOMY OF BONE CIRCULATION

INTRODUCTION

Bones, particularly long bones, must be considered as a composite of different tissues working together as a functional and anatomical unity. Bone functions in three vital areas. Firstly, the mechanical strength of the mineralized structure forms either a framework or a protection for the soft tissue organs of the body. This hard tissue is undergoing a continual process of renewal as well as responding to the changes of environmental stress. Bone also provides a constantly available source of calcium ions for metabolic needs, while the bone marrow provides for manufacture and release of the cellular elements of blood. These functions require an abundant blood supply, under strict neurohumoral control, adapted both to the various functional needs and to the different tissue elements of bone, combining to make an anatomical and functional entity.

HISTORICAL REVIEW

The study and knowledge of intraosseous vessels is several hundred years old. It can be reviewed as consisting of two distinct periods. During the first phase, anatomical studies on bone circulation were mainly descriptive and morphologic. Langer[263] was one of the first to describe the anatomy of bone circulation. Following his work, numerous authors increased the knowledge of the morphology of the bone circulation by techniques which are now well established, of which we will review only the essential characteristics. These investigations were carried out primarily on dead bone either before or after intravascular injection. The long bones of the lower extremity (femur and tibia) were most extensively studied. Most of the experimental work was performed on laboratory animals, particularly the rabbit and the dog. Products used in these intravascular injections consisted of dyes (India Ink, carmine blue, methylene blue, Berlin blue), heavy metals which were opaque to x-ray (lead oxide, colloidal silver iodine, barium sulphate, bismuth carbonate), and plastic materials (vinyl resins, methacrylate, polyesters). The method used to study these injected anatomical preparations included microscopic observation either with or without clearance of the calcium moiety (Spaltheholtz technique[422], microangiography, and corrosion). The injection of the smallest vessels, i.e., the capillaries, requires the injection of very fine particles sometimes smaller than one micron.

During the more modern period of study of the intraosseous circulation, attempts centered on recognizing a more functional element of the anatomy. This included documenting the location of vascular pedicles with their role in the distribution of the blood supply. The direction of blood flow was also studied. Initial research efforts consisted of studying the morphology of the intraosseous vessels in different experimental situations, e.g., following the ligation of a given vascular pedicle. DeMarneffe, Trueta, Ruthishauser, Brookes, and Rhinelander were among the names associated with this period of research during which time many useful facts were collected. The most recent period has allowed the study of bone circulation *in vivo*. The intraosseous or intra-arterial injection of radiopaque, water-soluble, contrast media followed by serial radiography or cineradiography has been employed for over 25 years and has greatly increased our knowledge of bone blood flow. It remains an important diagnostic tool. The most remarkable and original contribution of recent times was reported by Branemark[64] by direct intravital microscopy of bone marrow capillaries of the rabbit. His work is fundamental in uncovering the physiology of bone capillary blood flow.

BLOOD VESSELS

Any discussion of the vascular anatomy of long bones must take place in the framework of a firm understanding of the essential points of the functional element of that anatomy. Adjacent arterial pedicles are so profusely anastomosed that they are able to substitute for one another. In bone, there is no infarction because of the failure of a single arterial pedicle. The venous drainage network is of large caliber, insuring rapid emptying of blood delivered by the arterial tree. This is evidenced by the almost instantaneous appearance in the general circulation of a contrast medium injected into bone (less than one second). This wide open drainage system, providing for rapid evacuation, is essential in bone because of the semi-closed nature of the rigid, mineralized part of bone which forms a protective capsule for the hematopoietic elements. At the same time, it does not allow substantial changes in volume without producing dangerously elevated intraosseous pressures[265]. Since the marrow is largely responsible for the manufacture and release of the cellular elements of blood, its capillary and sinusoidal networks cannot be greatly disturbed without causing a serious threat to the function of the marrow. We will consider separately the three vascular components of the bone circulation: arterial, venous, and capillary.

ARTERIAL PATHWAYS

The arterial supply to bone is both rich and diverse. The numerous anastomoses only assume their final form after closure of the growth plate. The arterial supply can be divided into six groups of vessels designated according to their anatomical location (Fig. 1): 1.) diaphyseal or nutrient artery (1 or 2), 2.) proximal metaphyseal arteries, 3.) distal metaphyseal arteries, 4.) proximal epiphyseal arteries, 5.) distal epiphyseal arteries, and 6.) periosteal arteries. The given long bone, therefore, does not have a single arterial pedicle. However, the many different vessels can be placed in one of three systems: a.) the diaphyseal or nutrient system, b.) the epiphyseal-metaphyseal system, which is responsible

for the blood supply to the joint, or c.) the periosteal-cortical system, with multiple sites of entrance throughout the diaphysis.

Diaphyseal Arteries

The diaphyseal artery has a well-defined and constant anatomical course for each long bone. The canal through which the artery enters the bone (nutrient canal) is generally located nearest the most rapidly growing epiphysis and is directed toward the slowest growing epiphysis[49]. In its course through the nutrient canal, the diaphyseal artery gives no branches. Flow in the artery is regulated by a circular muscular sphincter[121]. Once in the marrow cavity, the diaphyseal artery divides into two main branches directed toward the two epiphyses. One branch obliquely continues the course of the main trunk while the other curves acutely in the opposite direction. Each of these branches divides serially, producing a host of parallel branches. The terminal branches of the diaphyseal arterial tree anastomose with the branches of the metaphyseal system. It is certain that either of the two systems can substitute for the other after a certain latency period.

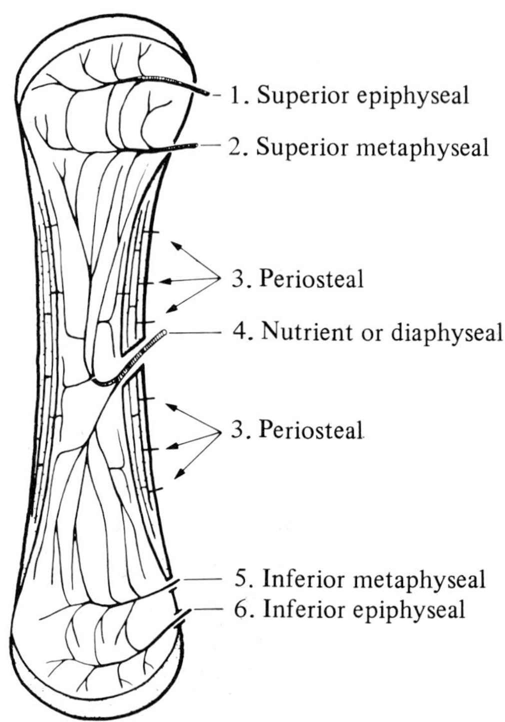

Fig.1.—Diagram of the arterial supply of a long bone with its six groups of vessels.

Beginning near their origin and all along the diaphyseal course, the two main branches of the diaphyseal artery give off transverse rami towards the endosteum where they anastomose to form an endosteal network. From this network, three types of cortical arteries arise (Fig. 2). The *short branches* penetrate to the middle third of the cortex. The *recurrent branches* penetrate only the inner quarter of the cortex before completing a 180° loop to return to the marrow cavity[65]. The *transfixing branches* traverse the entire cortex to anastomose with the periosteal vessels[71,359]. The nutrient artery supplies predominantly the diaphyseal marrow cavity as well as the inner third of the cortex.

Finally, the close relationship between the diaphyseal artery and the central venous sinus should be underlined. At times, the artery actually encircles the central venous sinus in a spiral, as described by Sick et al[413].

Metaphyseal-Epiphyseal Arteries

This group of afferent vessels is of the utmost importance, not only for the joint and its bony elements but also for the bone as a whole. The two kinds of

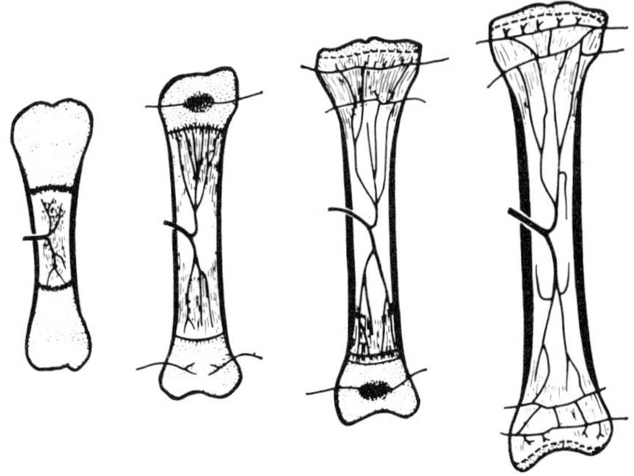

Fig.3.—Evolution of the arterial network with growth.

arteries, metaphyseal and epiphyseal, differ both by their point of entrance into bone and by their origin: The metaphyseal arteries are rami of the circulus vasculosus articuli of Hunter and enter the metaphysis through numerous vascular orifices. The epiphyseal arteries, in general, arise from the circumferential arterial network adjacent to the epiphysis, penetrating the epiphysis near the margin of the articular cartilage.

The epiphyseal plate represents the boundary separating these two systems during bone growth, although the barrier is not absolute. Certain metaphyseal arteries perforate the growth plates as has been shown by Trueta[445] and Tilling[437]. However, in the adult, the two systems are richly interconnected by abundant anastomoses, constituting a primary factor of vascular unity (Fig. 3).

Certain arteries destined for the epiphysis penetrate the metaphysis first, as is the case with the posteromedial retinacular artery to the femoral head. Metaphyseal and epiphyseal vessels can also arise from a common trunk, such as the posterior metaphyseal arteries of the femoral neck and the epiphyseal arteries of the femoral head, both coming from the medial circumflex artery[237]. For these reasons, all authors agree on the functional unity of the epiphyseal-metaphyseal system which constitutes one part of the articular arterial system.

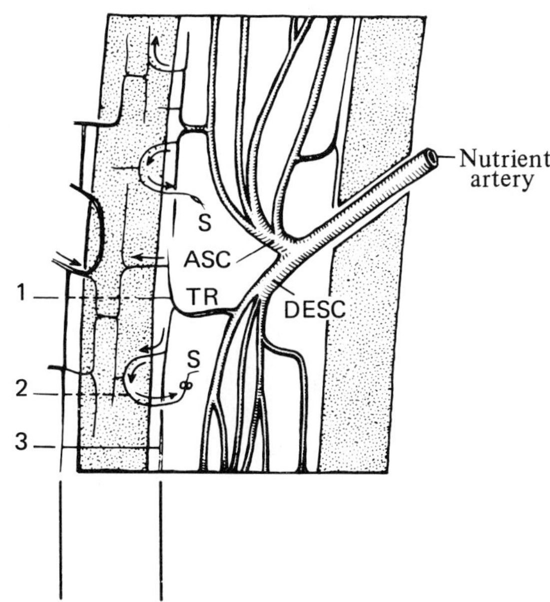

Fig.2.—Division of the diaphyseal artery into two branches with their cortical ramifications.

Periosteal Arteries

The periosteum is a well individualized and identifiable connective tissue covering which surrounds the diaphysis of the long bone. The outer fibrous layer does not appear to have any purpose other than to support and protect the periosteal vessels. The inner layer, which is in direct contact with the cortex, has an important osteogenic function[440]. The presence of an arterial network within the outer fibrous layer has been well documented. Annular vessels surround the diaphysis and metaphysis. These vascular rings are connected by longitudinal anastomotic chains. The vascular network is comparable in pattern to that encountered in other fibrous membranes such as the dura mater[75]. In its peripheral aspect, this network is in continuity with the neighboring muscular arteries, particularly in those areas where there is muscular attachment directly to bone.

On its deep surface, the network is connected to numerous thin-walled capillaries located in the osteogenic cellular layer of the periosteum. This latter network is itself connected with the intracortical circulation. Opinions vary regarding the morphology and specificity of these intracortical vessels. In the classical descriptions, numerous perforating arterioles arise from the periosteal arteries. These enter the cortex and anastomose with endosteal arterioles themselves arising from the nutrient artery. However, many authors, particularly Brookes[65] and Tillis[437], consider that only capillaries penetrate the cortex from the periosteum with no penetration of true arterioles.

VENOUS PATHWAYS

(Fig. 4)

The veins are more abundant in both number and volume than the arteries. The volumetric capacity of the venous system is six to eight times greater than the arterial system. The blood which enters bone may be drained either directly or indirectly. In the direct system, the emissary or perforating veins are without valves. They cross the cortex in a straight line to empty into the larger, deep venous trunks of the extremity. Most of the emissary veins are associated with arteries, commonly two veins per artery. The direct system consists of epiphyseal-metaphyseal veins and nutrient veins. At the proximal end of the femur, the epiphyseal-metaphyseal veins form four groups: two superior, ascending towards the hypogastric veins (gluteal veins and posterior femoral neck veins) and two inferior, descending towards the femoral veins, associated with the anterior and posterior circumflex arteries. At the distal end of the femur, they form horizontal rings which drain into the popliteal vein at different levels.

The indirect system consists of the large central venous sinus and its tributaries. This irregular afferent channel has very thin walls formed by a single, epithelial layer. A great number of venous capillaries or venules of short perpendicular course collect within the diaphysis which gives its characteristic

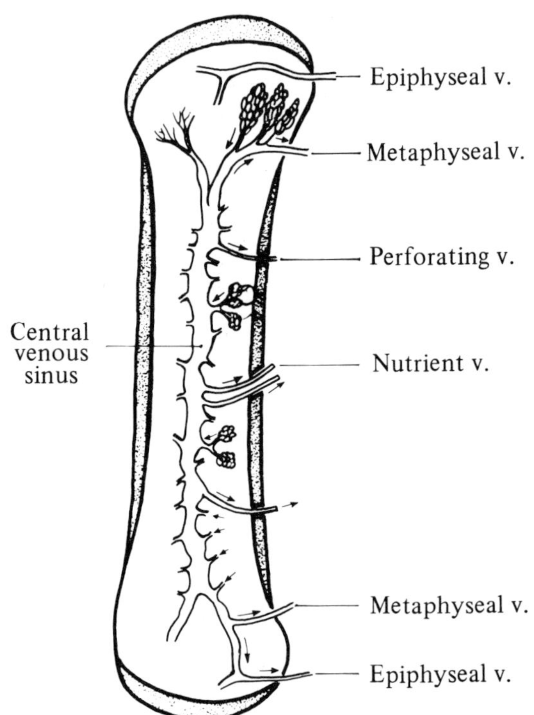

Fig.4.—Diagram of the venous drainage pathways of a long bone.

hairy, caterpillar-like appearance when injected. The large caliber and tortuosity of the central venous sinus is in marked contrast with the thin diameter and smooth walls of the nutrient artery. At the metaphyseal-diaphyseal junction, the central venous sinus receives several axial-metaphyseal veins which are more numerous in the proximal than in the distal metaphysis. The main drainage of the central sinuses is through the nutrient vein.

INTRACORTICAL VASCULARIZATION

Knowledge of the intracortical circulation is more recent, and its morphology is still under debate. The intracortical "vessels" travel through the channels which exist in the cortex, primarily the Haversian canal and, secondarily, Volkmann's canal. Classically, it has been stated that the Haversian canals have an axial orientation, parallel to the diaphyseal axis. In fact, we now know that they are oriented obliquely in the diaphyseal axis from the periphery towards the center of the diaphysis[68,94].

Trias and Féry[441], in a recent work on the adult femur of the dog, demonstrated the existence of two vascular systems within the cortex. The parenchymal system is formed by a regular network of capillaries which anastomose the medullary and the periosteal circulatory systems. The nutrient system of the cortex springs from medullary vessels which directly penetrate the cortex, being distributed in a radial pattern and subsequently dividing into equal branches. They are accompanied by satellite veins.

The diameter of the Haversian canals varies from 25 to 125 microns with an average of 50 microns. These canals anastomose with each other, forming, themselves, a real network. Although the larger canals contain two vessels, where some histologists have been able to recognize both vein and artery, most canals are narrower, containing a singular vascular channel of the capillary type and about 15 microns in diameter[71]. The direction of flow in these cortical capillaries is still under study and some dispute. Another characteristic of this cortical network is its constant remodeling, like the cortex itself. Remodeling of the Haversian systems requires vasculogenesis preceding and directing it. It should, therefore, not be regarded as a fixed system. The cortical vascular network provides an anastomotic system between the diaphyseal intramedullary circulation arising from the nutrient artery and the periosteal circulation. The importance of this connection becomes evident whenever there is suppression of the intramedullary-diaphyseal arterial system.

MARROW CAPILLARY SYSTEM

(Fig. 5)

The capillary system within the bone marrow is better understood and easier to study than the cortical capillary system. The pioneering work of Rindfleisch in 1880[363], Doan in 1922[122], and Sabin in 1922[381], form the foundations of our understanding of the marrow vessels. By his intravital microscopy in the rabbit tibia, Branemark[64] has made a remarkable contribution to our understanding of the dynamics of bone circulation in that he was able to visualize both direction and speed of circulatory flow.

There are three types of capillary vessels within the marrow: the arterial capillaries or true capillaries, the sinusoidal capillaries or sinusoids, and the venous capillaries or venules. Branemark has determined the relative size of these vessels to be 8 microns, 15 to 60 microns, and 12 microns, respectively. The arterial capillaries are easily recognized, as they follow a straight course and have an adventitial layer. They represent the last echelon of the arteriolar division, and they themselves redivide. They terminate in the sinusoids by an enlarged, conical, trumpet-shaped ending.

The sinusoids represent a unique element in the marrow circulation and are probably fundamental to bone marrow blood flow. The term "sinusoid" was first used by Minot in 1901[65]. The sinusoid differs significantly from the capillary in that it possesses no adventitial layer. The simple endothelial cells take on the form of surrounding structures: the marrow trabeculae, the marrow cells, and especially the lymphocytes. This explains the variable shape of the cells which may be spindle-shaped, ameboid, or hexagonal. It also explains the variable dimensions of the sinusoids which can be very large, dilated, or flattened and non-functional, "dormant[122]." The density of the sinusoidal network, which is profusely interconnected, varies considerably depending upon whether the marrow is active or at rest. Branemark confirmed *in vivo* that following bleeding the increased hematopoietic activity was associated with increased sinusoidal blood flow.

There are certain difficulties in determining whether an apparent space between two marrow lipocytes is actually a sinusoid with a true endothelial

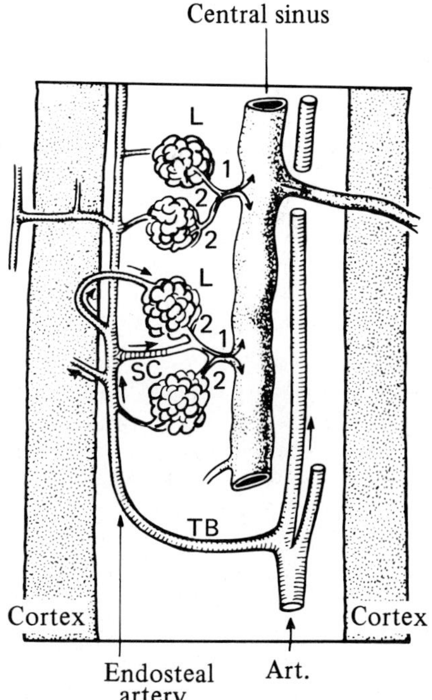

1:1st order venule   SC:Shunting capillary
2:2nd order venule   TB:Transverse branch
                         L :Lobular sinusoids

Fig.5.—Diagram of the intramedullary circulation.

lining. Even so, it is obvious that distention of these sinusoids within a rigid, cavity-like bone cannot take place unless other structures are reduced in volume. Branemark believes that it is the lymphocyte which adapts by diminution in volume. By observing the movement of red blood cells, Branemark observed that sinusoidal circulation can stagnate either by the cells simply coming to rest along the wall or by simply turning in circles in the sinusoidal network. It is possible that this relative stagnation is related to the manufacture of blood cells by the reticuloendothelial system present at the sinusoidal walls. Here one touches on the very important problem of hematopoiesis.

The venules are next in line in the capillary circulation. Several sinusoids are drained by a single, second-order venule. Several second-order venules then combine to form a larger or first-order venule which connects perpendicularly into the central diaphyseal venous sinus. In this manner, the circulation is distributed in zones. Each venule of the first order being responsible for the drainage of an arborization of profusely anastomosed sinusoids[134,143] (Fig. 6). There is, however, a second possibility for connection via a special connecting or shunting capillary[64].

Yoffey[470] has performed an important histological study of the bone marrow vessels from which the following points are worth emphasizing. There are two types of arterioles, one having a thick wall but short course; the other branches off the first type, having a thinner wall but a much longer course. Venules have a very thin wall of a single endothelial layer but with a lumen as much as 30 times larger than the neighboring arteriole. The sinusoids are permeable to blood elements. The polynuclear cells, formed outside the vessels, enter them by ameboid movement. It is thought that lymphocytes behave similarly.

INTEGRATION OF THE OSSEOUS CIRCULATORY SYSTEM

Diaphyseal and Intracortical Circulation

As we have indicated, the diaphyseal blood supply comes primarily from the nutrient artery and its branches. The periosteal arteries appear to play only a secondary role in the nutrition of the diaphyseal cortex. However, there is an important anastomosis in which the intracortical vessels integrate the two systems, insuring that either system can take over the nutrition of cortical bone should that become necessary (Fig. 7). Nonetheless, the understanding of this intracortical circulation is of recent origin and still the source of some discussion. There is not uniformity of opinion concerning the direction of blood flow in the intracortical system. Some investigators believe that the cortex is primarily nourished by the periosteal vascular system, either partly (the outer third according to Rhinelander[359]) or almost in its entirety, particularly in the young animal (Trias et al.[440]).

Brookes[75], however, believes the circulation to be centrifugal, since intra-arterial injection of barium sulphate into the nutrient artery fills the cortical vessels from within the marrow space. He believes that blood from the endosteal arteries flows across the cortex into the Haversian capillaries and drains into the periosteal and muscular venous networks. In this schema, the intracortical vascular network appears to be an intermediate capillary bed between the intraosseous arterial and the extraosseous venous systems. However, Brookes[75] himself agrees that, in pathological conditions, the periosteal circulation is

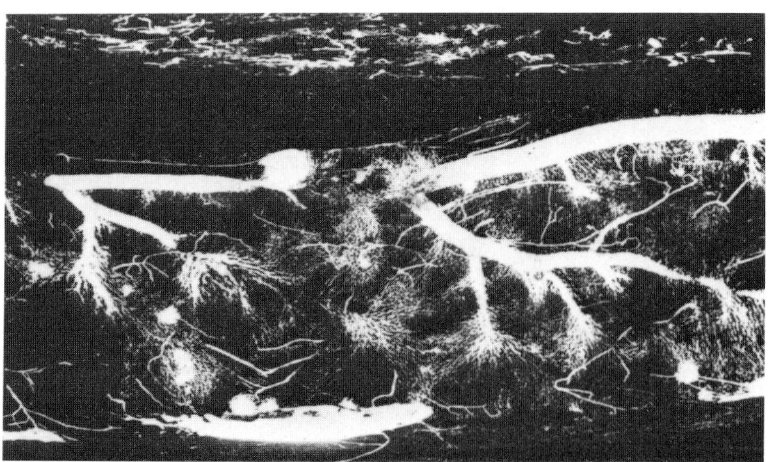

Fig.6.—Angiographic picture of the cortical circulation with its groups of sinusoids draining into a collector vein (humerus of a rabbit). Kindly supplied by M. Brookes.

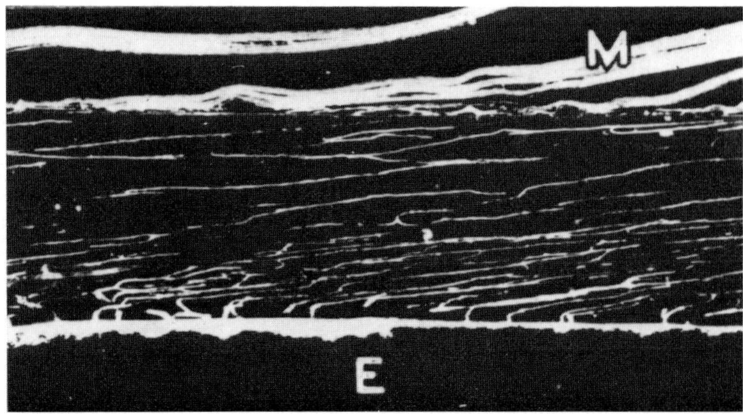

Fig.7.—Angiographic picture of the cortical circulation with its periosteal and endosteal contributions. Kindly supplied by M. Brookes. M: muscle bundle, E: medullary cavity

capable of compensating for deficient nutrient artery circulation. In this circumstance, it is presumed that there is a reversal of flow in the intracortical capillaries, which then would serve as an anastomosis between the periosteal arteries and the endosteal veins. Vascular neogenesis of periosteal origin is another potential compensatory mechanism. We would agree with Brookes that the intracortical vascular system is primordially formed by the Haversian capillary network. This is the functional circulation for the cortex, supplying both nutrition to the osteocytes and biochemical exchange between blood and bone. The direction of flow must be regulated by the pressure gradient between the medullary and the periosteal systems. This gradient may vary according to physiologic or pathologic conditions (Fig. 8).

The Articular System

The blood supply to the joint can be looked upon as the unifying system between the ends of two contiguous or adjacent bones. Such a unifying concept, concerning the blood supply, fits the fundamental concept of the joint as a functional entity. Two networks have been described. Firstly, the intermediate network represents the supply system which originates from the primary, large vessels of the extremities. It is made up of two perimetaphyseal circles of articular arteries. These two circles are united by a longitudinal anastomosis which crosses the joint line, thus forming an encompassing vascular cage. The second, the deep functional nutritive circulatory network, is made up of branches arising from the first system. These branches also travel in a circular peripheral route along the cartilage-synovial junction. This circle gives nutrient rami to the epiphyseal plate and the epiphysis itself, thus contributing to vascular unity particularly in regards to growth. This system was described by

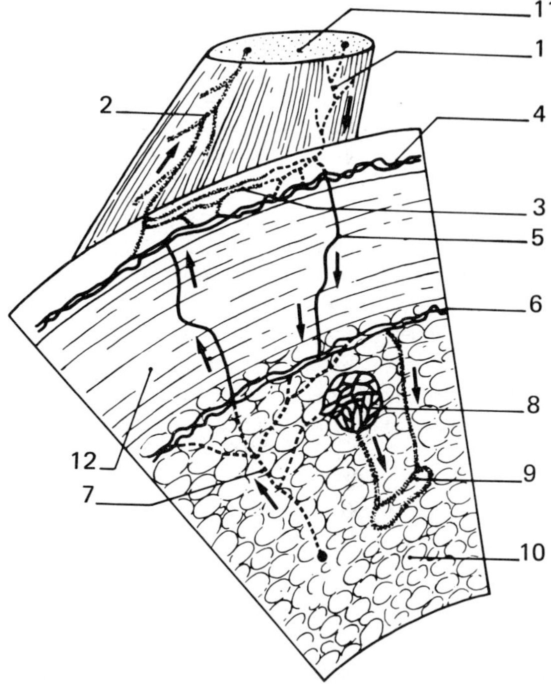

Fig.8.—Diagram of the cortical circulation with the capillary anastomosis between the endosteal and the musculo-periosteal circulation (transverse section).

1. musculo-periosteal arteriole
2. musculo-periosteal venule
3. superficial periosteal network
4. deep periosteal network (capillaries)
5. cortical capillary system, inter-connecting the periosteal and the endosteal networks
6. endosteal capillary network
7. medullary arteriole
8. cluster of sinusoids
9. medullary venous collector
10. diaphyseal marrow
11. muscle
12. cortex

Hunter[218] and later by Harris[197] as the circulus vasculosus articuli.

The anatomical delineation of the actual blood supply of the joint reinforces the concept of both physiologic and functional unity. This vascular unity plays a role, not only in the growth and development of the two adjacent epiphyses as they are molded to carry out their common locomotor function, but also influences the pathology which later involves the joint. This articular circulation can be schematized by the drawing adapted from Branemark[64] (Fig. 9).

Interrelationship Between the Two Systems

The vascular independence of the two bony segments, articular and diaphyseal-metaphyseal, even though each forms a separate system, exists only during the growth period. The epiphyseal plate closure brings about the interrelationship of the two vascular networks. The epiphyseal vessels develop anastomoses with their homologous metaphyseal vessels insuring, after the completion of growth, the continuity of the intraosseous circulation.

The metaphyseal region appears as a transitional zone between the epiphyseal and diaphyseal circulatory networks. Although the metaphyseal circulation is connected to the diaphyseal circulation prior to epiphyseal closure, it is more similar to the epiphyseal circulation in that both supply cancellous bone. The hemodynamic situation in cancellous bone differs from marrow circulation in the diaphysis and cortical circulation. Although it would appear that the metaphyseal system occupies an important determinant role in bone blood flow, this has not yet been worked out in detail as far as intraosseous hemodynamics are concerned.

LYMPHATIC PATHWAYS

This is a controversial subject. In the XIXth century, several German authors, especially Budge[79], observed what he thought to be lymphatic spaces around the intraosseous vessels. These observations, however, have not been confirmed by more recent works. It has been established that certain colored particles such as carbon (India Ink) and some radioactive markers have been recovered in the lymph nodes of the proximal extremity if they have been injected into the bone marrow. This implies that they have been transported from the bone to the lymphatic system, but it does not prove the existence of lymphatic pathways in bone.

The more recent works of Anderson[5] and Vizkelety[455,457] have demonstrated a periosteal lymphatic pattern on the surface of every bone but no intraosseous lymphatic pathways. The injection of In-

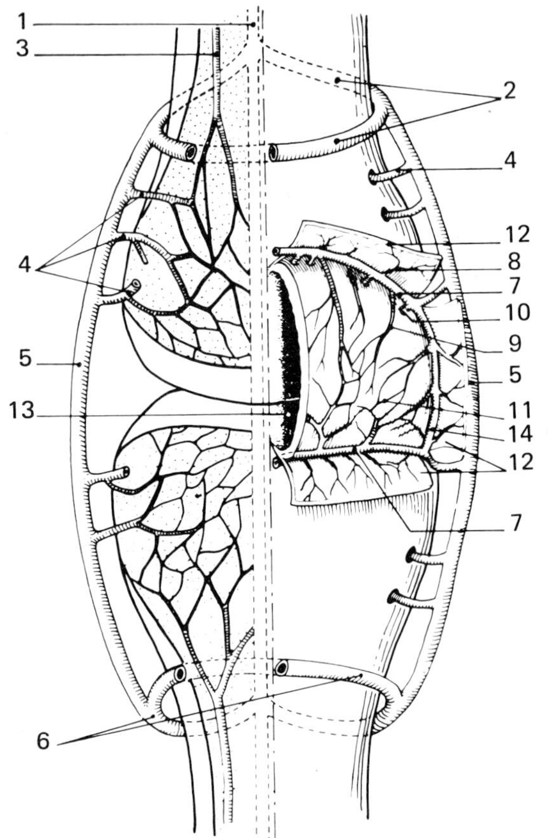

Fig.9.—Functional vascular diagram of an articulation. On the left: section demonstrating the intraosseous circulation. On the right: superficial extra-articular and subsynovial schema.

1. main artery to the limb
2. proximal metaphyseal arterial circle
3. terminal branches of the diaphyseal artery
4. epiphyseal and metaphyseal arteries
5. longitudinal anastomosis between the two metaphyseal circles
6. distal metaphyseal arterial circle
7. epiphyseal or deep arterial circle
8. capsular arteries
9. synovial arteries
10. bone epiphyseal arteries
11. synovial arterial network
12. retracted capsule showing the deep aspect of the synovium
13. articular cavity
14. anastomosis between the epiphyseal arteries

dia ink into the periosteum shows a fine network of lymphatic channels adjacent to the blood vessels, which join to form larger lymphatic channels before emptying into an afferent vein. When the India ink is injected into the bone marrow, the carbon particles accumulate inside the endothelial cells which line the vascular channels and inside the osteocytes, but no lymphatic vessels are visualized. Silver impregnation by an intravenous route visualizes a fibroreticular network surrounding vessels above a certain diameter, but fails to show any perivascular lymphatic space. Finally, experimental stasis produced by ligature of the femoral vein results in a dilatation of the extraosseous lymphatic pathways but does not result in visualization of an intraosseous lymphatic system. Although intraosseous capillaries become distended and perivascular edema appears, there is nothing suggesting lymphatics either in the marrow or the cortex.

THE NERVES OF BONE

More than a century has passed since nerves were first histologically visualized within bone marrow[191] According to Sherman[404], the first well-documented work is that of Variot and Remy in 1880[449]. They observed, both in man and other animals, nerves of 10 to 100 microns in diameter containing both myelinated fibers of 7 microns in diameter and non-myelinated fibers of 1 to 3 microns. These authors emphasized that the nerves were often adjacent to vessels, hypothesizing that they were either sensory or vasomotor nerves. Twenty years later, Ottolenghi[335] reported identical observations in human and animal femora and tibiae. He distinguished three types: one forming a network in the arterial walls between the media and the adventitia, the second surrounding capillaries, and the third type terminating in the parenchyma. DeCastro[84] finally demonstrated the presence of delicate, annular nerve endings around the parenchymal cells of the marrow and around the osteoblasts in contact with the endosteum. In a series of experiments using selective degeneration of nerve fibers, Kuntz and Richins[259] determined the nature and function of various nerve fibers present in bone. The efferent fibers, essentially non-myelinated and from the sympathetic system, were perivascular and vasoconstrictive in function. The afferent myelinated fibers also form a peri-

vascular network from which individual fibers go into the parenchyma, some of which are sensory conductors. The same authors attribute a third function to the nerves of bone marrow, that of stimulation and regulation of hematopoiesis. Foa[163] also agrees with these functions of the nerves within bone marrow.

Other works have shown the existence of a perisinusoidal plexis (Bohr, 1945 sited by Branemark[65]). Cooper[97] demonstrated non-myelinated fibers in intimate association with the vessels in the Haversian canals of cortical bone. Bohr believes that the central nervous control of the medullary circulatory system lay in the wall of the third ventricle at the level of the paraventricular and thalamic nuclei.

Weiss and Root[461], the general review of Serratrice and Eisinger[388], and others have contributed to our understanding of the role of the sympathetic nervous system in the control of erythropoiesis. They traced the sympathetic fibers from bone marrow through the peripheral nerves, to the main nerve supply to the extremity, and to the sciatic nerve in the case of the femur and tibia. It is possible that the control of the release of red blood cells from the marrow is regulated by vasoconstriction of the intramedullary arteries. Certainly, the control of intraosseous flow is by means of vasomotor fibers surrounding the vessels. Branemark[64] was able to observe, directly, *in vivo*, the slowing of blood flow and vasoconstriction brought about by electrical stimulation of the lumbar sympathetic plexis. He noted that the effect was less noticeable in the cortical circulation. A similar phenomenon was observed after the injection of adrenalin into the nutrient artery while the administration of a sympathetic blocking agent immediately accelerated intraosseous flow.

The facts, which we have reviewed, emphasize the complexity and vitality of the bone marrow which is both richly vascularized and innervated. There is a close interaction between the bone marrow, with its hematopoietic function, and the calcified tissue which encloses and protects it, acting, as Branemark notes, as its capsule[65].

CHAPTER II

THE PHYSIOLOGY OF BONE CIRCULATION

INTRODUCTION

The intraosseous circulation has not been well understood for two reasons; firstly, the complex nature of the organ system itself, and secondly, the inadequacy of methods of investigation. Because the connections to the body are multiple and complex. Bone as an organ cannot be isolated for study as other soft tissue organs. Furthermore, the multiplicity of afferent and efferent vessels and the absence of a single vascular pedicle considerably hinder the study of blood flow. Even with the recent addition of radioactive tracers, methods of exploration are either difficult to apply or of doubtful reliability. These factors account for the late start in physiological studies on bone circulation. Two groups of pioneer workers deserve credit for beginning the study of the dynamics of bone blood flow. Drinker and Drinker[123], in 1916, perfused the nutrient artery of the dog's tibia, demonstrating neurovascular control of osseous blood flow. It was more than twenty years later (1938) when Larsen[265] demonstrated the effect of vasoactive drugs on intramedullary pressure and, at the same time, made the important observation of the ischemic role of increased intramedullary pressure (IMP). One may wonder why these pioneering and remarkable studies did not have a stronger impact among the specialists of bone pathology. At the time that these experiments were carried out, they seemed to have little direct application to human pathology. Moreover, many believed the measurement of intramedullary pressure (IMP) was not a reliable parameter, and that methods of measuring blood flow were more complex and, at the time, inadequate. We undertook to re-evaluate the proposed methods and to apply them to investigation of human intraosseous circulation, comparing the findings with clinical and radiological data. For this reason, a large portion of this chapter is devoted to the practical aspect of available investigational techniques and to the results observed on man.

INTRAMEDULLARY PRESSURE

GENERAL CONSIDERATIONS

When a trocar is introduced into the bone marrow space and is connected to a manometer, a positive pressure can be recorded. We prefer the term intramedullary pressure (IMP), as also used by Arnoldi[26]. Shim[411] has used the term "marrow cavity pressure of bone," which is a more precise term than intraosseous pressure (Azuma[32]), since this recording is not taken within the mineralized tissue. The term "bone marrow pressure" is also used, but we feel it is too precise a term for the usual investigational conditions. The needle is usually somewhere within the heterogeneous medullary tissue. It is, in fact, a tissue or interstitial pressure but is not the exact pressure exerted by the bone marrow tissue as a whole as thought by Held and Thron[201]. These latter authors placed the tip of the needle on the surface of the bone marrow just at the endosteum, thus measuring "the tissue pressure of bone marrow." Wilkes and Visscher[466] also measure this medullary pressure proper by placing a tonometer in contact with the endosteum. However, this technique is too complex to be adapted to human investigation (Fig. 10).

In Chapter III, we will describe in detail the technique for measuring intramedullary pressure. However, before discussing the physiological factors which affect this pressure, it is useful to consider four practical matters concerning its measurement.

1. Since there is a positive pressure within bone, the outershell (cortex) is under pressure. Any perforation of this shell brings an immediate fall in pressure. Therefore, in measuring intramedullary pressure, there must be a water-tight fit at the outer cortex to avoid leakage.

2. The transmission of intramedullary pressure as registered in a manometer is sometimes artifactually low because of obstruction of the lumen of the trocar by blood clot or tissue fragments. This can be partly avoided by filling the trocar and cannulae with heparinized saline (50 mg/100 ml).

3. Because of the heterogeneity of the intramedullary tissue, it may be argued that the tip of the needle may be placed in a variable and unpredictable tissue environment from one examination to another. In fact, in normal cancellous bone, it is not possible for the tip of the needle to be completely buried in a bone trabecula or in the lumen of a vessel as the opening of the needle is too large for such an occurrence. On the

other hand, the needle can be partially obstructed by a fragment of bone which can be moved with an obturator stylus.The tip of the needle could also be in contact with an intraosseous arteriole which would then register a higher pressure than a true tissue pressure. Probably what happens more frequently, as reported by Polster[348], is that a vascular injury is produced by the needle tip with the production of a small hematoma around the tip, resulting in artificial elevation of intramedullary pressure due both to local distension and to the transmission by this fluid medium of the neighboring arteriolar pressure.

These facts probably account for the lack of immediate IMP stability in the first few seconds or minutes. The IMP sometimes rises slowly but more frequently descends to a plateau from the initial pressure. However, in all cases, in less than five minutes, the monitored IMP reaches a stable, relatively fixed value which lasts for the duration of the investigation. This fundamental point, which allows the IMP measurement to be clinically useful, has been confirmed by most authors who use our techniques.

4. Ideally, these measurements should be carried out under the best physiologic conditions, particulary avoiding general anesthesia, as this increases intramedullary pressure, according to Petrakis[342]. This is difficult to accomplish in animal experimentation but on the other hand is quite easy in man, using local anesthesia.

NORMAL VALUES
OF INTRAMEDULLARY PRESSURE

IMP in the Laboratory Animal

Table I summarizes the main data in this field taken from the literature. The dog, cat, and rabbit have been primarily investigated. The long bones of the extremity have been most frequently investigated, and the femur, tibia, and humerus have been studied in descending order of frequency. The pressure was recorded most frequently in the diaphysis, i.e., the medullary cavity of bone, but has also been recorded in the metaphysis and epiphysis, i.e., the marrow of the cancellous bone. The diversity of values recorded by different authors is alarming with measurements from 0 to 120 mm Hg. It must be noted, however, that most reports (with the exception of Azuma[32]) report the range of values and sometimes the average but not all of the measurements obtained. Unfortunately, this does not allow plotting of a frequency curve. In viewing

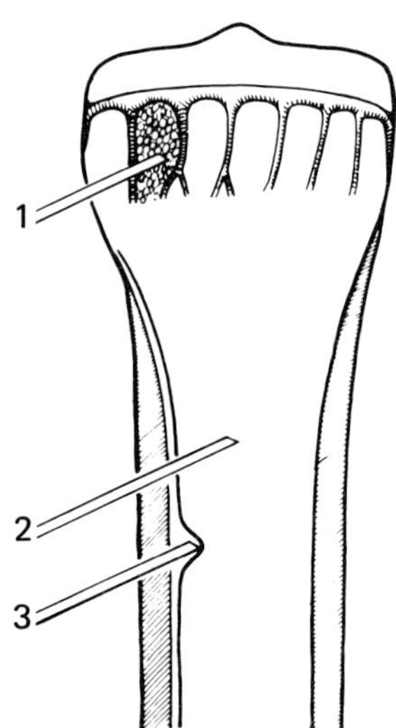

Fig.10.—Diagram showing the different sites for taking intramedullary pressures.
1. Pressure in the epiphyseal or metaphyseal marrow (IMP)
2. Pressure in the diaphyseal marrow or the medullary cavity.
3. Tissue pressure, strictly speaking (Held and Thron).

TABLE I

IMP–EXPERIMENTAL ANIMAL

Date	Author	Animal	Bone	Region	Range of measurements mm Hg	Mean
1938	Larsen	Dog	Femur	Inferior metaphysis	30–40	
1951	Kalser et al.	Dog	Femur	Diaphysis		41 Diast. 52 Syst.
1952	Bloomenthal et al.	Dog	Femur	Diaphysis	20–115	50
1957	Stein et al.	Adult dog	Femur	Diaphysis		32 (max.)
				Inferior epiphysis		18.8 (max.)
		Adult dog	Tibia	Diaphysis		51.7 (max.)
				Superior epiphysis		12 (max.)
1959	Herzig et al.	Cat	Femur	Diaphysis	24–114	
1959	Weiss et al.	Dog	Femur	Diaphysis	75–90	
1963	Shaw	Cat	Femur	Diaphysis		37 syst.
1964	Azuma	Adult rabbit	Tibia	Diaphysis Epiphysis	4–70	10 to 30 (60% of cases)
1964	Cuthbertson et al.	Dog	Tibia Humerus	Diaphysis	2–182 cm H_2O	
1972	Shim et al.	Dog Rabbit	Femur Tibia	Diaphysis Diaphysis	40–120 20–60	

the diversity of this data, it is tempting to conclude with Polster[348] that IMP is not reliable, either because it is too labile to be meaningful or because measurement methods are inadequate. However, we have seen that the causes of technical error are few but easy to understand and to avoid. Even under experimental conditions, those who have used IMP have not had trouble with the stability of the pressure measurement at any given point during the period of investigation. Shim[41] noted that "the IMP is remarkably constant during the control period." Held and Thron[201] emphasized that "the homogeneity of the results in all of the investigations indicate that the measured pressure is determined by anatomical and physiological conditions which are sufficiently constant."

It is necessary to try to understand the reasons behind the large range of values in laboratory animals. First of all, pressure distribution curves must be determined. Azuma[32], working on the anesthetized rabbit, noted that 60% of the pressure measurements in the tibia ranged from 10 to 30 mm Hg. The range of recorded pressures appears to be larger in the dog than in the rabbit. Age and possible diseases in the animals have to be taken into account,

particularly with dogs which tend to be old and in ill health. It is also important to emphasize that the IMP varies with the animal, the bone examined, and even the region examined. Specifically, the IMP is not the same in the diaphysis, metaphysis, and epiphysis. This relative independence of the IMP demonstrates the relative independence of regional circulation within a given bone. In this respect, however, there is some confusion in the literature, since the gradient of pressure between diaphysis, metaphysis, and epiphysis is not always recorded as being in the same direction. Stein et al.[423], working on the femur and tibia in the adult dog, and Azuma[32], in the adult rabbit, recorded diaphyseal pressures higher than epiphyseal pressures. However, Shim et al.[410] reported unequal diaphyseal and metaphyseal pressures without constant relationship. Cuthbertson et al.[109] recorded metaphyseal pressures higher than diaphyseal pressures, while Michelsen[312] recorded distal metaphyseal pressures higher than proximal metaphyseal pressures (in the rabbit). Our own observations in man correspond to those of Cuthbertson.

Since the IMP is influenced by both the sympathetic nervous system and vasoactive agents, as well as by local conditions of oxygenation and pH levels, pressures which are not "normal," can be recorded if these factors are active in an abnormal way during the course of an experiment. In summary, in the experimental animal, IMP has a stable value for each region of the given bone during a long period of observation. In the femoral diaphysis, the average peak pressures observed are fairly close between different authors varying from 32 to 52 with Larsen[265], Shaw[399], and Bloomenthal[54] recording intermediate values. It is likely that the pathological conditions within an animal or the experimental circumstances associated with a particular type of investigation account for a certain disparity of the reported average values.

IMP In Man

IMP in normal man has obviously been recorded much less frequently than in the experimental animal. However, these measurements are much more in agreement (Table II). In man, considerable variation exists in different bones and in different regions of a given bone. The first order of difference is between the long bones and the membranous bones. In the flat bones (sternum, ilium, spinous processes), the IMP is near atmospheric pressure, particularly in the sternum where it is characteristically less than 10 mm Hg. Measurements of the long bone have been determined primarily for the tibia and femur. In the tibia, the most important reference work is that of Kabakele[241], done under general anesthesia. This author reported on 220 measurements in children (3 to 17 years old) and 40 in adults (20 to 45 years old). Tables III and IV demonstrate that the range of the recorded pressure is small. However, there is a significant difference between diaphyseal pressures and epiphyseal-metaphyseal pressures with the latter higher.

IMP in the femur (Table II) recorded in the trochanteric region or the femoral neck in man are very close from one author to the next. Thus, the average values of 17 mm Hg in our cases, 18.7 in Arnoldi's[29], and 12 to 15 in Simon's[417], substantiates the reliability of this measurement. Our own work records femoral head pressures higher than the trochanteric and femoral neck regions with the head being in a range of 25 mm Hg. The pressures within

TABLE II

NORMAL IMP IN MAN
Long Bones

Date	Author	Bones	Site	Range of Values mm Hg	Mean mm Hg
1955	Miles	Adult femur	Epiphysis	30−37	
1960	Simon	Adult femur	Sup. metaphysis	12−15	
1964	Shaw	Infant tibia			Approx. 25% of systemic arterial pressure
1968	Arlet et al.	Adult femur	Sup. metaphysis	12−26	17.2
1972	Kabakele	Infant tibia	Sup. epiphysis Sup. metaphysis Diaphysis		23 20 10
		Adult tibia	Sup. metaphysis		18
1972	Arnoldi et al.	Adult femur	Neck of femur		18.7

Flat Bones

Date	Author	Bones	Site	Range of Values mm Hg	Mean mm Hg
1940	Tocantins	Sternum		3.7−8.9	
1954	Petrakis et al.	Sternum Ilium		−2−+17 2−63	
1972	Arnoldi	Spinous process		2.2−12.9	8.3
1972	Mayer et al.	Sternum		0−8	
1973	Eisinger et al.	Ilium			19

the femur are then not uniform throughout the bone with higher pressures recorded at the ends of the bone rather than in the diaphysis, contrary to the observation of some in the dog. Statistical analysis of

TABLE III

NORMAL IMP IN HUMAN IMMATURE ADULT TIBIA
(in cm. of H_2O)

Region Explored	Number of Measurements	Range	Mean
Epiphysis	25	25−67*	36.7
Superior metaphysis	60	24−32	30.3
Inferior metaphysis	10	25−44**	31.4
Proximal 1/3 diaphysis	32	13−25	19.1
Middle 1/3 diaphysis	75	9−38***	17.6
Distal 1/3 diaphysis	18	10−29	16.4

*Apart from one measurement of 67, all other measurements were between the range of 25 and 36.

**Apart from one measurement of 44, all other values were between 25 and 32.

***Apart from one measurement of 38, all other values were between 9 and 30.

TABLE IV

NORMAL IMP IN HUMAN ADULT TIBIA
(in cm. of H_2O)

Region explored	Number of Measurements	Range	Mean
Diaphysis	26	9−22	16
Metaphysis	14	20−36	27

our recorded data marks 30 mm Hg as the upper limit of normal. Above this figure, the IMP can be considered abnormally high, a point to which we will return in Chapter III.

SPONTANEOUS PHYSIOLOGICAL VARIATIONS OF THE IMP

Pulse Pressure

When recording IMP, a pulse pressure can be observed which is synchronous with cardiac contraction. The upper and lower values represent systolic and diastolic pressure. This pulsation confirms that the needle is within the bone marrow tissue. The absence of pulsation is due either to technical error in placing the tip of the trocar or constitutes a pathological finding. The height of the pulse pressure is small being in the order of 2 to 7 mm Hg in our experience. In the femoral neck in normal controls, Arnoldi[29] registered pulse amplitudes of 2 to 11 mm Hg with an average of 4 mm Hg. The intramedullary pulse is directly related to the intraosseous arterial pulse. The intratibial pulse disappeared after ligation of the femoral artery at the base of the leg, as recorded by Stein et al.[123]. In man, the pulse pressure recorded either in the trochanter or the femoral head disappears when the femoral artery is compressed in the groin (Fig. 11). Simultaneous recording of femoral artery pressure and IMP in the trochanteric region shows a slight delay in the peak of the pulsation in relation to the arterial pulse (Fig. 12). The effect of femoral vein compression on pulse pressure has not always been found the same by different authors. Our findings confirm the observation of Bloomenthal et al.[54] that the pulse pressure decreases, although this was not found by Azuma[32].

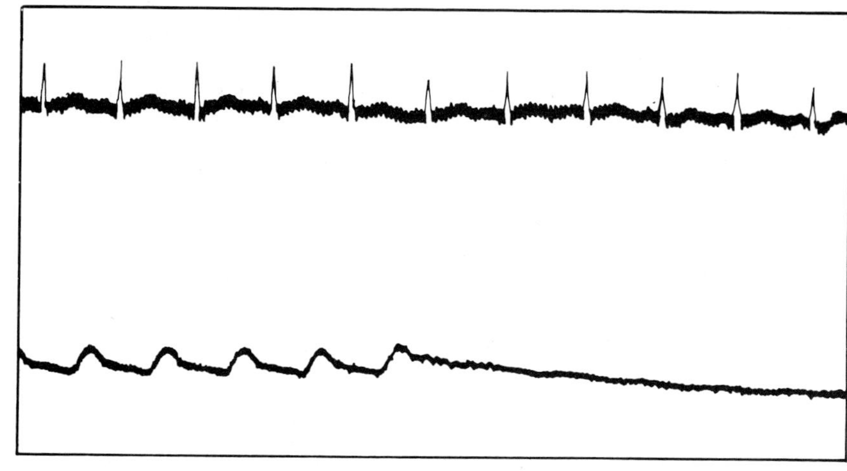

Fig.11.—Simultaneous recording in man of the trochanteric IMP and of the ECG, demonstrating the disappearance of the bone pulsation when the femoral artery is compressed.

Variations In IMP In Relation To Respiratory Movements and Coughing

The IMP exhibits a second type of periodic undulation, in relation to breathing (Fig. 13). In the dog, rabbit, and man (Fig. 14 and 15), the IMP decreases with deep inspiration and increases with expiration[423,32]. A similar finding can be recorded in the extraosseous, systemic venous pressure in general. By facilitating the venous return, the inspiration lowers the peripheral venous pressure while expiration hinders venous return, increasing venous pressure in the large venous trunks at the extremities. This has also been observed during the Valsalva maneuver[342]. This is probably the mechanism whereby coughing produces an important rise in IMP (Fig. 16). However, Shaw[399] observed the opposite in the cat, i.e., a rise in IMP with inspiration.

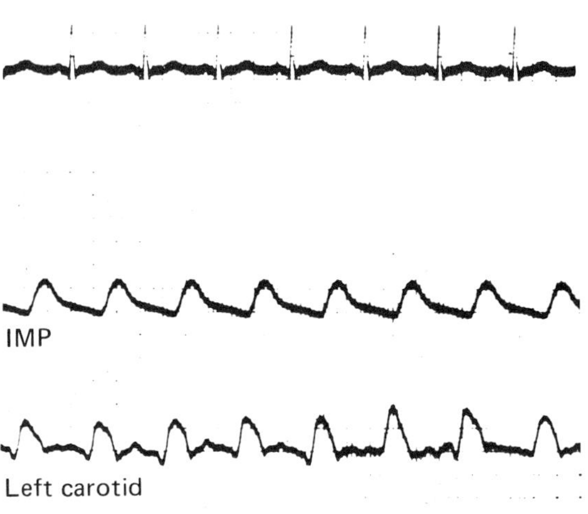

Fig.12.—Simultaneous recording in man of the trochanteric IMP, the ECG, and the carotid pulse.

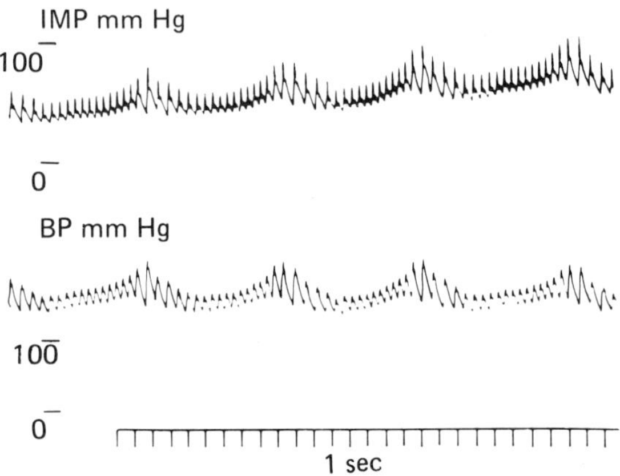

Fig.13.—Simultaneous recording of the IMP and the arterial blood pressure. Periodic undulation in relation with the respiratory movements in both curves.

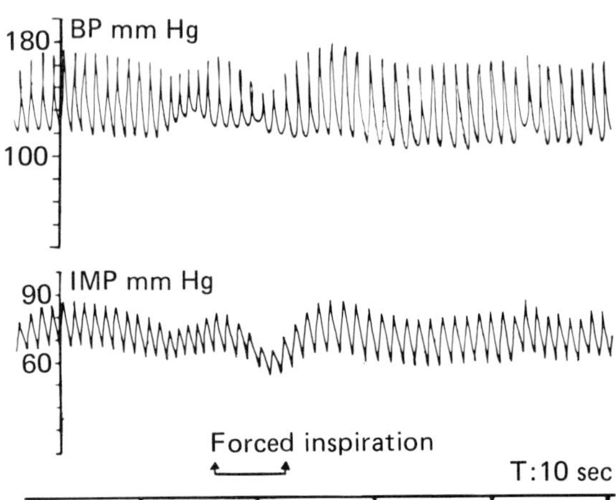

Fig.14.—Simultaneous recording of the IMP and the arterial blood pressure in man. Increase of the IMP during forced inspiration.

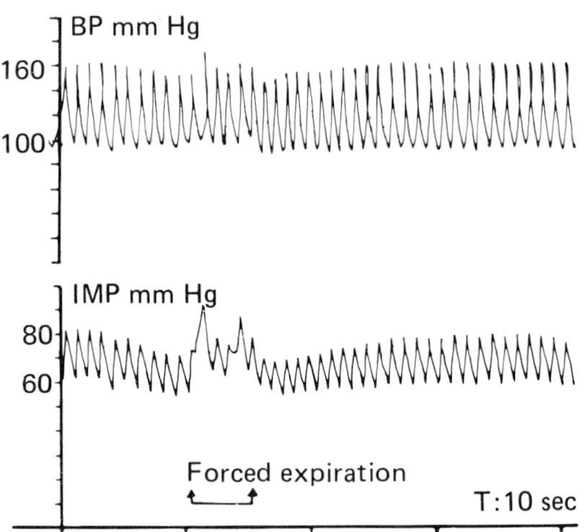

Fig.15.—Simultaneous recording of the IMP and the arterial blood pressure in man. Increase of the IMP during forced expiration.

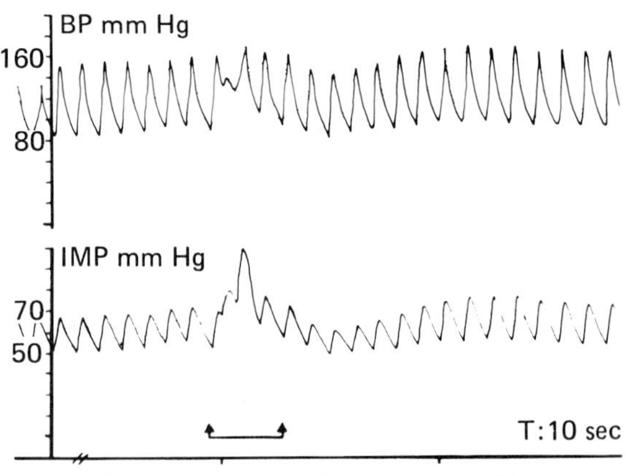

Fig.16.—Simultaneous recording of the IMP and the arterial blood pressure in man. Increase of the IMP by cough.

Variations In IMP With The Systemic Arterial Pressure

Kalser et al.[242] failed to find a clear relationship between general arterial and intramedullary pressure in the dog. In man, we have statistically analyzed 100 consecutive measurements of the systemic blood pressure and IMP showing a direct correlation. This may explain why the IMP is statistically higher in patients over 60 years of age[360]. However, even though the IMP is slightly higher in the hypertensive than in the normotensive subjects, the difference is small and general arterial hypertension does not bring about abnormally or dangerously high IMP. Later in the chapter, we will see that vasoactive drugs can act simultaneously on the general arterial pressure and the intramedullary pressure either in the same or in opposite directions. In man, the simultaneous monitoring of brachial artery pressure and intramedullary femoral pressure allows us to see that any sudden change in arterial pressure has an immediate effect on the femoral IMP, usually in the same direction. The contraction of the iliopsoas and quadricep muscles (slight elevation of the leg in extension) produces a hypertension of 10 to 20 mm Hg in the bone marrow associated with a concommitant rise in the femoral arterial pressure. There is, therefore, a dual correlation between general arterial pressure and IMP. In man, there is a statistical correlation with the ambient level of systemic blood pressure, and there is also a consistent correlation between fluctuations in the general arterial pressure effecting parallel changes on the IMP.

INDUCED PHYSIOLOGICAL VARIATIONS

Muscular Contractions Induced by Electrical Stimulation in the Animal

MacPherson and Shaw[292] were the first to observe that the stimulation of muscle contraction produced an immediate rise in IMP in contiguous bone, which persisted for the duration of the contraction and disappeared with its cessation. Shim et al.[411] made the same observation on intratibial pressure when the quadriceps were electrically stimulated. Since they were studying blood flow in the nutrient artery, they were also able to detect an increase in this flow. It can be argued that muscular contractions block the cortical drainage and produce an intraosseous venous congestion. This compressive effect leads to increased outflow in the large venous trunks. Mac Pherson[292] has suggested that muscular contraction increases marrow tissue pressure, which mechanically reinforces the trabeculae and cortex. In this way, it could function as a protective mechanism during vigorous physical activity.

Voluntary Muscle Contraction in Man

Since most of our intertrochanteric IMP measurements are done under local anesthesia, it is possible for the patient to voluntarily contract his muscles. If the patient effects a straight leg raising, contracting the psoas and quadriceps, we see an immediate rise of intertrochanteric IMP in the order of 5 to 30 mm Hg. When the muscle contraction is released, the pressure first falls slightly below and then quickly returns to the baseline. Although we do not have reasons to refute the explanations of MacPherson[292] or Shim[411] as outlined in the previous section, we must emphasize that simultaneous recordings of general arterial pressure in the brachial as well as the femoral artery demonstrates that this systemic arterial pressure rises simultaneously with the IMP during quadriceps contraction (Fig. 17). This hypertensive effect of effort is well known by the physiologists, and the role of this increase in arterial pressure in the production of the IMP rise cannot be excluded.

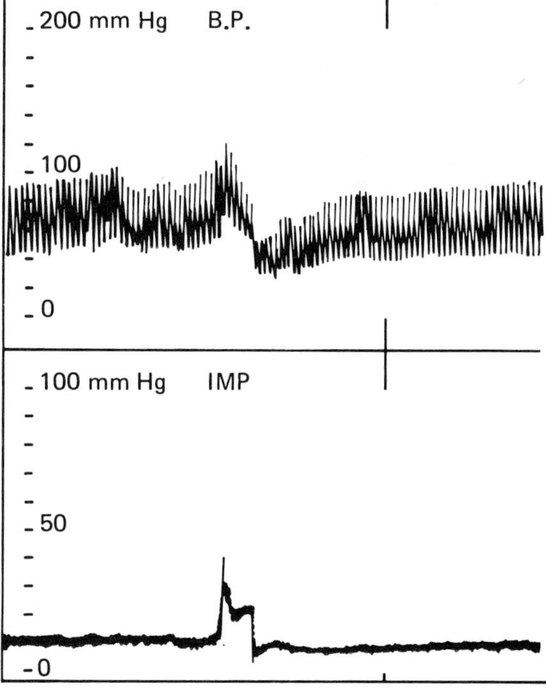

Fig.17.—Simultaneous recording of the IMP and the arterial blood pressure in man. Increase of the IMP and of the arterial blood pressure during voluntary contraction of the quadriceps.

Effect Of The Occlusion Of Regional Vessels

In the experimental animal, most authors have studied the effect on diaphyseal IMP in the tibia and femur by more or less complete occlusion on the femoral artery either by ligation or progressive cerclage. Held and Thron[201] have shown that the IMP decreases proportionally to the decrease of the femoral arterial pressure without ever reaching zero. Under these conditions, all authors have noted the disappearance of pulse pressure as well as the pressure undulations with respiration[411]. There are two interesting observations associated with this maneuver. When the compression is released, a transient rise of the IMP is observed above the level prior to compression. Shim[411] refers to this as a hypertensive reaction to the ischemia while Brookes[76] thinks of this as a vasomotor reaction, secondary to the acidosis associated with the ischemia. Secondly, when the occlusion is prolonged by complete and definite ligature of the femoral artery, the IMP regains the base line level, probably accounted for by the opening of anastomotic pathways[201]. In man, we have observed that digital compression of the femoral artery in the groin produces a clear decrease in the trochanteric IMP of approximately 50% and a disappearance of the pulse pressure (Fig. 18).

The occlusion of the femoral vein conversely produces a strong rise in the diaphyseal IMP of the tibia and femur. Shim[411] notices, at the same time, an increase in outflow of the nutrient vein but a decrease in the inflow of the nutrient artery (Fig. 19). Under these circumstances, there exists an acute intraosseous venous congestion due to shunting of systemic venous blood through the open intraosseous pathways. This increase is not completely compensated for by the increase in the outflow, resulting in actually hindering arterial inflow and in ischemia. This is a demonstration of the ischemic role of the obstruction of the large venous trunks, which we believe is fundamental to the understanding of the phenomenon observed in human pathology.

Effects Of Vasoactive Drugs

The effects of the drugs listed below have been studied in experimental animals by numerous authors and are now well understood[54,411,424].

Adrenaline—injected intravenously in doses of 0.1 to 1 microgram/kg/min produces a rise in the general arterial pressure and a reduction in the IMP of 33%, according to Shim[411]. The pulse pressure vanishes and the flow decreases by 29%. This effect is seen both in the diaphysis and in the epiphysis (Fig. 20). The vasoconstrictive effect of adrenaline has been observed *in vivo* in the rabbit tibia by

Branemark[64] and is responsible for the fall in IMP. A return to normal circulation occurs within five to ten minutes after the cessation of the drug infusion.

Noradrenaline—identical to epinephrine and neosynephrine.

Isoproterenol (Isuprel)—produces a parallel reduction in systemic arterial pressure and of venous outflow of the nutrient vein.

Ephedrine (also Benzedrine and Nicotine)—increases both systemic arterial pressure and IMP.

Acetylcholine—injected intra-arterially, producing a fall of both IMP and osseous blood flow[400].

Histamine—lowers both arterial pressure and IMP.

Neurogenic Variations Of IMP

Stimulation of the peripheral ends of the splanchnic nerve precipitates a fall of IMP in the tibia and a rise in general arterial pressure[203]. Stimulation of the peripheral ends of the vagus nerve occasions simultaneous fall in IMP and systemic arterial pressure. Stimulation of both the sciatic nerve and the lumbar sympathetic plexus produces a fall in IMP[411]. Ader, Geral, and Arlet[2] have also observed, in the dog, the same dissociation between the effects of stimulation of the sympathetic plexus on the general arterial pressure that rises and the IMP that lowers by an indirect, but very elegant, method consisting of sectioning of the splanchnic nerves (Fig. 21).

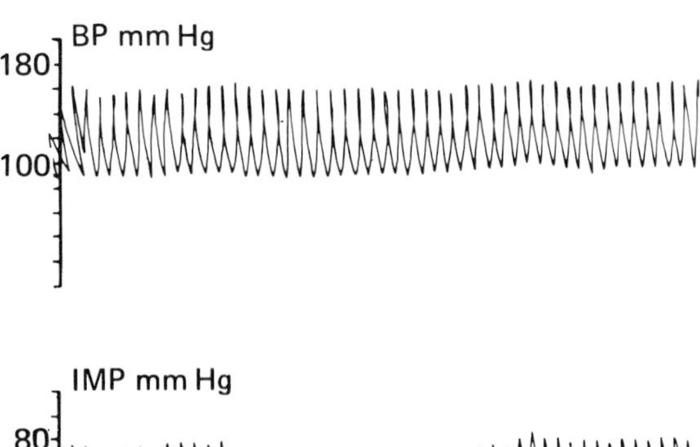

Fig. 18.—Simultaneous recording of the trochanteric IMP of the humeral arterial blood pressure in man. Fall of an abnormally high IMP from 70 to 30 mm Hg after compression of the femoral artery. The pulsation also disappears.

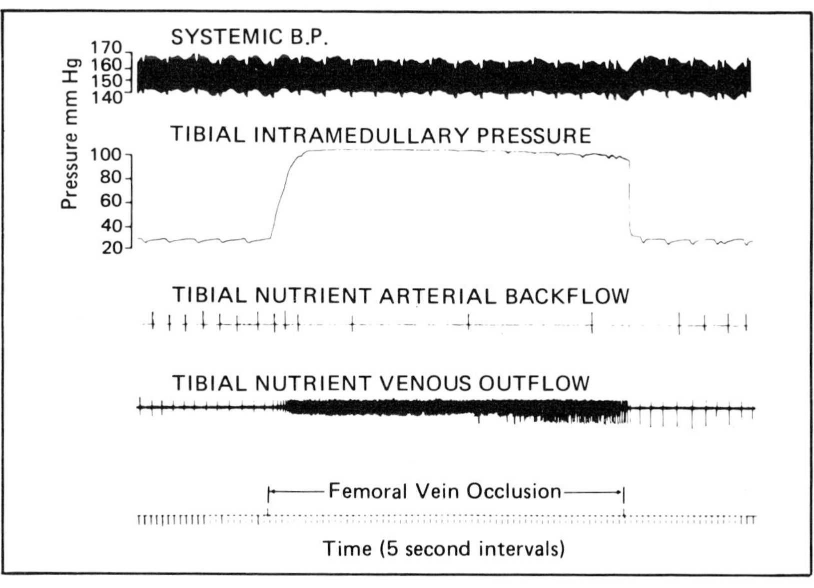

Fig.19.—Effect of the occlusion of the femoral artery in the dog. Increase of the tibial IMP associated with a decrease of the nutrient artery flow. It is interesting to note that the flow of the nutrient vein increases a lot during the same period (from Shim[411], reproduced with permission).

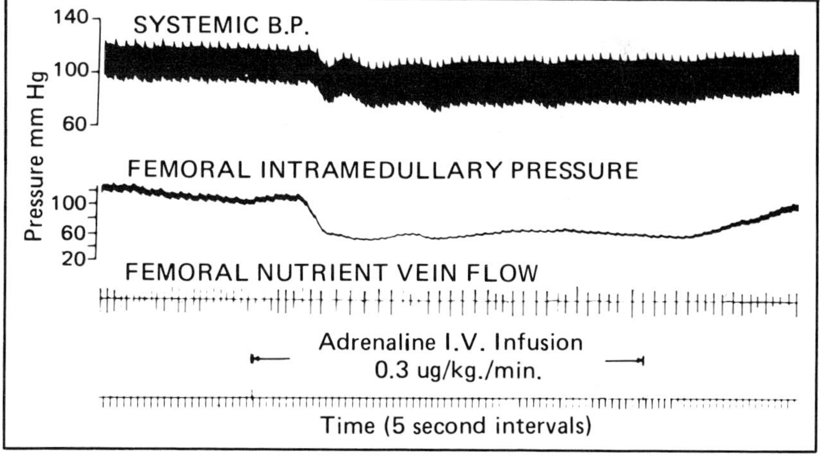

Fig.20.—Effect of intravenous adrenalin perfusion in the dog. Fall of the femoral IMP associated with a fall of 50% of the nutrient vein flow (from Shim[405], reproduced with permission).

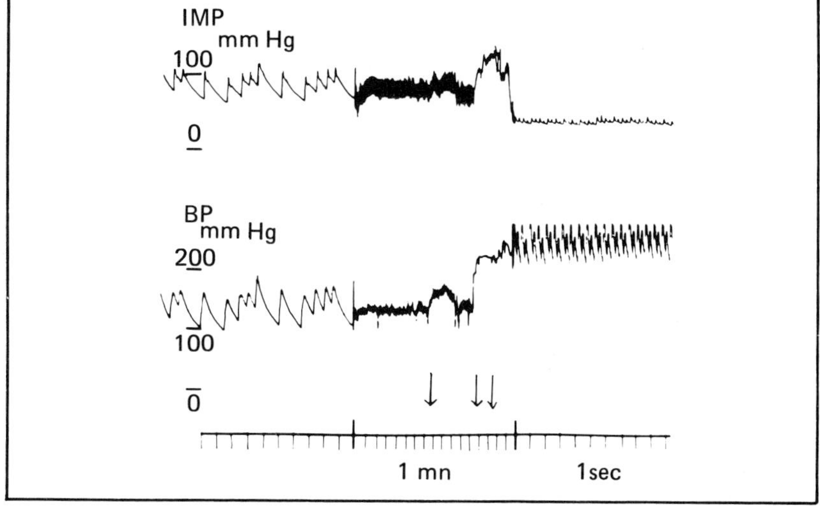

Fig.21.—The IMP and the arterial blood pressure are independent in the course of hypertension produced by defrenation in the dog. The arrows indicate the moment when both Hering nerves and both vagi are sectioned.

The Interpretation Of The IMP

Normal values of the IMP for cancellous bone in the proximal human femur are always higher than pressures recorded in the femoral vein and are clearly always lower than the pressure in the femoral artery. In fact, the IMP is usually one-third to one-fourth of the arterial pressure. It is, therefore, neither a venous nor an arterial pressure but rather a tissue interstitial pressure, probably near to the pressure existing in the capillary. In man, the capillary pressure is between 32 mm Hg on the arterial side and 12 mm Hg on the venous side. The diagram from Kita et al[252] illustrates the location of this pressure as measured in the bone marrow (Fig. 22). The IMP can be considered a precapillary pressure. On the one hand, the interstitial spaces are separated from the capillary blood by a thin, semi-permeable membrane which permits both nutrient exchange and the equalization pressures from one side to the other of this membrane. On the other hand, the needle must open capillaries and create at its tip a small hematoma which communicates with capillary blood. We believe, as do most authors, including Azuma[32], Polster[348], and Shim et al[411] that what is measured is the pressure within a small hematoma situated at the tip of the needle which has produced vascular injury. It is possible that the pressure measured in this way may be a function either of the type of vessel which is injured or of the vasomotor reaction caused by the injury. Nevertheless, the IMP is dependent upon intraosseous blood flow and accurately reflects the hemodynamic changes within bone[411].

If the IMP reflects the pressure existing within the capillaries, it does not directly inform us of either arterial or venous intraosseous pressures. The pressure within the intraosseous arterial system decreases rapidly before reaching the capillary level, probably in part due to the tortuosity of the nutrient artery and to its branches which are at right angles to the main trunk. This protects the thin-walled sinusoids from excessive pressure. The pressure within the main venous drainage is probably higher than that of the large venous trunks of the extremities since substances injected into the marrow rapidly pour into these large extraosseous trunks. Michelsen[312] likens this pressure differential across the cortex to a waterfall. He simultaneously measured IMP and emissary vein pressure first in "free flow" and then after ligature proximal to the catheter. The pressure within the extraosseous emissary vein then rose rapidly to reach the level of the IMP. He concluded that IMP and the pressure in the intraosseous venous system are very close, a finding which has been confirmed by Wilkes and Visscher[466].

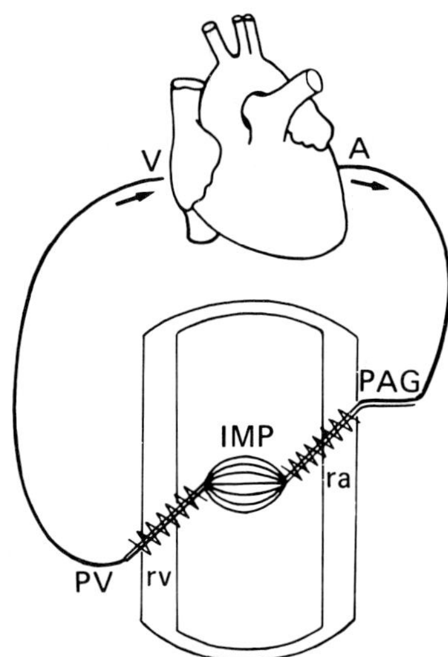

PAG: General arterial pressure
PV: Venous pressure
IMP: Intramedullary pressure
ra: Arterial resistance
rv: Venous resistance

Fig.22.—Diagram adapted from Kita[252]. The sinusoidal capillary system is located between two vascular systems of high resistance where the pressure gradient is high.

If the pressures within the intraosseous vessels are different from one level to the other, the gradients of pressure between the three types of vessels—arterioles, capillaries, and veins—will be less than in soft tissue organs. The central venous sinus in the diaphysis operates perhaps as a pressure regulator. It should also be noted that the nervous system of bone vessels plays an essential role in the regulation of intraosseous pressure, changing the caliber of these vessels, and insuring a relative independence of the intraosseous pressure from systemic pressure.

BONE BLOOD FLOW

THE TECHNICAL PROBLEMS

Blood flow through a vessel is defined as the quantity of blood which flows per transectional area per unit time. The blood flow to an organ is the quantity of blood that passes through that organ during a unit of time (generally one minute). The bone blood flow to a particular bone would, therefore, be the amount of blood which flows through that bone per unit time. In principle, the quantity of blood which goes into bone must also come out. This is probably an essential characteristic for a rigid organ system like bone, while for a soft and distensible organ some of the blood flowing in could be retained. If an organ system has a single or a few well-defined arteries, the inflow is theoretically easy to measure. One could also measure venous outflow when there is a single or a few veins. Measurement of bone blood flow is complicated because of the multiplicity of afferent and efferent vessels (Fig. 1). This fact represents the most serious difficulty in measuring bone blood flow, making it virtually impossible to directly measure total blood flow to a given bone.

METHODS FOR MEASURING BONE BLOOD FLOW

The direct methods consist of collection of blood from one or several afferent or efferent vessels. Indirect methods which are those usually used are numerous and represent a testimony to the imagination and ingenuity of researchers interested in bone blood flow. Most indirect methods consist of studying the intraosseous transit of either a radiopaque or radioactive substance. Other methods include measuring temperature changes within bone or gas concentration changes in blood removed from bone[467].

Direct Methods

The most commonly used direct method in the experimental animal is the drop-counting method from a cannulated vein which drains from the bone. Although a reliable estimate of bone blood for a given bone cannot be claimed with this method, Cumming[105] took advantage of the special arrangement of the nutrient vessels of the rabbit's femur in isolating the superficial femoral vein between two ligatures and ligated the deep femoral vein and circumflex veins. He then concluded that all blood draining throughout the isolated fragment of the superficial femoral vein must come from the femur. Cannulizing this segment with a T-tube, he counted the drops of blood which he then returned to the animal. On 33 measurements done on the rabbit in these conditions, he estimated a bone blood flow of 52 ml/100 gm of fresh bone. These values, which are close to those of cerebral blood flow, are much higher than those considered as normal with other methods. Nevertheless, this method of "drop-counting" has been used by numerous authors since Drinker and Drinker[123] catheterized the femoral nutrient vein and tibial vein of the dog. Although this method does not allow precision in estimating total flow of a given bone, it represents an interesting model to study flow variations of the nutrient vein under several different physiologic stimuli. Cumming[105] himself demonstrated, in this way, the spectacular action of adrenaline on the nutrient venous outflow, which decreased by 75%.

Indirect Methods

Most of these methods consist of studying either the dilution, clearance, or fixation of a colorant, a radiopaque substance or a radioactive compound during its transit through bone. These become measurements of clearance rates more than flow, which apply to a section of bone rather than the entire bone. Total flow must then be extrapolated. Details of those methods we find most interesting follow.

Cr[51] red cell dilution—This method was first used by White, Ter-Pogossian and Stein[465] and reaffirmed by Brookes[75]. Fifteen minutes following the injection of 0.5 ml of packed red cells tagged with 100 microcuries of Cr[51] injected into the epigastric vein of a rat, the tail is amputated and a drop of blood collected on a slide to measure radioactivity. The time from injection to sampling allows proper mixing of the marked cells with the host red cells. The rat is sacrificed by freezing, the bones removed, fixed in formalin, and, after weighing, sectioned into pieces which are measured for radioactivity. In this way, the circulating red cell volume is calculated for a given specimen and expressed in volume/100 gm net weight of tissue.

Clearance of a radiopaque compound—Iodinated compounds are used in intraosseous venography to estimate flow by calculating rate of disappearance of the compound. Matumoto and Misuno[301] developed a simple method using a densitometry technique of great precision to estimate flow in man. Three to 15 ml of 40% Urografin is injected directly into the femoral head through an anterior approach under general anesthesia. The speed of disappearance is analyzed by serial radiographs. The authors studied 264 hips in this way, of which 67 were in Perthes' disease where the flow was considerably reduced.

Clearance of a non-bone-seeking radioactive isotope—Iodide is also used in this technique as I[131] Sodium Iodide (NaI). Petrakis et al[341] have used this technique in leukemic patients since 1954. Brown-Grant and Cumming[77] injected this material into the femoral diaphysis and followed the decreasing level of radioactivity over the injection site by counting at five second intervals for at least one minute. Under normal conditions, half clearance time is 20 to 25 seconds. This rapid clearance is related to circulation and is a function of blood flow. No clearance occurs in conditions of no flow. Semb[386] repeated this technique using labeled Iodoantipyrine, which we have also used (Fig. 53). Kane and Grim[243] using the same fundamental concept have also used K[42] and Rb[86].

Clearance of a bone-seeking isotope—The first use of this method was in 1950 by Tucker[448] using P^{32} in man to study the viability of the femoral head after fracture. Frederickson, Honour, and Copp[170] used the clearance of $Calcium^{45}$ to measure bone blood flow in the rat. However, it is the work of Shim et al[406] which finally defined the experimental conditions of bone blood flow by this method, in this instance using $Strontium^{85}$. Bone fixes the radioisotope circulating in the blood, thus removing it from the general circulation. If the concentration of the circulating isotope is known for a given period, for instance five minutes, as well as the quantity of fixed strontium during that same period (i.e., in number of counts), then the blood flow to a given bone can be calculated in accordance with Fick's formula:

$$D = \frac{Q}{A - V}$$

Q = amount of Strontium fixed in the bone in one minute.

A - V = arteriovenous difference of strontium radioactivity.

Shim, Copp, and Patterson's experimental protocol details the following steps[515]:

1. Catheterization of the carotid artery connected to a syringe which automatically aspirates arterial blood. The radioactivity of five pooled blood samples is to be determined.

2. Injection of 8 to 10 microcuries/kg of $Strontium^{85}$ into the jugular vein.

3. The animal is sacrificed by cardiac arrest five minutes after the injection. The bone to be studied is dissected free, weighed wet, and then ashed and measured for radioactivity. The obtained values are divided by the average radioactivity of one ml of blood to calculate the clearance in five minutes and then redivided by five to give the one minute clearance. Since the bone does not completely clear 100% of the strontium from the blood which is circulating through it, the results are less than actual blood flow. The extraction coefficient is of the order of 75%, while in the method of calculation, venous radioactivity is considered as negligible.

Shim et al[403] were able to apply this methodology in the human to one case of amputation. Estimated blood flow in several of the skeletal pieces examined vary from 1.3 ml/min/100 gm in the fibula to 6.9 ml/min/100 gm in the patella, with an average in the total skeletal parts of 2.43 ml/min/100 gm. If a correction related to the rate of extraction is applied, the calculated value would be 4.8 ml/min/100 gm.

Thermocouple technique—This original indirect method was devised by MacPherson et al[292]. Two thermocouples are placed in opposition near each other so that the temperature of the tissue in which they are inserted does not modify the electromagnetic force between the probes. One of the thermocouples is heated slightly above the temperature of the tissue. The dissipation of heat is a function of the blood flow. Therefore, any change in blood flow produces a change in the electromagnetic forces and the generated electrical current. This method has the disadvantage of studying only a small portion of the bone and may represent only changes in local flow.

NORMAL VALUES FOR BONE BLOOD FLOW

The average value proposed by Shim et al[410] of 10 ml/min/100 gm of fresh bone appears reasonable. This is an average value taken from several bones in the dog and rabbit. Values given from different authors vary from 3 to 30 ml/min/100 gm (Table V). Within this range, total skeletal blood flow would be between 4 and 10% of the resting cardiac output (Ray et al[354]) or 500 ml for a cardiac output of 5 liters/min. Skeletal weight represents approximately 10% of body weight. This blood flow rate is very similar to average tissue blood flow. Recently, Shim, Patterson, and Copp[410] in measuring $Strontium^{85}$ clearance from the rabbit's femur found variable average flows in different sites of the bone, recording 7 ml/min/100 gm in the diaphysis, 18 ml/min/100 gm in the femoral head, 10 in the trochanteric region and 12 in the condyle. It is interesting to compare these results with those of the IMP. They confirm a certain independence and regionalization of local flow areas within a given bone. According to these authors, flow is higher in the femoral head than in the trochanteric region.

REGULATION OF BONE BLOOD FLOW

There are three types of regulatory mechanisms for controlling bone blood flow: nervous, humeral, and metabolic.

Nerve Control of Bone Blood Flow

Drinker and Drinker[123] were first to demonstrate nerve control of bone circulation. Shim and Patterson[407], using the rabbit femur, measured flow directly in the diaphyseal vein by catheterizing and counting the drops electronically. This direct method of measurement of flow in the nutrient vein produced very steady readings, allowing several factors to be studied. Stimulation of the sympathetic plexus to the extremity lowered flow while producing generalized elevation of arterial pressure. It appeared that selective bone arterial vasoconstriction occured

TABLE V

MEASUREMENT OF BLOOD FLOW: RESULTS OF VARIOUS METHODS

Authors	*Method*	*Subject*	*Results in ml/min/ 100g. bone*
Edholm et al., 1945.	Plethysmography	Man	1.9–5.9
Ray et al.,1955.	Sr^{90} (clearance)	Dog	5
Frederickson et al.,1955.	Ca^{45}	Rat	10–30
Weinman et al., 1963.	Ca^{45} Sr^{85} (both clearance)	Dog	5.6 *adult dog* / 7.7 *immature dog*
White el al., 1964.	Cr^{51} labelled RBC's (dilution)	Rabbit (tibia)	16
Kane and Grim 1964.	K^{42}, Rb^{86} (clearance or disappearance curve)	Dog	12
Matumoto and Misuno, 1966.	Iodine (disappearance curve), radiologic densitometry	Man	3–7
Brookes, 1967.	Cr^{51} labelled RBC's (dilution curve)	Rat	18–30
Shim et al., 1971.	Sr^{85} (clearance)	Dog	10.15
		Rabbit	9.6
Shim et al., 1971.	Sr^{85} (clearance)	Man	1.3–6.9
Semb, 1971.	Iodoantipyrine labelling (disappearance curve)	Dog	8.9 ±1.9

(Fig. 23). Electrical stimulation of the peripheral nerve also lowered flow rate (Fig. 24). Conversely, Trotman and Kelly[443] demonstrated that sympathectomy increases bone blood flow in the dog. Sectioning of the peripheral nerve (containing most of the sympathetic fibers to the limb) increased bone blood flow to the tibia, fibula, and calcaneum. Stimulation of the vagus decreased bone blood flow but also produced a general decrease in blood pressure and IMP. It is likely that these experimental findings reflect actual physiologic phenomena and that bone blood flow is regulated by vasomotor nerves to the intraosseous vessels. Rapid changes in the caliber of intraosseous vessels have been visualized *in vivo*, particularly at the level of the sinusoids[64].

Hormonal Control Of Bone Blood Flow

Drinker and Drinker[123] had already demonstrated in 1916 that perfusion of the nutrient artery of bone with adrenaline produced a dramatic reduction of nutrient vein outflow. Blood outflow through cortical veins decreases or stops in the dog after the administration of adrenaline[405]. One microgram of adrenaline decreases flow from 25 to 75%[405,467]. These studies lead one to the conclusion that vasopressive hormones also influence bone blood flow. Noradrenaline is the chemical mediator of the sympathetic nervous endings. Semb[387] using the clearance of Xenon[133] from the dog tibia demonstrated that adrenaline, noradrenaline, and acetylcholine injected into the femoral artery on the same side produced a decrease in xenon clearance. Since the amount of adrenaline injected intra-arterially was very small, no change in systemic blood pressure occurred, while hypertension was produced by the noradrenaline and hypotension with acetylcholine. Bradykinine and histamine also decreased xenon clearance. However, if histamine was injected directly into the bone, xenon clearance increased as if the histamine produced a direct vasodilatory effect on the intraosseous vessels. Vasodilators increase bone blood flow only if they are directly injected into bones. Bone blood flow is decreased if they are injected into the femoral artery, probably by diverting blood to the muscular vessels which have a greater capacity to dilate. Semb[381] emphasized that the effect of these drugs on muscle circulation may have repercussive effects on bone circulation.

Metabolic Control

Three factors which have been studied include acid metabolites, such as lactic acid, blood and tissue pH, and O_2 concentration in the circulating and bone blood. Injection of acid preparations such as N/15 lactic acid[467] or weak hydrochloric acid into the femoral artery or nutrient artery of the dog tibia increased flow. Inhalation of air with high concentrations of CO_2 or low concentrations of O_2 also increased bone blood flow[106, 407].

Temporary reduction of bone blood flow by occlusion of the femoral artery is followed upon release of the occlusion by a two to three fold increase in bone blood flow over the control. A hyperemia or vasodilatation of the intraosseous vessels occurs,

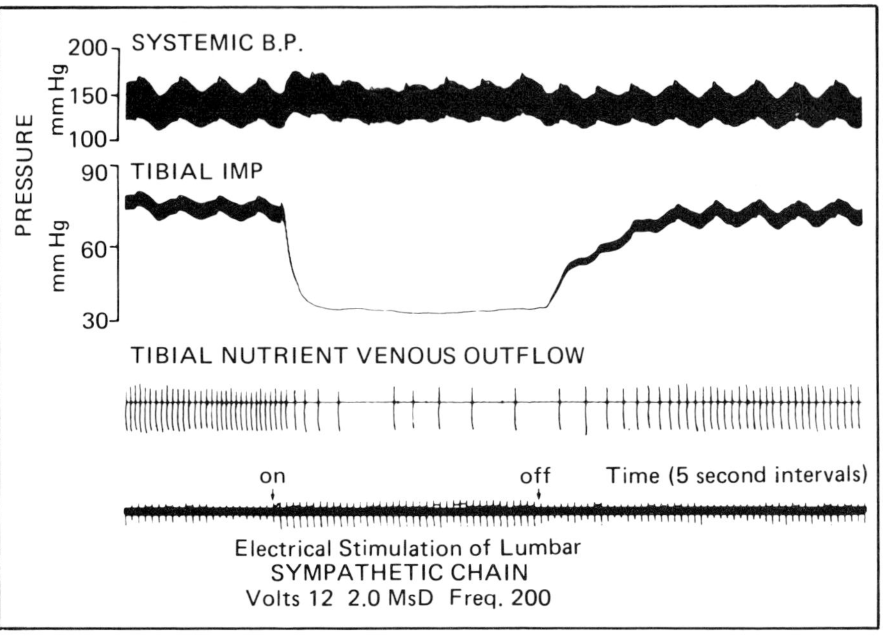

Fig.23.—Effect of electrical stimulation to the lumbar sympathetic system in the dog: fall of the tibial IMP associated to an important decrease of the blood flow. On this curve, the blood flow is expressed by the recording of the venous flow from the catheterized nutrient vein (from Shim[407], with permission).

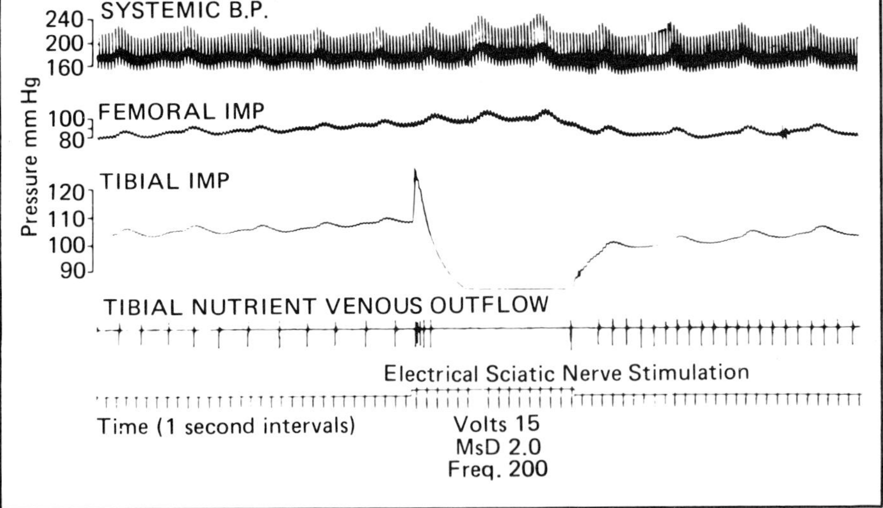

Fig.24.—Effect of the electrical stimulation of the sciatic nerve in the dog: fall of the tibial IMP associated with decrease of the tibial nutrient vein flow (from Shim[408], with permission).

which is not dependent upon the nervous system, since it is observed on denervated bone and is not changed by adrenaline injection. It, therefore, appears that this vasodilator or hyperemic reaction is related to changes in some of the blood constituents since bone blood flow during this time has a higher concentration of hydrogen ions and CO_2 and lower concentrations of O_2. In summary, hypoxia, hypercapnea, and acidosis increase bone blood flow.

Miscellaneous Factors Influencing Bone Blood Flow

A decrease in total cardiac output reduces bone blood flow but to a lesser degree than the skin. Systemic hypotension will decrease bone blood flow, but systemic hypertension may also decrease bone blood flow as is seen with the injection of adrenaline. A variety of local factors may reduce bone blood flow, including fractures, dislocations, arterial damage, obstruction of intraosseous vessels, and increased intra-articular pressure. The latter was demonstrated by Salter and Bell[382] in immature pigs. They showed that a rise in intra-articular pressure of more than 70 mm Hg can result in epiphyseal necrosis. Shim[412], working with the rabbit, showed that subcapital fracture brought about a reduction in femoral head blood flow of 83% on the average

TABLE VI

SPONTANEOUS AND PROVOKED VARIATIONS IN BONE BLOOD FLOW, INTRAMEDULLARY PRESSURE (IMP) AND SYSTEMIC ARTERIAL PRESSURE (SAP)

Factors	*Flow*	*IMP*	*SAP*
Sympathetic stimulation	↘	↘	↗ →
Sciatic stimulation	↘	↘	→
Vagal stimulation	↘	↘	↘
Epinephrine	↘	↘	↗ →
Norepinephrine	↘	↘	↗
Acetylcholine	↘	↘	↘
Histamine	↘	↘	↘
Femoral artery occlusion	↘	↘	
Sympathetic transection	↗		
Sciatic transection	↗	↗	
Benzedrine		↗	↗
Acid metabolytes	↗		
pCO2	↗		
Femoral vein occlusion	vein ↗ artery ↘	↗	

CORRELATIONS BETWEEN, BONE AND MUSCLE FLOW

Shaw[401], using a thermocouple technique, was able to simultaneously study bone and muscle blood flow. Although there are certain limitations inherent in this technique in that the flow measurements are done only on a limited area around the tip of the thermocouple probe, certain correlations between two adjacent circulation areas can be made. The measurements were made in the proximal third of the femoral diaphysis and in the overlying quadriceps. When the quadriceps was contracted by intermittent stimulation of the femoral nerve, it could be seen that each muscle contraction produced a temporary decrease in muscle blood flow, but a simultaneous increase was produced in both intramedullary pressure and diaphyseal blood flow of short duration. When the muscular contractions were repeated, however, both muscle and bone blood flow rose while intramedullary pressure decreased. Conversely, the vasodilatation of muscle vessels can bring about a decrease in bone blood flow, probably being one of the explanations for reduction in bone blood flow by acetylcholine[411] and perhaps also adrenaline. We have reported in an earlier section the observation of muscle contraction on intramedullary pressure in man. These contractions produced an elevation in systemic arterial pressures as well which must be included in accounting for the change.

CORRELATIONS BETWEEN BONE BLOOD FLOW AND INTRAMEDULLARY PRESSURE

The most important studies have been carried out by Shaw[399], studying local flow with a thermocouple implanted into bone in the cat, and Shim, Hawk, and Yu[411], using a venous and arterial collection method in the dog and rabbit by catheterization of the diaphyseal vessels. Both of these investigators, using divergent techniques, demonstrated that in physiologic conditions of short duration both parameters vary in the same direction. For example, the occlusion of the femoral artery produces a simultaneous fall of both intraosseous blood flow and IMP (Fig. 25). Other factors which produce simultaneous changes in pressure and flow include intra-arterial injection of adrenaline which produces a drop in nutrient artery flow and diaphyseal vein flow with a drop in IMP. The systemic hypertension and increase in muscle blood flow with adrenaline administration also demonstrates the independence of the osseous vascular system. IMP then seems to be a post-arteriolar pressure (Fig. 22). Stimulation of the sympathetic chain produces a similar response. Shim et al.[411] have demonstrated that quadriceps con-

while a base of neck fracture reduced flow by only 52%.

There are several factors as well which increase bone blood flow. Pharmacological agents such as Benzedrine causes an increase in intramedullary pressure as well as systemic arterial pressure. Unknown factors operative in pulmonary disease produce increased bone blood flow in hypertrophic osteoarthropathy. Mechanical factors such as arteriovenous fistula results in increased tibial flow[354]. Proliferative diseases, such as Paget's disease and malignant bone tumors increase blood flow.

Several factors may cause venous congestion within bone, particularly occlusion of the vein of the extremity. This produces increased IMP[224] and a decrease in arterial flow. Cuthbertson et al[110] believed that in these circumstances, the intraosseous veins represent collateral pathways for the venous return. All of these physiological variables are summarized in Table VI. The effect of muscle contractions, or the lack thereof, on bone blood flow is not well established. Immobilization with a constricting plaster cast, however, does reduce bone blood flow.

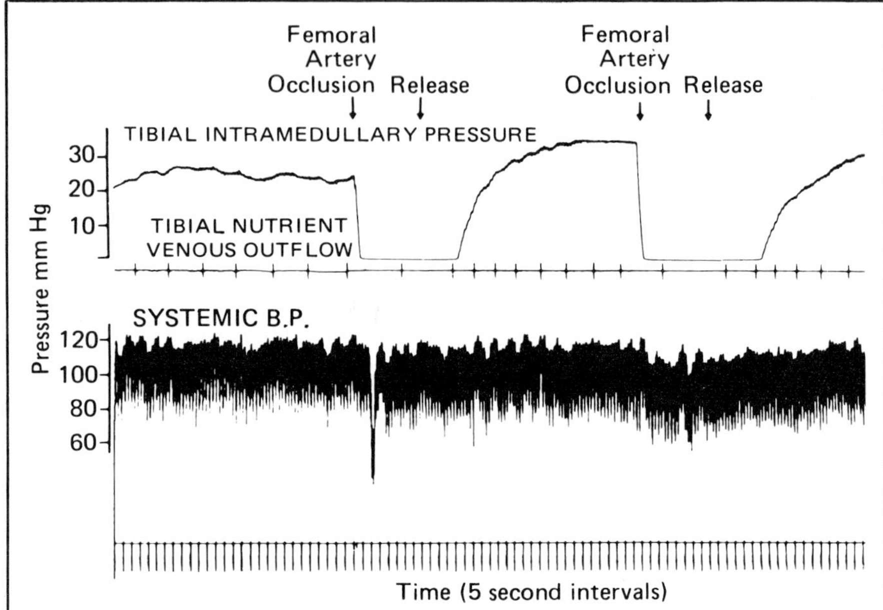

Fig.25.—Effect of the occlusion of the femoral artery in the rabbit. The tibial IMP rapidly falls at the same time as the nutrient venous flow (from Shim[408], with permission).

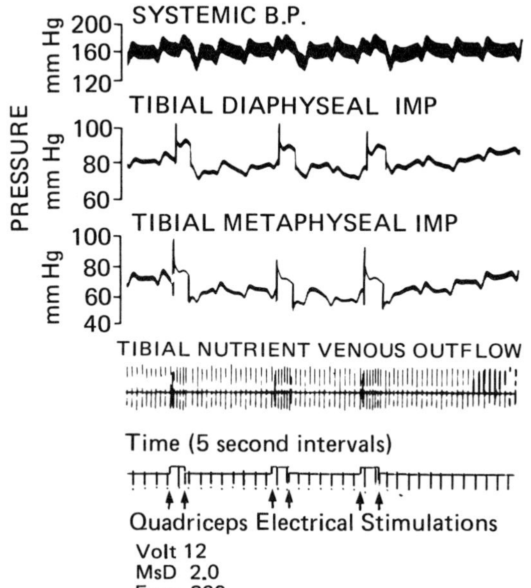

Fig.26.—Effect of the quadriceps contraction in the dog: it produces an increase of the IMP and of the nutrient venous flow. It is interesting to note in this curve that for each quadriceps contraction there is a corresponding small elevation of the systemic arterial pressure (from Shim[408]).

traction by electrical stimulation increases IMP and osseous venous outflow (Fig. 26). Azuma[32], using a bone perfusion technique, was able to control flow, showing that blood flow and IMP always moved in the same direction.

Manipulation of the venous side of the circulation produces more complex changes. Occlusion of the femoral vein produces intraosseous hypertension and acceleration of outflow in the diaphyseal vein, probably due to the fact, that under these conditions, part of the venous blood of the lower extremity is diverted through this "collateral" pathway[110]. However, if all of the draining veins to bone are occluded, the IMP increases, but the intraosseous blood flow decreases. Here we see a new phenomenon of increased IMP and decreased bone blood flow. Bone which is congested cannot receive arterial blood. This is the fundamental role of stasis in initiating the process of ischemia and in a dissociation of blood flow—IMP relationships in pathological conditions. We conclude that in physiologic circumstances, there is a real parallel between flow and pressure, but this parallel may disappear in pathologic circumstances.

CORRELATION BETWEEN THE ANATOMY AND PHYSIOLOGY OF BONE BLOOD FLOW

INDEPENDENCE OF DIFFFERENT VASCULAR NETWORKS

We have already emphasized several times the unitarian and connective characteristics of the different intraosseous vascular pathways. However, the anastomoses that join these different systems do not provide either anatomically or physiologically a completely free communication. Although these different vascular pathways may substitute from one another at time of a crisis, under normal circumstances each of these networks assumes a precise role with a specific distribution which does not overlap the neighboring one. This regionalization is very clear cut with regard to the arterial vessels but also exists within the venous network.

Anatomical regionalization—Occlusion of each pedical brings about definite and well limited ischemic lesions. Ligature of the diaphyseal artery, for example, produces necrosis of approximately the inner half of the cortex. Ligation of periosteal arteries produces necrosis of approximately the outer half of the cortex. Occlusion of the retinacular arteries produces necrosis of the femoral head. Moreover, intraosseous phlebography also demonstrates preferential drainage pathways which exist for each region. Metaphyseal injection demonstrates drainage through the metaphyseal veins. Epiphyseal injection is less selective and the drainage routes are more numerous. For example, in the hip, the ligamentum teres is demonstrated as well as the epiphyseal veins. Intraosseous injection in the diaphysis fills the central venous sinus first.

Functional regionalization—The most striking example of this is a difference in pressure existing between metaphysis, diaphysis, and epiphysis. Notwithstanding the direction of this gradient, its existence presupposes the presence of adaptable barriers and permanent differences in neurovascular control. Although the growth cartilage disappears in the adult, a difference in metaphyseal and epiphyseal pressures persists indicating that a physiologic barrier to free circulation continues. Not only do large functional sectors exist, but there is also regionalization on a much smaller scale. Each medullary space or even each capillary-sinusoidal cluster has its proper existence. This can explain the findings of Jacqueline[220] of lesions of stasis origin first producing heterogenous and disseminated lesions.

INTERDEPENDENCE OF THESE NETWORKS

In the previous section, we have seen that a certain regional autonomy exists, both in the anatomical and the functional levels. However, this is not absolute, and the autonomy is only relative. Following closure of the epiphyseal plate, vascular continuity does exist between the metaphysis and the epiphysis. This is evidenced by the transmission of a provoked increase in pressure from one region to another of a given bone[141, 142].

Evidence has also been presented favoring the functional unity of the articulation and particularly its vascular unity. This existence of a unitarian vascular network accounts for hemodynamic repercussion from one epiphysis to the other (Fig. 9). Provoked intraosseous hypertension in one epiphysis may produce a similar response in the opposing epiphysis across an articulation. We have seen such responses, particularly in reflex sympathetic dystrophy. Nevertheless, such transmission of provoked intraosseous hypertension is not always seen across an articulation as there is undoubtedly considerable damping by extraosseous drainage pathways. The vascular unity between two adjacent bone ends may be extended via epiphyseal-metaphyseal anastomoses and metaphyseal-diaphyseal anastomoses to proximal and distal joints, creating a central intraosseous and periarticular axis. In certain pathological states, this may provide additional drainage or supply pathways which are of considerable importance. Drainage through these alternate pathways is sometimes seen on intraosseous venography in pathologic conditions.

<h1 style="text-align:center">CHAPTER III</h1>

<h1 style="text-align:center">FUNCTIONAL INVESTIGATION OF BONE
UNDER NORMAL CONDITIONS</h1>

INTRODUCTION

In the preceding chapters, we emphasized the difficulties in investigating the intraosseous circulation. Intraosseous arteries are of small caliber and their visualization by contrast medium is considerably hampered by the opacity of the bony structures which encompass them. The flow measurement of the blood that enters and exits from bone is practically impossible, except in circumstances which are not clinically very applicable, e.g., amputations[409]. All of this may seem somewhat discouraging, but, in fact, such restrictions are applicable to most diagnostic methods. Even x-rays, which are so valuable in the diagnosis of bone pathology, have serious limitations and uncertainty of interpretation.

Even though we do not possess a complete knowledge of the intraosseous circulation in man, we do have many paraclinical methods which are both simple and safe. These methods allow us to investigate bone as a living organ and to detect alterations in its vascularity. It is possible, then, to carry out a truly functional investigation of bone blood flow. This third chapter is devoted to the methods of functional evaluation. Some have been used for a long time and are easy to carry out. Their reliability has been established, and they should be used for diagnosis similar to the way in which we use x-rays. We will refer to these as the basic methods. They include IMP measurements, intraosseous venography, radioisotope scintigraphy and scintimetry, and most important, the biopsy. Other methods are more difficult to carry out or are too difficult to interpret to be employed in all cases.

BASIC METHODS OF ASSESSING BONE CIRCULATION
HEMODYNAMIC METHODS
Measurement of Intramedullary Pressure

We have seen earlier that the IMP is devoid of specific significance and without absolute value in terms of bone blood flow. However, when it is measured with the same instruments, the same technique, and in identical experimental conditions, it represents, in spite of its relativity, a true biological constant, useful as a fundamental and reliable reference. After extensive use of this parameter of measurement, we have found that 30 mm Hg represents the upper limit of normal values.

Instruments - Stainless steel trocars, 3 mm in diameter with a Luer lock, proximal end for fitting with a syringe, come in lengths of 8 and 15 cm. In order to facilitate manipulation, there are two short transverse projections which form a type of handle. The obturator has a pointed distal end which protrudes exactly 1 mm, while the proximal end is attached to a steel cylinder with a knurled handle. This permits inserting the trocar into bone with a mallet without damage to the Luer lock fitting (Fig. 27). Polyethylene catheters, such as those used in a physiology or a cardiology laboratory, are used to connect the trocar to the pressure transducers (Fig. 29). Several types of pressure transducers are commercially available; we have used the Statham type (Fig. 28). A pen recorder with pre-amplifier connected to the pressure transducer completes the electromanometer used to record the pressure curve (Fig. 30).

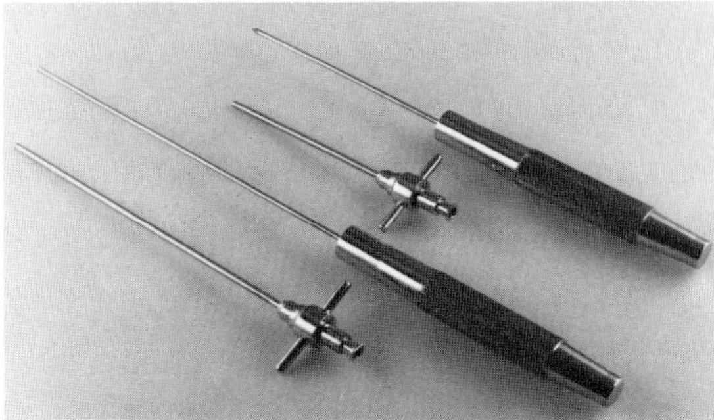

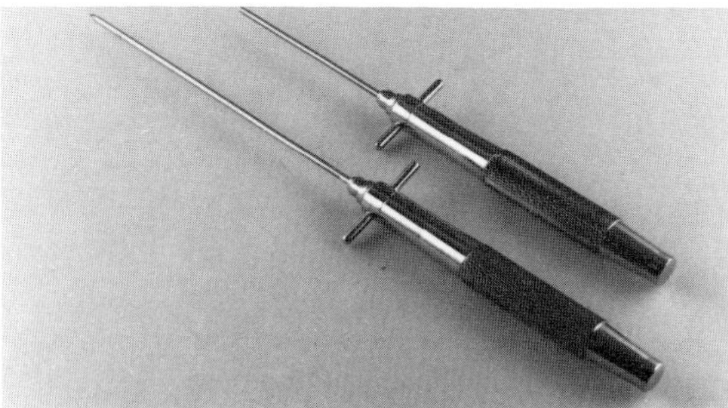

Fig.27.—Photographs of the trocars which we used for the measurement of IMP. Above: the long and short trocars with obturator attached to a knurled handle. Below: the assembled trocars, ready to be hammered into place. The Luer lock ends are protected.

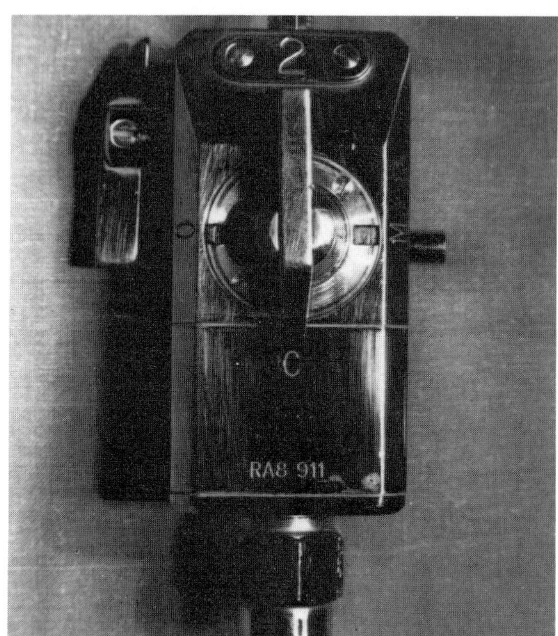

Fig. 28.—Statham pressure transducer with built-in three-way stopcock.

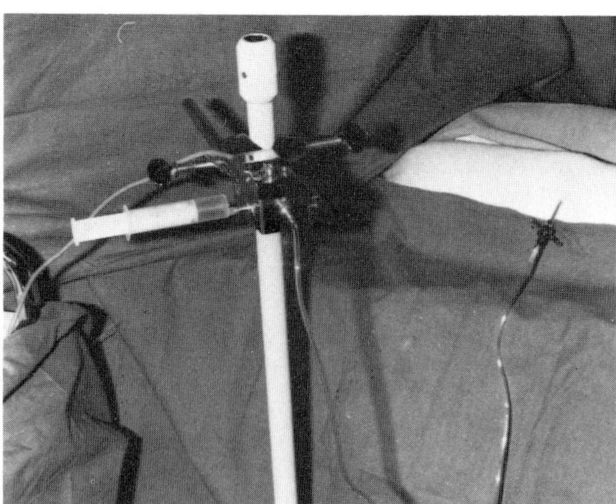

Fig.29.—Transducer and recorder connected to the intraosseous trocar by a flexible but thick-walled polyethylene catheter.

Technique - The IMP can be taken at any given point on the skeleton with direct insertion of the trocar into the epiphysis or the metaphysis. For the diaphyses, it is better to make a drill hole into the cortex without penetration of the endosteum using a drill bit slightly smaller in diameter than the trocar. The actual technique of pressure measurement is extremely important if reliable and reproducible results are to be obtained. Under local anesthesia with the patient in the supine position, the region over the greater trochanter is prepped and draped as for a surgical procedure. Positioning of the trocar is assisted with an image intensifier. Local anesthesia is infiltrated from the skin, down to and including the periosteum. A small stab wound is made into the skin, and the point of the trocar is placed 1.5 cm proximal to the proximal margin of the vastus lateralis origin. The trocar is oriented horizontally and perpendicular to the long axis of the body (Fig. 31). It is then inserted 2 to 3 cm into the greater trochanter with a mallet. It is critical that the first placement be correct, since a second hole in the bone brings an immediate fall in the IMP. If a second trocar is desired for a different position, the first trocar should be left in place with the obturator inserted.

The pressure transducer is placed on a verticular post at the same height as the trocar. The catheter is

connected to the transducer to which a three-way stopcock and 20 cc syringe filled with heparinized saline are attached. It is important that the connecting catheter and the transducer contain no air locks. Under normal circumstances, with the removal of the obturator from the trocar, a drop of medullary blood mixed with fat fills the space, if not, the trocar should be filled with heparinized saline using a long, thin spinal needle. It is important that there is continuous fluid filling of the entire system. Luer lock fittings on the cannula assure a water-tight fit.

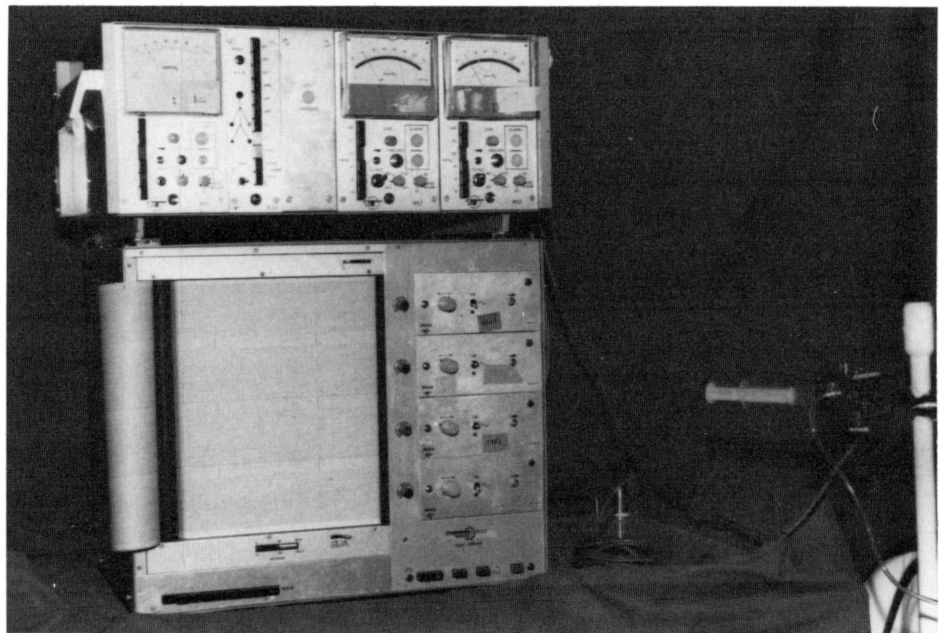

Fig.30.—Electromanometer strip-chart recorder.

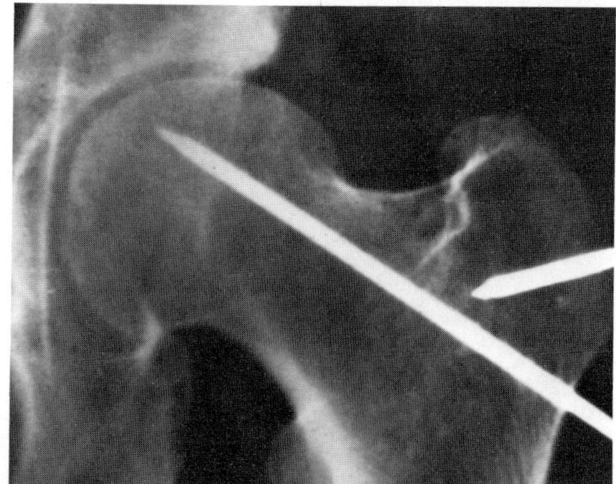

Fig.31.—Trocars placed for IMP measurements in the trochanteric region and in the head.

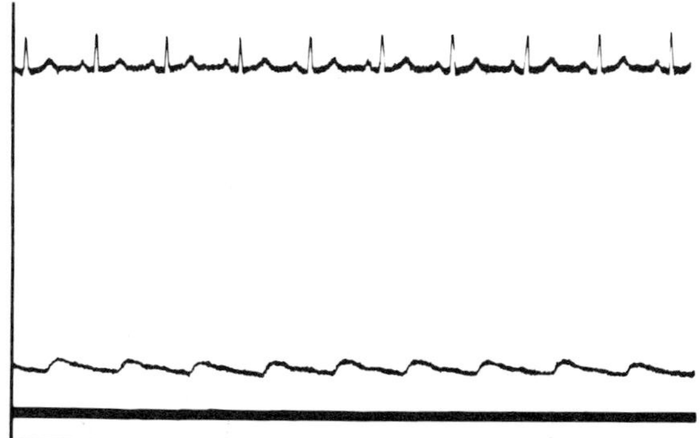

Fig.32.—Recording of normal IMP (below) showing correlation with the EKG (above).

Each recording system will have its own method for calibration. It is important that the system be individually calibrated before each recording to be sure that reliable and absolute values can be read from the pen recording paper. After calibration of the transducer, the three-way stopcock is open to air and the pen recorder set at zero with the positioning switch. This does not alter sensitivity or change the calibration. The three-way stopcock is then turned to connect the patient to the transducer, and the recording begins.

Variable speeds on the pen recorder may be used at different times in the recording in order to better evaluate specific aspects of the curves (Fig. 32). Generally, several minutes are required until the IMP reaches a level plateau. We have found that taking the pressures recorded five minutes after the beginning of recording is generally sufficient for baseline stabilization. We have found that in many recordings an average IMP of 20 mm Hg corresponds to normal conditions of bone at rest. The recorded pressure should show both the synchronous undulation of arterial pulse (pulse pressure) and some undulation with respiration. This may be small but is characteristic of IMP. During the investigation, we monitor the general arterial pressure by indirect reading with a blood pressure cuff or, in some cases, by means of arterial catheterization.

The stress test (Fig. 33) - This represents a hemodynamic test of the capacity of the vascular bed of the bone marrow. It is carried out by injecting 5 ml of physiologic saline into the intertrochanteric trocar. The three-way stopcock is turned to shut the pressure transducer "off" and open the cannula to the syringe. It is important that this be correctly done, since most pressure transducers can be damaged by excessive injection pressures. Immediately following the injection, the three-way stopcock is again turned to connect the cannula to the transducer. Several types of information can be gained from this test. First of all, one should note the resistance to injection of the solution. Normally, this is no more difficult than intravenous injection. In fact, the intraosseous route has been used therapeutically as a substitution for the intravenous route when the latter is unobtainable. For example, intramedullary injection can be used for a Pentathol injection to induce anesthesia. This ease of injection is a demonstration of marrow tissue permeability, of the extent of venous drainage pathways, and of the speed of osseous transit which takes less than one second. In this way, bone marrow can be considered similar to a peripheral vein. One should also note the pain which may or may not be experienced during injection. As long as the injection is slow, it is normally painless. Finally, the effect of the injection on the intramedullary pressure is studied on the pen recording. Within a few seconds of the injection, the pressure curve has returned to the baseline. However, occasionally the curve will demonstrate a peak of variable magnitude which rapidly falls to near the baseline value. Usually, we will wait five minutes for the pressure to return to the baseline, although it has returned to normal in a much shorter time. Any pressure which remains 10 mm Hg above the baseline after five minutes must be regarded as pathological, in which case, the test is positive. To conclude that the circulatory state is normal, the stress test must be negative.

The stress test is invaluable because it allows us to detect latent pathology which is not sufficiently advanced to produce changes in rest pressure within the bone marrow, but which is evident when the circulation of the marrow is overloaded. It, therefore, reveals pathology which would not be otherwise detected and demonstrates a derangement of drainage of the bone and predicts intraosseous stasis.

Measurement of femoral head pressure - This usually requires general anesthesia. It can be carried out either by transcutaneous insertion of the trocar, using a technique similar to intra-articular injection, by direct insertion into the head during a surgical approach to the hip, or by introducing the 15 cm trocar in the central axis of the femoral neck through the trochanter. The progression of the trocar is monitored using the same technique as with an insertion of an internal fixation device. This is greatly facilitated by the image intensifier, taking both AP and frog-leg view. If an image intensifier is not available, the level of the femoral head is marked on the skin with a radiopaque object, taking into account the femoral neck anteversion, the angle of inclination of the femoral head and neck, and the rotation of the lower extremity. Using this technique, pressure can first be recorded 3 cm in from the initial osseous insertion then 5 cm in the mid-portion of the femoral neck and then at approximately 8 cm within the femoral head. The trocar can be directed to that section of the femoral head which shows radiologic change. Pressures then can be successfully taken in the trochanter, the neck, and the head, or one can simultaneously monitor both head and trochanteric regions by inserting a second trocar into the greater trochanteric region (Fig. 34). With the trocars in place, they are connected to two separate monitoring systems. We have sometimes introduced a third trocar into the acetabular roof to simultaneously monitor three pressures from both sides of the joint. To do this, one needs three pressure transducers and

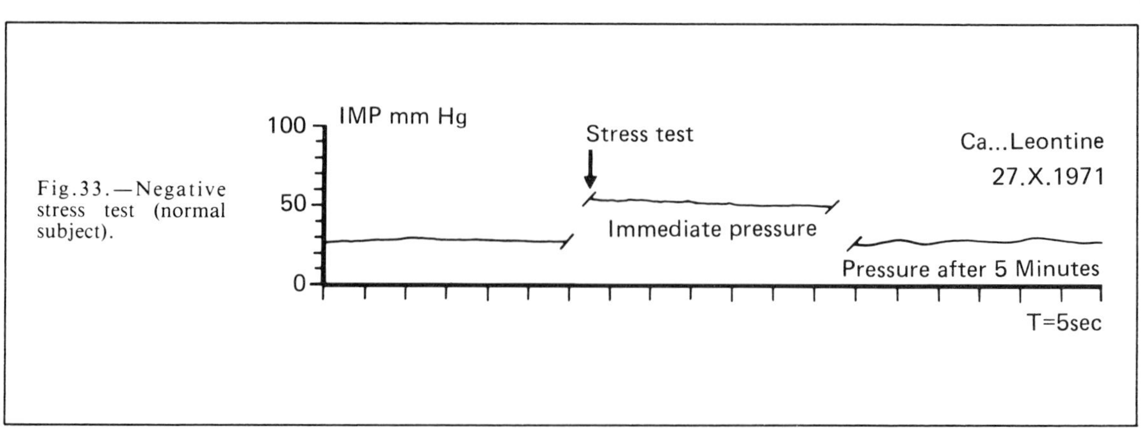

Fig.33.—Negative stress test (normal subject).

a three pen recorder for simultaneous measurement on the same chart. The stress test can then be carried out in the head as well as the trochanteric region at different points in time, noting the influence of the stress test in adjacent areas of bone. These observations give some insight into the interconnected nature of the bone marrow bed and of the general repercussion on other areas of an induced, localized increase in pressure.

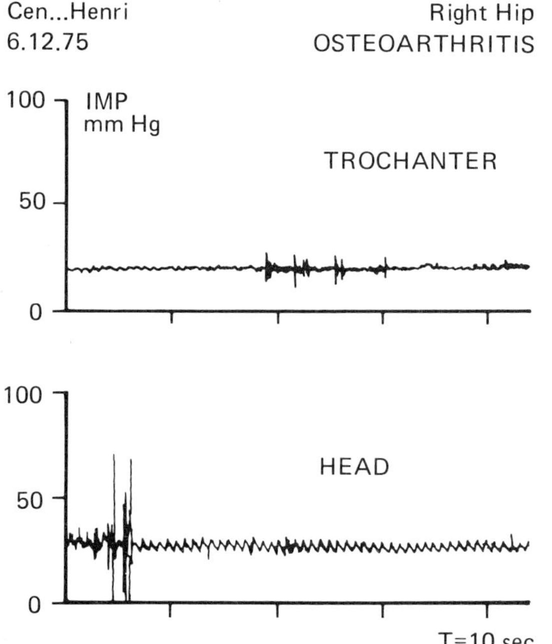

Fig.34.—Simultaneous recording of the IMP in the trochanteric region and in the femoral head.

Results - According to all the studies performed in the normal hip[10,21,29,241,417], the obtained values are fairly constant at about 20 mm Hg as we have already seen in Chapter I. We have adopted the upper limit of normal as 30, in order to have a sufficient margin of error. It should be noted, however, that the pressure within the femoral head is always higher than the trochanteric pressure with a differential of approximately 5 mm Hg. The pen recording also allows precision in recording the pulse pressure within bone which is slightly delayed in relation to that of ventricular systole. The normal amplitude is about 3 to 7 mm Hg (Fig. 32).

The hemodynamic test of Raynal and Levy[355] These two authors studied the IMP under epidural anesthesia, e.g., with perfect circulatory stability. The test consists of studying the changes in the IMP, both in regard to the ambient level of pressure and to the change in characterization of the pulse pressure under the influence of change in the general circulation. Under these circumstances, the injection of a vasodilator into the general circulation results in an increase in limb blood flow as measured by plethysmography. Other drugs increase both blood flow and systemic general arterial pressure. Under normal circumstances, this enhanced circulation results in both a rise in IMP and an increase in pulse pressure. This is particularly true when the arterial pressure was low to begin with (Fig. 34B). The amplitude of the pulse pressure increases in a parallel fashion to the plethysmographic oscillation.

This test is of interest in the necroses. In suspected femoral head necrosis after a fracture, a clear improvement in the IMP and its pulse pressure can be obtained by "improvement" of the general circulation, indicating that the circulation of the femoral

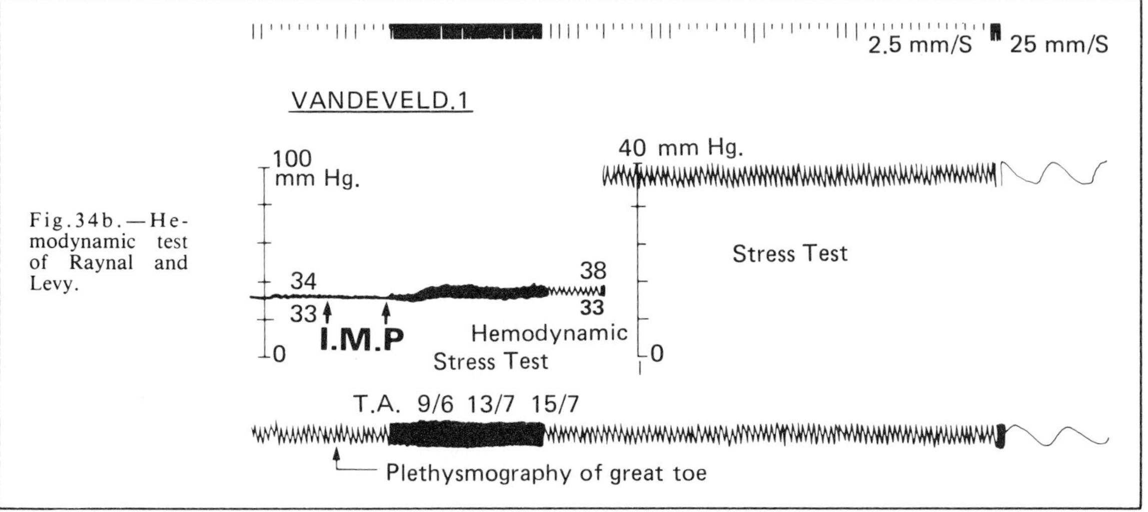

Fig.34b.—Hemodynamic test of Raynal and Levy.

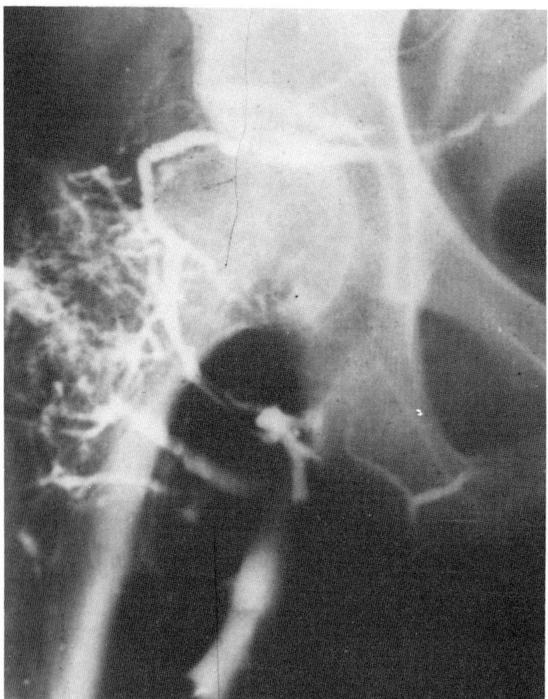 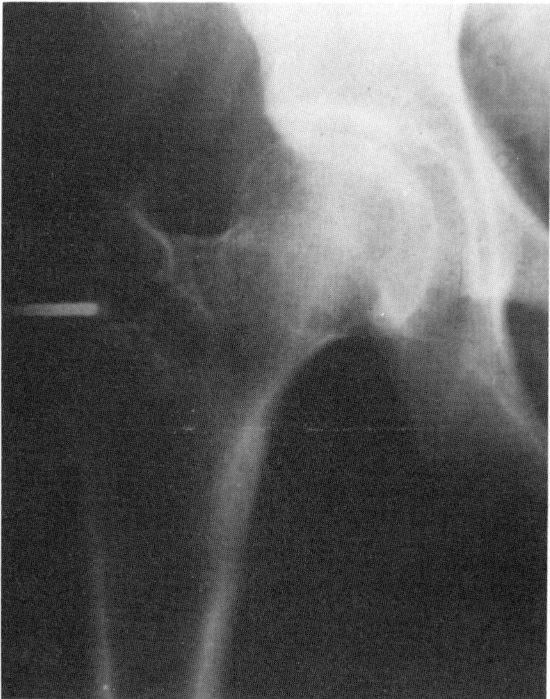

Fig.35.—Normal pertrochanteric venography. Visualization of the two main pedicles, superior or ischiatic and inferior or circumflex. No evidence of reflux or stasis 15 min. later (film on the right).

head is well preserved. The same thing can be measured in terms of intraosseous temperature. On the other hand, in non-traumatic necroses, there is no appreciable change in either the level or the morphology of the pulse pressure.

INTRAMEDULLARY VENOGRAPHY

This test consists of observing the intraosseous and extraosseous drainage pathways of contrast material injected into the bone marrow[15,150]. This was originally used by the Toulouse school for visualization of the pelvic veins[43,126,127]. We have integrated this technique within the concept of a functional exploration of bone, restoring it to its original significance in the study of marrow circulation. In coupling it with the measurement of intramedullary pressure and the histologic examination of biopsy tissue, this technique is applicable to all forms of hip disease.

Intertrochanteric phlebography - Ten ml of contrast material is injected into the marrow in the intertrochanteric region through the same trocar used for taking the IMP. Its intraosseous course and evacuation is studied through serial x-rays, with an image intensifier, or with cineradiography. Intramedullary venography requires general anesthesia, since the in-

jecting compound produces significant discomfort, particularly if an obstruction to its evacuation exists. The injection is performed manually and slowly to avoid traumatizing the tissues with a hemodynamic rush of fluid with potential effects on the histopathology of the specimen which is to be taken later. Films are taken serially at the termination of injection, five and fifteen minutes later. Occasionally, additional films at one and six hours later or even the following day are taken if necessary. These films give a fairly clear idea of the venous drainage of the bone marrow (Fig. 35). Cineradiography films the pathway of the radiopaque substance from the time of its injection until its evacuation from bone, giving a living and dynamic image of the venous drainage. This can also be followed on an image intensifier.

Under normal circumstances, the radiopaque material is quickly evacuated via normal efferent vessels of the metaphysis best seen in the first film. Four main veins drain the proximal femoral metaphysis. The two superior pathways join the hypogastric system. The intergluteal vein ascends between the gluteus medias and maximus to enter the pelvis posteriorly. The posterior vein of the neck initially has a horizontal course before changing direction to join the internal iliac vein. The two inferior pathways running parallel in an inferior medial direction con-

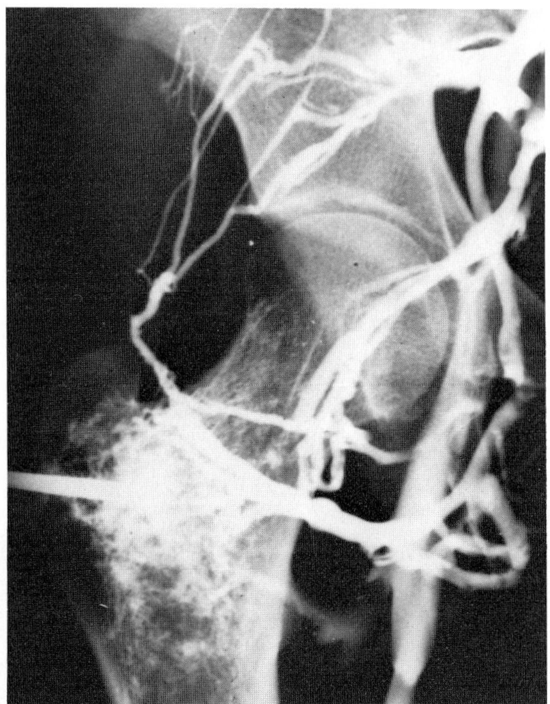

Fig.36.—Intramedullary venography demonstrating the four normal efferent pathways of the upper femoral metaphysis: intergluteal, ischiatic, anterior and posterior circumflex.

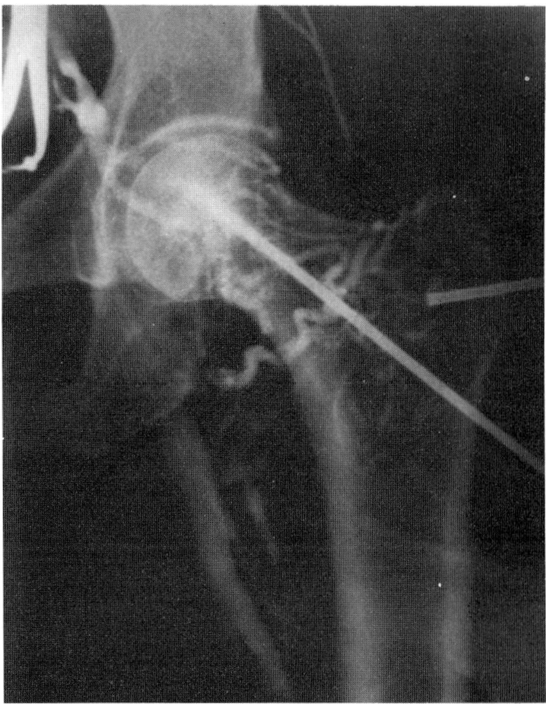

Fig.37.—Intra-capital venography shows the retinacular veins and the ligamentum teres or obturator vein.

sists of both the posterior and anterior circumflex veins. The former runs along the intertrochanteric line while the latter, often doubled, crosses the lesser trochanter to empty into the femoral external iliac vein. Their course is fairly straight, and their caliber is regular. The primary veins of the system, however, are the posterior vein of the neck and the posterior circumflex vein (Fig. 36). Under normal circumstances, rapid drainage occurs resulting in no diaphyseal or epiphyseal reflux; and, at the end of five minutes, there is no metaphyseal stasis of injected contrast material. The intraosseous metaphyseal network is revealed by a fine reticulated image of a small network of vessels constituting the origin of the principle veins. When observing this on the image intensifier, one has the impression of an immediate drainage from the tip of the needle to the cortex, as if the origin of the efferent vessel had been injected directly. We have often observed, however, that at the junction between the metaphysis and diaphysis near the level of the lesser trochanter a radiopaque spot, more or less regular in outline, remains visible for some time. This gives the appearance of a buffer reservoir between the two circulations, metaphyseal and diaphyseal.

The extraosseous venous trunks which collect these efferent vessels are the deep and common femoral veins on the one hand and the internal and common iliac veins on the other. They immediately fill and quickly empty. As viewed with cineradiography or under the image intensifier, these trunks normally exhibit contractions (venous peristalsis). These dynamic observations give the impression that osseous transit is normally of very short duration from the emergence at the tip of the needle to the exit from bone (in the order of one second). This can be accurately measured by cineradiography. The intramedullary venogram, apart from its measurement of bone transit, also gives a dynamic vision of functional continuity and morphology of the extrinsic drainage system which is of interest from a pathophysiologic point of view.

Intramedullary venography of the femoral head - Similar to intertrochanteric venography, this consists of injection of 10 ml of radiopaque material through the trocar used to measure intramedullary pressure in the femoral head. The film technique is identical. However, the film demonstrates an extra vein, that of the ligamentum teres, which drains into the obturator vein and the internal iliac vein (Fig. 37). Any intraosseous phlebography allows a stress test which is even more sensitive than the stress test performed with saline, since the liquid is more viscous and intensifies the effect on the vascular bed. Because of this, we usually measure the IMP following venography. The increase in pressure is usually higher and the return to the normal value delayed, but, in normal circumstances, there is little difference between this and the test with saline. On the other hand, as we shall see in the section on pathology, these values are much higher than the test with saline under abnormal circumstances. There is a problem of choice between these two techniques. In our experience, we can say that intertrochanteric venography gives the best pictures, and that it is usually sufficient in most pathological cases. On the other hand, if this phlebography does not reveal any abnormality, it may be useful to do a second venography, using an injection in the femoral head.

Complication Iodine shock—We have only observed one such case under local anesthesia, and it was not serious, characterized by generalized and transient erythema. Perhaps general anesthesia acts as an inhibitor to these reactions since under any other circumstances it has not been observed. Venography is contraindicated in cases with a positive iodine test or history of intolerance. Intramedullary venography has been the object of prior criticisms for producing changes that could invalidate the biopsy interpretation. For this reason, we have carried out a series of 100 biopsies without venography. The histologic changes in these cases were indistinguishable from those with venography, thus obviating this potential criticism. The pathology of these cases compared to those with venography, thus circumventing this potential criticism. Moreover, Enria and Ferrero[137] and Susse[432,433], who studied these marrow changes observed only minimal and reversible alterations consisting of very small areas of localized fibrosis. Schobinger[385], five days after venography, described a small area of fatty necrosis in the lateral malleolus in an arthritic amputee, but he himself commented that he could hardly see any difference with the contralateral, medial malleolus which had not been injected. Since the sample is taken only a few minutes after the injection, there is little time for changes to occur.

HISTOLOGIC METHODS OF INVESTIGATION

The Core Biopsy[144]

The goal of this method is to obtain a cylindrical specimen of bone and bone marrow from the whole length of the upper femur, from the lateral cortex to

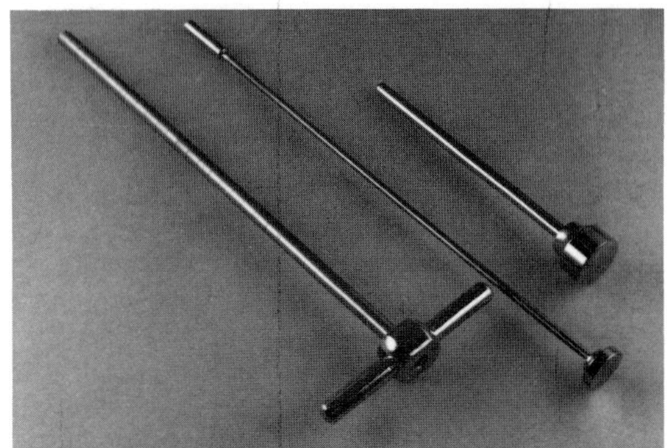

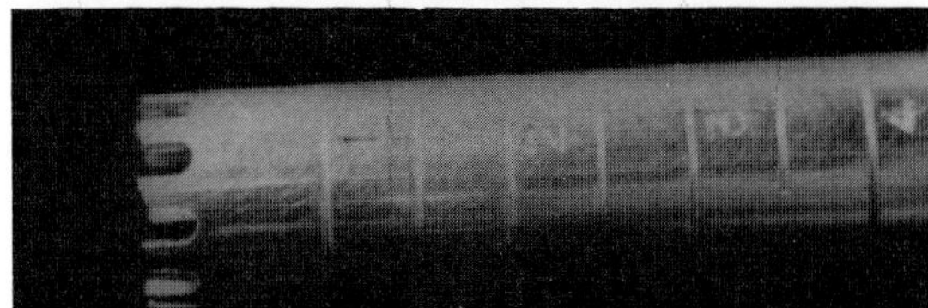

Fig. 38a.—The 8 mm core biopsy trephine, the most commonly used, showing the serrated cutting end.

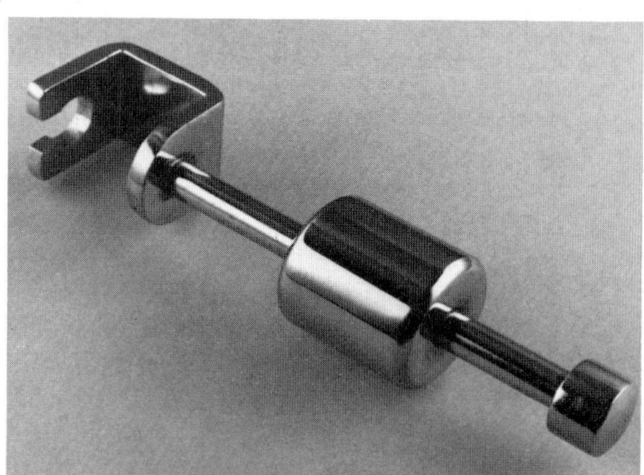

Fig. 38b.—Extractor for the trephine and trocar.

the femoral head as near as possible to the cartilage surface with a margin of safety. We believe that this biopsy is essential to determine exactly the condition of the bone in all hip pathology, particularly where its cause or consequences has a major vascular component.

Instruments - To obtain the specimen, we have devised a 35 cm long, hollow trephine with a serrated distal end and a transverse handle at the proximal end to facilitate manipulation. The trephine is calibrated to allow direct measurement of the distance of insertion[144] (Fig. 38a). Three diameters are available: 6, 8, and 10 mm. Each is equipped with two obturators, a short one which allows the trephine to be inserted with a mallet without deforming the outlet and a longer 36 cm one which allows the bone biopsy to be removed.

Technique (Fig. 39) - With the patient in the supine position and under general anesthesia, the IMP measurements and venography are first carried out if indicated. The lateral aspect of the trochanter at the level of the trochanteric flair is exposed by a short mid-lateral longitudinal incision. The fascia lata and vastus lateralis are split in the direction of their fibers. Anterior and posterior retractors expose the lateral femur. With a gouge or a Smith-Peterson Nail Starter, a piece of the lateral cortex is removed to allow the trephine to be inserted. This should be at the point of prolongation of the femoral neck, the site for most hip pinnings, in the mid-lateral plane. The trephine is inserted with continuous, rotational movement, directing it towards the superior part of the head which has been marked with a cutaneous mark during the scout films. Anteversion must be accounted for. The technique is much simpler if image intensification is available, since the progression of the instrument can be observed in both the AP and frog-leg projections. If the femoral head is very sclerotic, the trephine may not advance by simple, manual pressure and rotation. In these cases, it has to be very carefully hammered in using the short ob-

turator to avoid damage to the trephine opening. Distance of insertion can be exactly determined by the scale on the trephine. We recommend that the biopsy proceed to within 4 to 5 mm of the subchondral plate which, of course, is easier to see with the image intensifier (Fig. 39b). When the final insertion has been reached, the trephine is rotated several times at that level and then slowly withdrawn with continous rotation with the short obturator in place. Since the friction at the side walls of the trocar and specimen surface is greater than the tension between the specimen and the contiguous bone, the specimen is usually extracted in this manner. The specimen is removed with the extraction obturator and placed in a biopsy container with 10% buffered formalin (Fig. 40). We sometimes carry out a second biopsy with the small trephine to take a bone sample from a different site of the neck or the head, either because the first biopsy was not correctly oriented or because one wants to sample an area with a distinct radiologic appearance. The core channel is irrigated with saline and left open. We have abandoned the metal rings intended to prevent the closure of the cortical orifice as well as the pedicle muscle transplants which we did

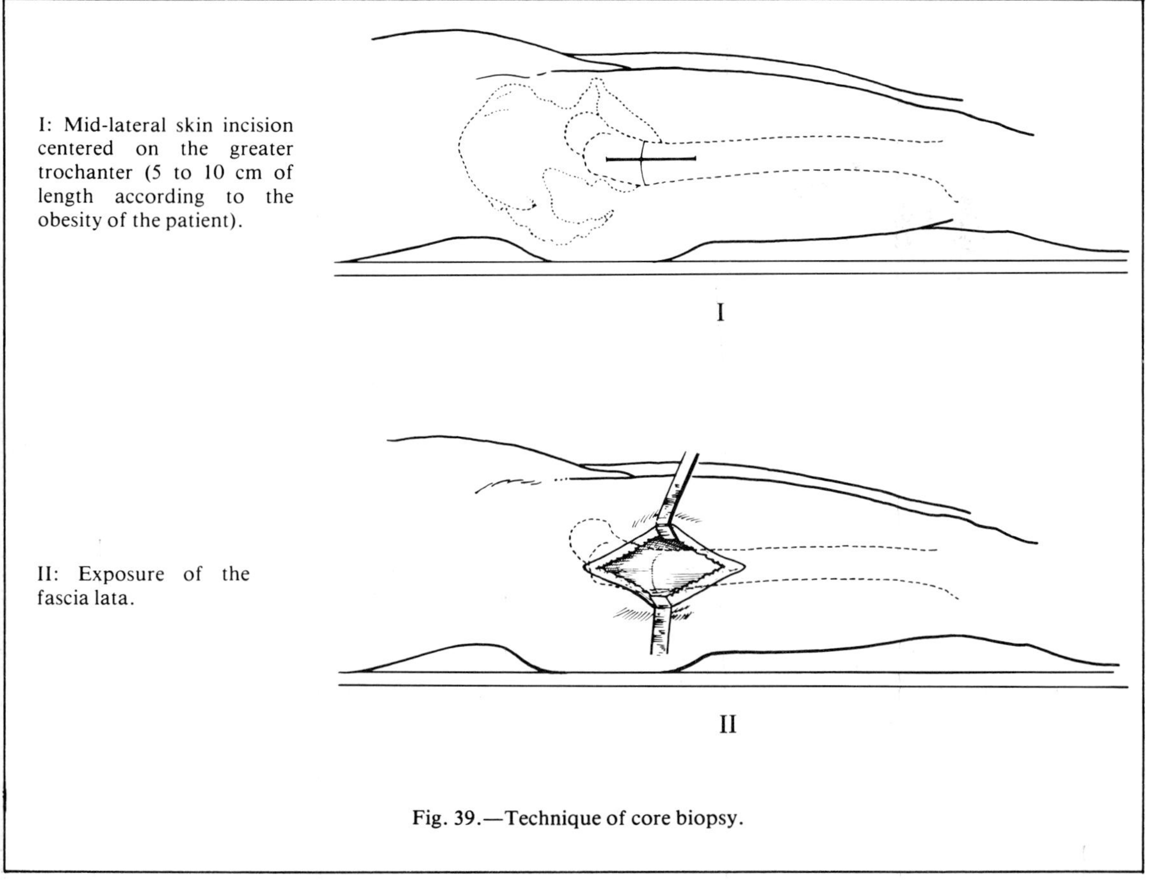

Fig. 39.—Technique of core biopsy.

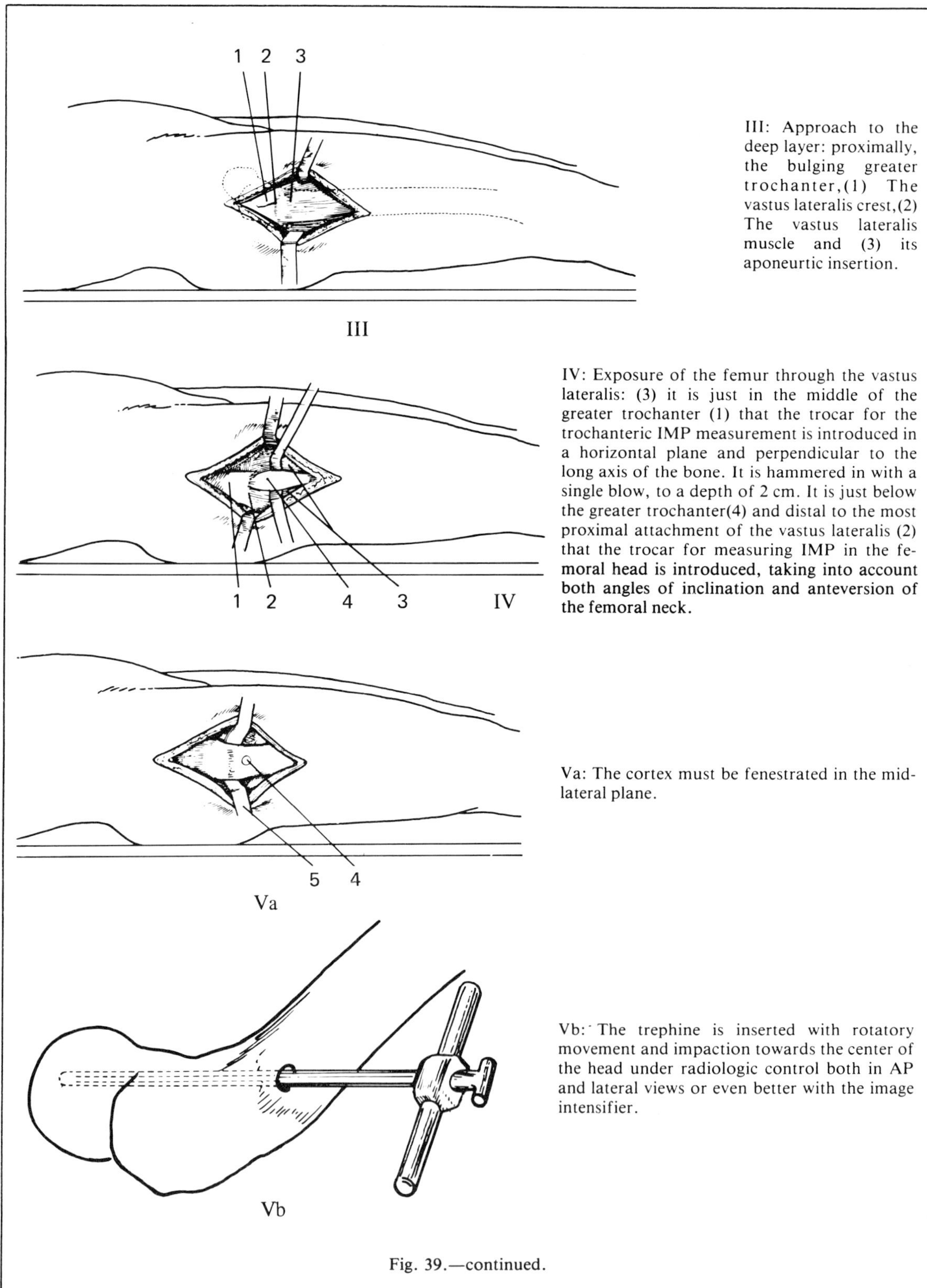

III: Approach to the deep layer: proximally, the bulging greater trochanter,(1) The vastus lateralis crest,(2) The vastus lateralis muscle and (3) its aponeurtic insertion.

IV: Exposure of the femur through the vastus lateralis: (3) it is just in the middle of the greater trochanter (1) that the trocar for the trochanteric IMP measurement is introduced in a horizontal plane and perpendicular to the long axis of the bone. It is hammered in with a single blow, to a depth of 2 cm. It is just below the greater trochanter(4) and distal to the most proximal attachment of the vastus lateralis (2) that the trocar for measuring IMP in the femoral head is introduced, taking into account both angles of inclination and anteversion of the femoral neck.

Va: The cortex must be fenestrated in the mid-lateral plane.

Vb: The trephine is inserted with rotatory movement and impaction towards the center of the head under radiologic control both in AP and lateral views or even better with the image intensifier.

Fig. 39.—continued.

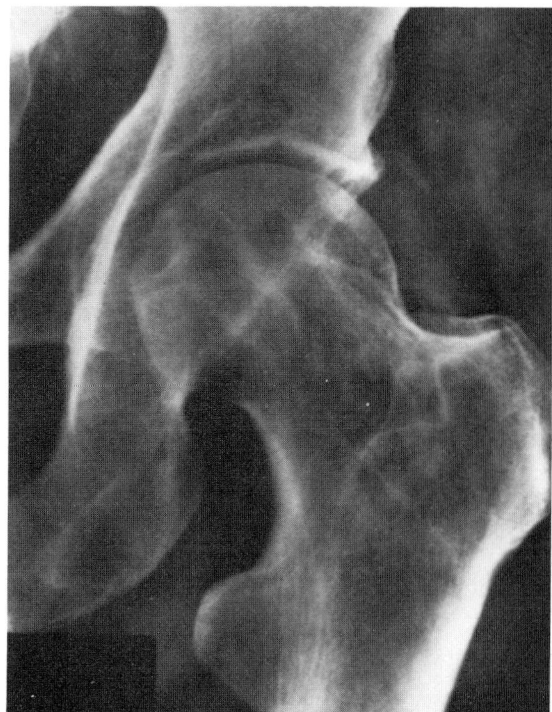

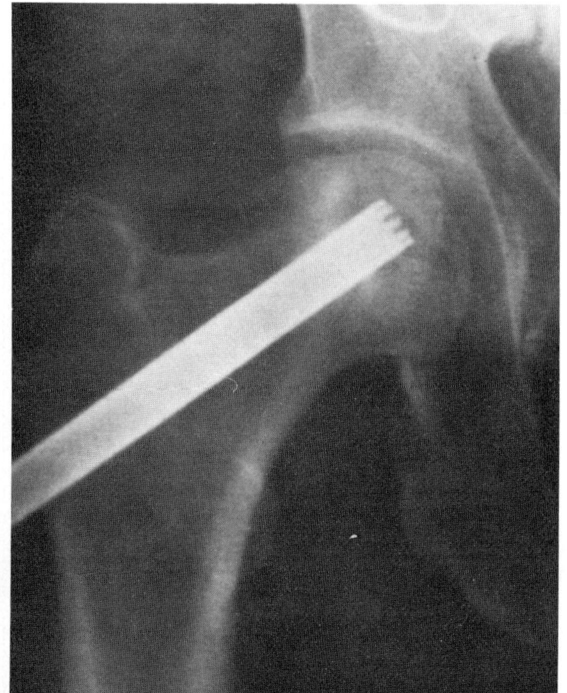

Fig. 39b.—Trephine in situ.

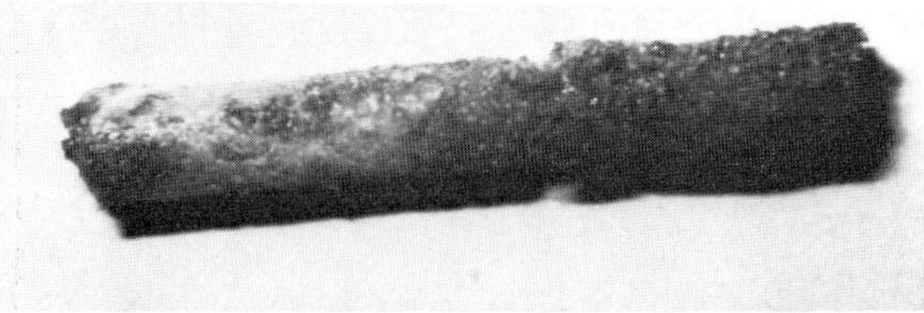

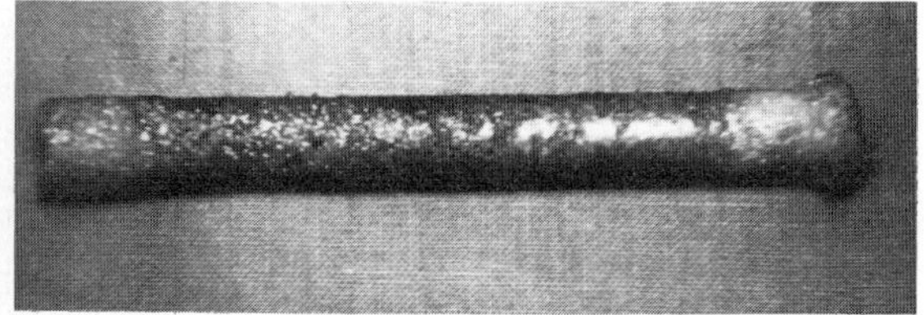

Fig. 40.—Biopsy specimens removed from the trephine.

Fig. 41.—Core tract.

initially (Fig. 41). The vastus lateralis, fascia lata, and skin are sutured in layers over a single, small suction drain.

Postoperative care—Bed rest for several days is followed by immediate mobilization. Protected weight-bearing is carried out for several weeks, although this may be extended depending upon the radiologic state of the femoral head.

Comment - This core decompression is not at all like those previously advocated. Some authors, such as Graber-Duvernay[189] have recommended it for osteoarthritis, mainly for its antalgic effect. However, this was quickly abandoned because the initial favorable effects did not last. The coring produced only venous decompression for a few months. As it was then performed, a drill was used, and no biopsy sample was obtained. Others, as we have seen carried out by Phemister[345] and later on by Bonfiglio[55,56], insert a tibial graft in the core channel. These authors reserve this procedure for advanced cases of osteonecrosis with the idea of supporting the head to avoid or minimize its collapse. Our method is, therefore, fundamentally different from three points of view. From the diagnostic point of view, it produces a specimen which includes cancellous tissue of the femoral head, which is important in the early stages of hip pathology. From the pathophysiologic point of view, it represents an irreplaceable means of breaking the vicious cycle of the ischemia by reducing intramedullary hypertension, producing a drainage pathway for stasis and facilitating the revascularization of the femoral head. From the therapeutic point of view, because of its physiologic basis, it acts on the natural history of the disease, relieving pain and permanently arresting some of the ischemic processes. (See Chapter X)

It does not appear logical to us to block the core channel with a graft which both increases the dead material to the already dead or dying bone and obviates the buffer reservoir role that the core channel can play in the face of a congested circulation. For this reason, we like this channel to remain open as long as possible. Its diagnostic, physiologic, and therapeutic goals have little in common with the blind or mechanical concepts of the past.

Variations in the basic technique - Core biopsy with the four-part trephine (Fig. 42). This set differs from the previous trephine in that there is an outer metal tube with a serrated distal end similar to the previous tube, but the proximal end has stepped off indentations in the proximal ring. The inner metal tube is made out of thin metal with a transverse han-

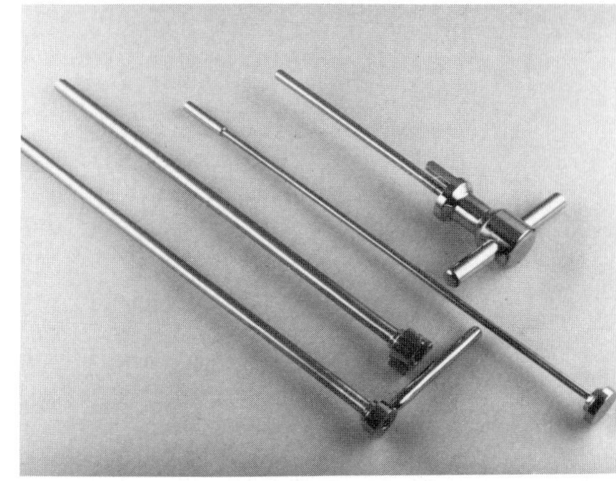

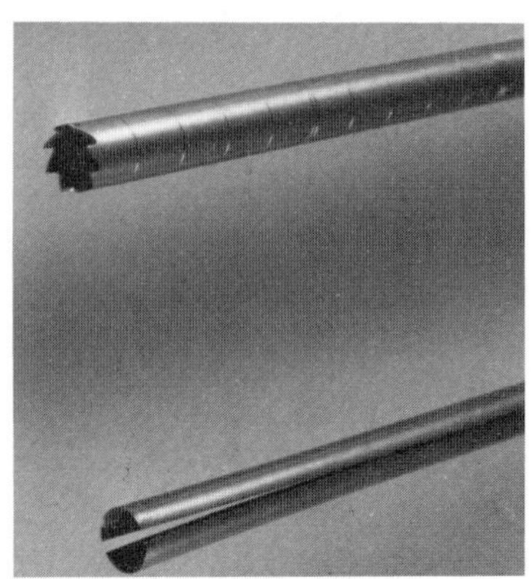

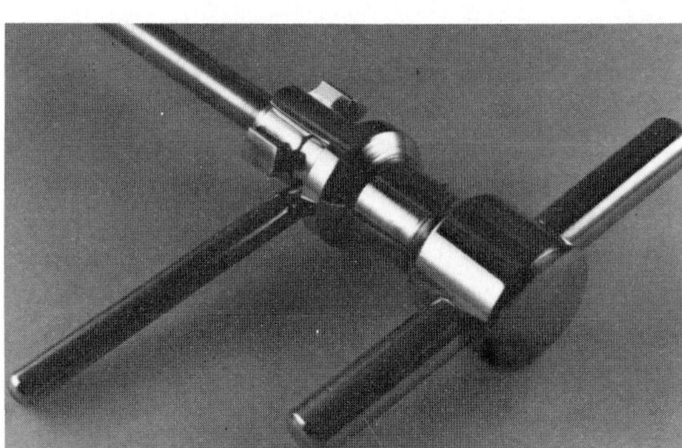

Fig. 42.—Four-part trephine system with slotted inner sleeve for soft bone.

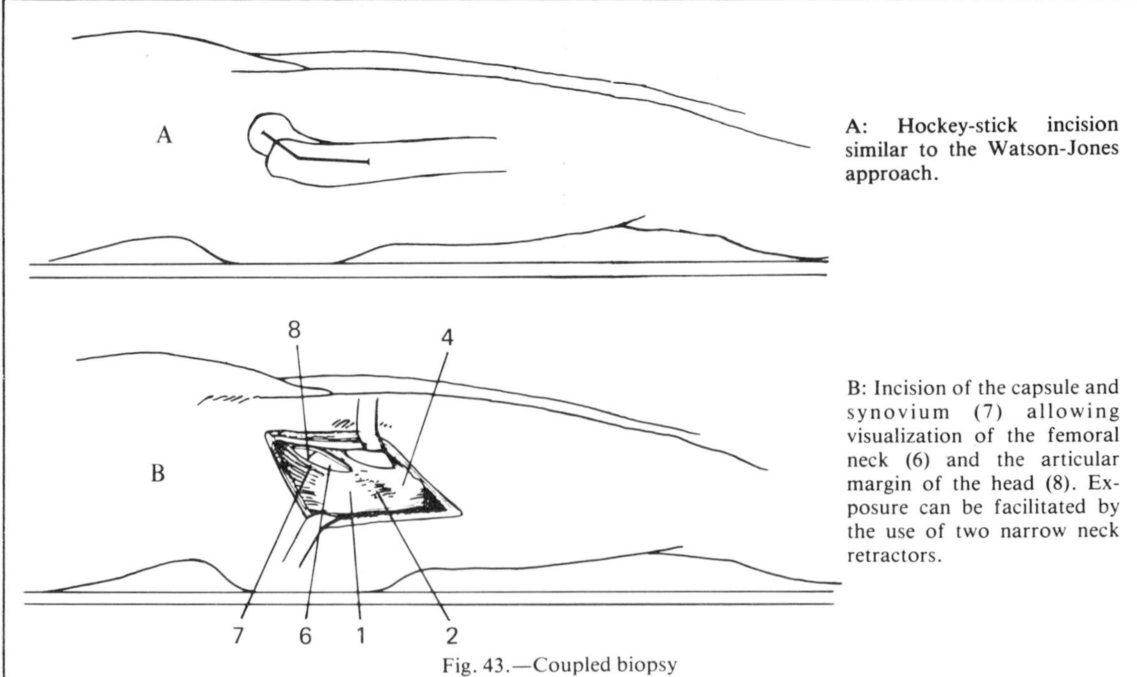

A: Hockey-stick incision similar to the Watson-Jones approach.

B: Incision of the capsule and synovium (7) allowing visualization of the femoral neck (6) and the articular margin of the head (8). Exposure can be facilitated by the use of two narrow neck retractors.

Fig. 43.—Coupled biopsy

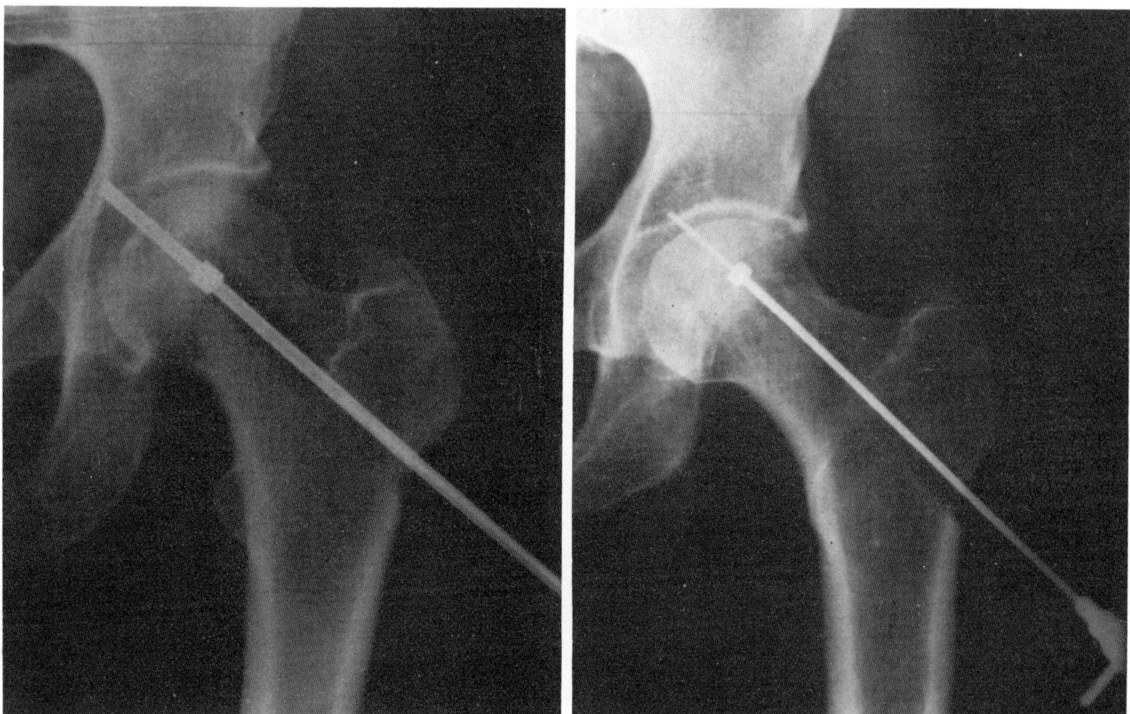

Fig. 44.—Hip chondrotomes in situ, allowing the removal of acetabular and femoral head articular cartilage with subchondral bone in the same specimen.

dle on the proximal end, while the distal end is slotted for a length of 6 to 8 cm. The short obturator contains a handle which allows the outer tube to be turned by engaging the stepped indentations of the outer trephine. It also allows the trephine to be inserted with a mallet without damaging the proximal end of the inner tube. The fourth part is the extraction obturator. The trephine is inserted by turning the outer tube with the short obturator while holding the handle of the inner tube to prevent rotation. The outer sleeve then, in effect, cuts the tract while the inner, non-rotating sleeve allows the biopsy specimen to slide down the channel without creating artifact. The specimen can also be extracted from the inner sleeve, non-traumatically, since the sleeve is slotted. This method is best for osteoporotic or soft bones. It cannot be used for bone which is sclerotic.

Combined Biopsy (Fig. 43)

By extending the incision proximally in a hockey-stick fashion similar to the Watson-Jones incision, retractors can be placed around the femoral neck between the gluteus medius and the tensor fascia lata. The capsule and synovial membrane are incised on the anterior aspect of the neck after first inserting a needle in the joint to aspirate any existing synovial fluid. The entire joint can be inspected, noting any macroscopic pathology. Capsular and synovial biopsies are taken by sharp dissection. The capsular incision can be enlarged. With hip flexion, the most inner and inferior portions of synovia can be reached. By placing the retractors inside the joint around the neck, the cartilaginous borders of the head can be easily visualized. The synovial membrane is left open and the other layers closed.

Core biopsy with Cartilage biopsy (Fig. 44)

The biopsy of the cartilage constitutes, in our opinion, a method with a great future through advances in biochemical and electron microscopic techniques. Together with the bone and synovial biopsy, it gives precise and complete information on the condition of all the articular tissues. Application of such a technique could greatly change our diagnostic concepts.

Technique - This can be carried out through either an intra- or extra-articular approach. By the intra-articular approach, this can easily be done at the time of arthrotomy. The lower extremity can be positioned so as to uncover any peripheral portion of the head. The sample comes from a more or less marginal area and is performed at the same time as synovial biopsy. For the extra-articular approach, we have developed a personal technique for use with the core decompression. First, the typical core tract is made with extraction of the core biopsy specimen. Next, a long chondrotome is introduced into the core tract. The chondrotome has a short obturator so that it can be driven with a mallet through the subchondral bone and cartilage of the head and through the acetabulum and into the cancellous bone of the acetabulum. It is then possible to extract the specimen which contains cartilage and subchondral and cancellous bone from both the femoral head and the acetabulum from the weight-bearing area. The chondrotome is similar to that which we have developed for patella biopsy. There have been no technical complications. The purpose of these biopsies is to complete the functional investigation of bone and to study the effect of ischemia on cartilage. Since the identification of the ischemic coxopathy, we have naturally been led to this technique (See Chapter V). However, the greater risk of open biopsies limits their indications.

Complications of Core Biopsy

Maldirected trephine - If one adheres to a strict technique, the maldirection of a trephine should never occur, particularly if it is monitored with an image intensifier on both the AP and frog-leg view. However, with older techniques, two different sorts of errors could occur. Maldirection of the trephine in the anterior/posterior plane may produce either anterior or posterior perforation of the femoral neck. Insertion of the trephine too deeply could produce an articular wound with excision of a cartilaginous fragment.

Dense bone - In some exceptional and usually pathological cases (bone sclerosis of several sorts), it is not possible to introduce the trephine, even with heavy hammering. Because of the danger of femoral neck or head blowout fractures, it is best in these cases to stop the progression. This has only happened to us four times in almost 700 cases.

"Empty biopsies" - When the middle or sometimes large trocar is used, it may happen in some cases that no bone is found in the trocar when it is removed. This may happen, particularly in hard heads or where there had been insufficient penetration of the trephine. This is a rare occurrence, and one simply needs to change the trephine for the smaller 6 mm trephine which always produces a sample. We have only had an "empty" trephine with the small trephine on a very demineralized hip with a totally liquified marrow. Examination of the small

fragments taken with a curette permitted confirmation of the diagnosis of osteonecrosis.

Hematoma - These are unusual and usually consist simply of blood infiltrating the vastus lateralis, demonstrated by tenderness along the lateral aspect of the thigh which disappears in a few days. This can be avoided by use of a suction drain. In a few cases, however, the hematoma may discharge itself through the wound, which brings about a slight danger of secondary infection.

Phlebitis - This has become much less frequent since we have shortened the time of immobilization in bed. It is best to allow the patient to get up on crutches as soon as possible to encourage active mobilization and muscle contraction with physical therapy the day after surgery. In our first published series, we reported phlebitis in 6% of the cases. These are now rare occurrences.

Skin necrosis - In three patients with femoral head necrosis, we observed necrosis of the borders of the skin incision, probably produced by prolonged compression of the retractors on poorly vascularized skin. The excision of sloughed skin edges may be necessarily followed by secondary suture.

Acute or subacute arthritis - This has been observed in three cases. One case healed with conservative treatment without sequelae. The second case healed with stiffness and collapse of the superior pole of the head. The third case, with malignant tumor, required resection of the femoral head. On the other hand, we have never encountered an infection in the biopsy canal.

Normal Histology of the Biopsy Specimen

The specimen represents a cylinder of bone, approximately 5 to 7 cm in length, slightly shorter than the total penetration of the trocar. The difference occurs because a cortical hole is first made with a gouge. There is some compression at the trochanteric end of the specimen during extraction, even if this is protected by a small cushion of air between it and the distal end of the extraction obturator (Fig. 40). In the section which follows, we will be referring specifically to the structure of the bone tissue of the epiphyseal and metaphyseal region of the adult femur, as it is in these regions that most of our samples have been taken.

Macroscopic aspect - The surgeon performing the biopsy should describe the exterior aspect of the structure, the density, and the color, as well as the consistency of the specimen. Normal bone is red in the neck region, and yellowish with a sprinkling of

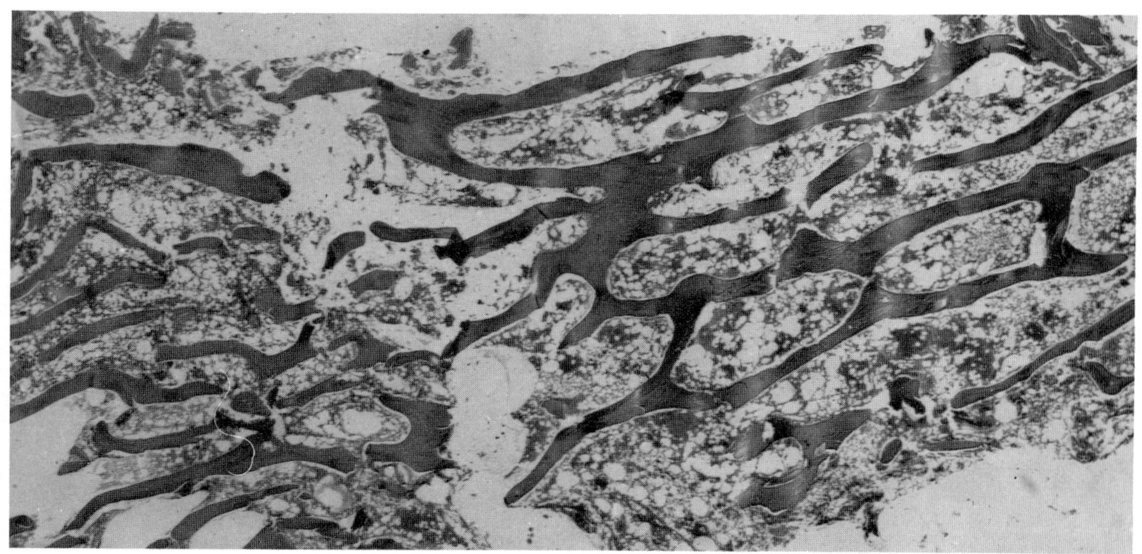

Fig. 45.—Histological aspect of a core specimen in the area of the supporting trabeculae.

red in the head. It is denser in the distal head portion than in the proximal neck portion. The specimen is fairly resistant to compression but would be crushed if compressed between two fingers. Some pathological bone specimens are as hard as wood; conversely, some are nearly liquid. An example of the latter is the medial femoral condyle in cases of severe reflex sympathetic dystrophy. Histologically, the hard tissue in the sample is represented by trabecular bone. In the upper end of the femur, since the forage is done in the axis of the femoral neck, one sees parallel trabeculae which diverge distally but are easily seen in the proximal part of the specimen (Fig. 45). At the distal end, the trabeculae are thinner, oriented less regularly, and weaker. They are sometimes fractured either by the biopsy technique or during the histologic sectioning.

Trabeculae of cancellous bone - Like the cortical bone, they are formed by lamellar bone in which the circular organization of the osteon is less evident and can only be observed in some of the larger areas, such as where several trabeculae come together (Fig. 46). Haversian canals of this region are quite rare. The trabeculae appear to be formed by segments of

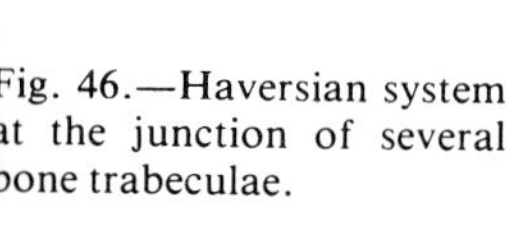

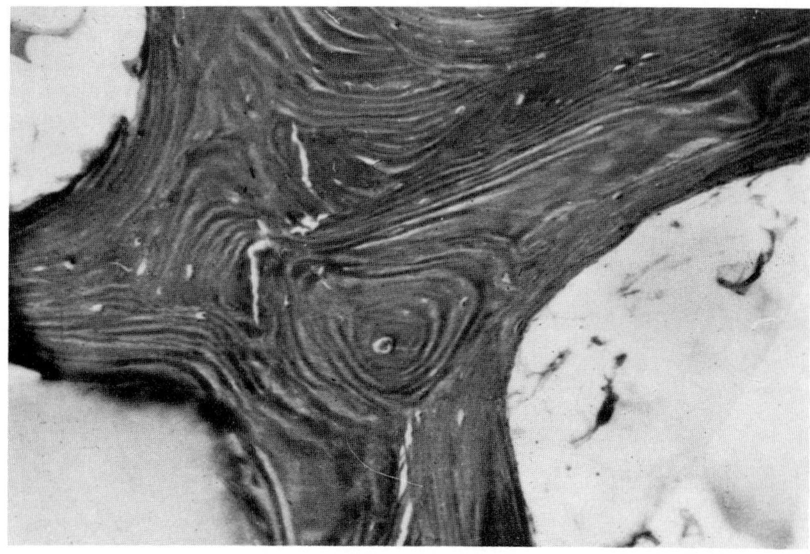

Fig. 46.—Haversian system at the junction of several bone trabeculae.

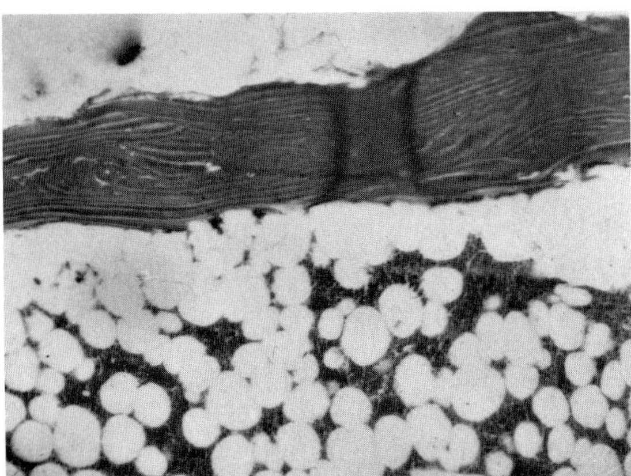

Fig. 47.—Lamellar appearance of a cancellous bone trabeculae.

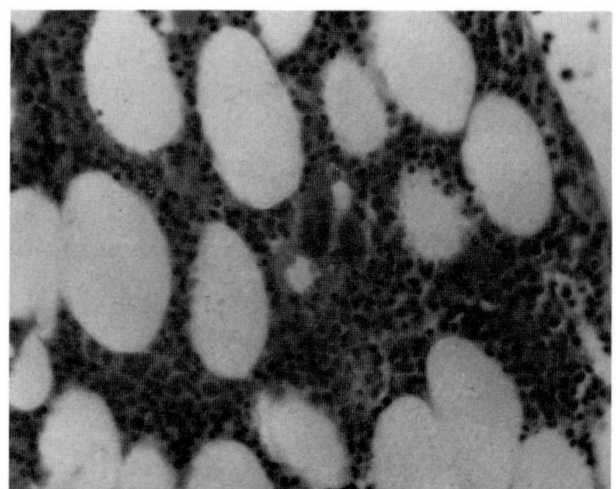

Fig. 48.—Mixed fatty and hemopoietic marrow.

osteons, and the bony lamellae are oriented in arches which vary from place to place along the trabeculae. Cement lines may be occasionally encountered (Fig. 47). The thickness of a given trabeculae varies from .1 to .5 ml, and they are separated by marrow spaces of thicknesses varying from .5 to several mm. Signs of cellular activity of the surface are uncommon. Active resorption lacunae with osteoclasts (Howship lacunae) are encountered only exceptionally. The inactive resorption lacunae (without osteoclasts) represent only a very small percentage of the surface. There are no resorption lacunae within the trabeculae, and osteoblastic activity is seldom observed. The osteocytes are fairly evenly distributed throughout the trabeculae, each occupying its own lacunae. Some lacunae are empty, either because of the thinness of the histologic cut, allowing the loss of the osteocyte during preparation, or due to cellular death. However, in general, no more than 30% of the lacunae are empty at the age of our patients[172].

Osteocytes, in fact, are visualized by their nuclei which occupy only a part of the lacunae. The nucleus of the osteocyte is sometimes very large, well defined, and centrally located. In other places, it may be pycnotic, indistinct, and eccentric. Standard techniques do not allow us, in these cases, to confirm or deny cellular death. The quality of the slides usually does not permit visualization of the cellular cytoplasm.

Bone marrow - This consists of four distinct elements: hematopoietic cells, fat cells or adipocyte vessels, as we have already described, and a few connective tissue elements occupying a smaller surface. These latter include collagen fibers around the vessels, reticulum fibers, and reticulum and histiocytic cells in small numbers. Hematopoietic tissue

(red marrow) rarely occupies the whole marrow space. It is usually mixed with fatty tissue (mixed marrow, Fig. 48). Vascular channels in a loose connective tissue matrix are always present. Hematopoietic tissue can be recognized by its spotty aspect and, occasionally, cells with very large multi-nuclei, the megakaryocytes. On good quality slides, it is possible to study, in detail, the cytology of marrow cells, but it is difficult to count them as it is usually done on a blood smear.

Fat cells are by far the most abundant. We have already said that among other functions, it is probably a filling tissue with variable volume that can adapt readily to changes of volume of other marrow elements. The adipocytes of bone marrow are very large cells with a flat nucleus, marginally located, and sometimes difficult to visualize or even invisible on thin cuts. The shape of the adipocytes is round when they are surrounded by hematopoietic cells or vessels, and polygonal where they form large areas of purely fatty tissue. Their volume varies between the fairly strict limits of 25 to 100 microns in diameter. Electronmicroscopic studies, particularly those of Oberling[334], demonstrated that like any cell they possess a cytoplasm, mitochondriae, endoplasmic reticulum, and Golgi apparatus. This organization confirms their metabolic activity. As we have previously mentioned, the great number of blood vessels or vascular spaces differentiates bone fat from subcutaneous fat. The adipocytes are separated from each other by intercellular capillaries which are sometimes flattened and non-functional, while at other times are dilated and active. This adaptation of the sinusoidal, intercellular capillary network is equilibrated by the opposite adaptation of the fat tissue which increases or decreases in volume, probably by hydration or dehydration. These tissues, side by side, are interdependent and form a unity. In special circumstances (e.g., bleeding), the adipocytes and the capillaries increase at the same time. In other circumstances (stasis), the interstitial capillaries are distended, and the adipocytes suffer atrophy. Some authors have asserted that the fat cells came from the reticular cells of the adventitia of the vessels. In any case, some of the lipocytes of bone marrow are supported and protected by a reticular network. The morphologic and physiologic connections between fat cells, reticular cells, and endothelial cells deserve emphasis, since they certainly play an important role in the physiology and the pathophysiology of bone marrow.

RADIOISOTOPE METHODS

There are already numerous applications of radioisotope methods of investigation of bone tissue. There are two basic types of investigation, one using isotopes without any particular affinity for bone and the other, bone seeking isotopes. In the first instance, the purpose of the investigation is to study intraosseous circulation, as reviewed in Chapter II. These have been of little value in studying clinical conditions in humans, with the exception of the case of femoral neck fractures. In this particular circumstance, the problem consists of determining the quantity of bone blood flow reduction in the femoral head and, therefore, to be able to predict its viability. The isotope is injected into the femoral head itself and the clearance of the isotope taken as a function of blood flow. We believe that this is a useful method and can be used in man for studying the circulation in a given region of bone. The technique will be presented later in this chapter.

The second type of investigation, which is now well recognized as clinically useful, is scanning of bone temporarily marked by an isotope injected by the intravenous route. With this method the intraosseous circulation is not directly measured but rather the bone metabolism, as emphasized by

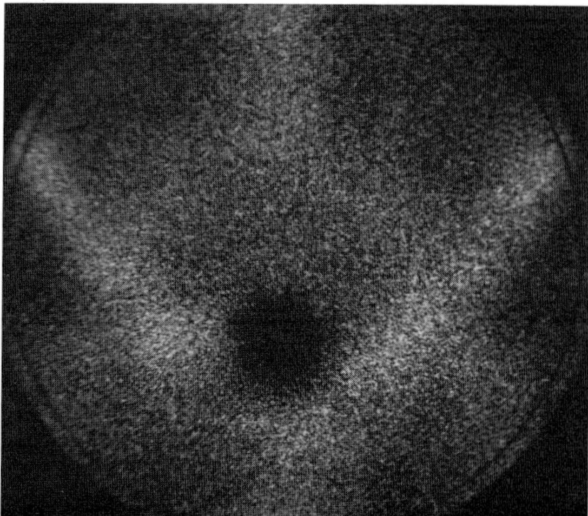

Fig. 49.—Scanning of a normal pelvis using Technetium99m labeled pyrophosphate.

Chewitz and Hevesy[89] already in 1935 and later by Bauer, Carlsson and Lindquist[38]. This has become a frequent method of investigation and indirectly allows recognition of bone lesions of vascular origin. The principle is quite simple. A bone seeking isotope is fixed on the trabecular surface during the time of mineralization of the bone. The first radioisotopes used have been Calcium[45,47] and Phosphorus[42]. However, most of the important works have been done with Fluoride[18] and Strontium[85,87].

Presently, the polyphosphates, pyrophosphates, and diphosphonates tagged with Technetium[99] have been substituted for other isotopes because of their cost and availability. All of these elements (with the exception of Calcium[45]) generated gamma rays whose intensity and topography are detected by a gamma camera. Table VII reviews the respective advantages and disadvantages of various isotopes. We will review, in detail, the techniques which are best known to us using Strontium[85,87]. It is generally agreed that strontium becomes incorporated in the bone trabecula-like calcium, forming bone crystals in substitution for calcium. In principle, the intensity of radiation is proportional to the speed of fixation, which itself is dependent upon the speed of mineralization. It is true, however, that in some bone necroses, there is increased uptake which might appear paradoxical but represents a method of investigation which is quite useful for early diagnosis of necrosis of bone. We will discuss later in this section the mechanism of fixation.

Technique of Investigation

The isotope is injected by the intravenous route.

TABLE VII

ADVANTAGES AND DISADVANTAGES
OF PRINCIPAL BONE SEEKING ISOTOPES

	Ca 47	Sr 85	Sr 87m	Te 99m
Half Life	4.7d	65d	2.8h	6h
Waiting time after injection	3 to 7d	3 to 7d	1 to 2h	2 to 5h
Irradiation (in RADS)	0.72	1.6	0.02	0.03

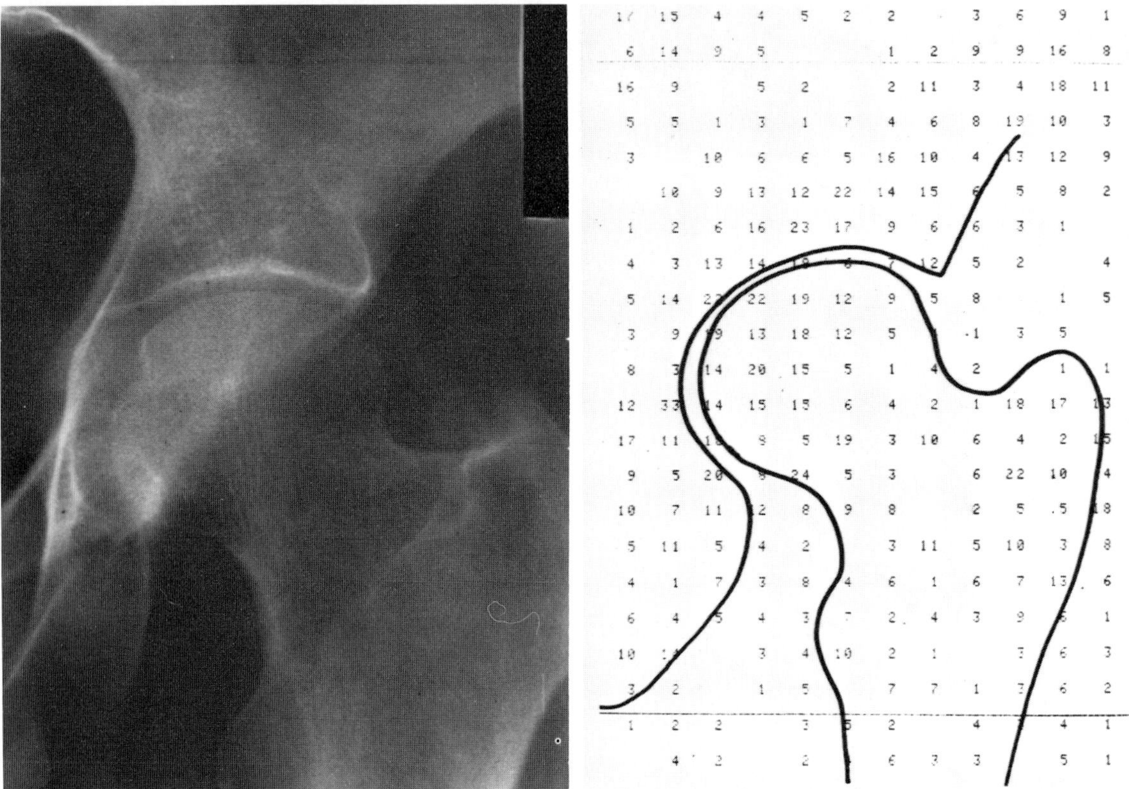

Fig. 50.—Scintimetry of a normal hip with Strontium[85] using the technique of Bauer. Notice the small number of counts per channel ranging from 1 to 33. Compare this scintimetry with that of Fig. 79 on the opposite hip of the same patient affected by osteonecrosis. (courtesy of Prof. G. Bauer)

Strontium[87m] is injected at a dose of 1 to 2 microcuries per kilogram of body weight. Its presence and concentration are detected by its gamma radiation. The radiation is detected by a gamma camera or by a moving scintigraph and transcribed either as points on a photographic film (Fig. 49) or in a more precise way by numerical countings in relation to a given region. This last technique developed by Bauer[41] using Strontium[85] produces a scintimetry with a remarkable topographical precision that is quite interesting (Fig. 50). In France, Gillet et al.[182] have produced similar topographic countings. It is generally agreed that the intensity of the fixation is proportional to the degree of bone nutrition in each of the respective regions scanned or at least to the speed of metabolic exchange. We will see, however, that this working hypothesis does not explain all the data. In general, the observed abnormalities are essentially abnormalities of increased fixation either in absolute terms, in terms relative to neighboring regions or to symmetrical regions on the opposite side of the skeleton. With the counting scintimetric method, one should also be able to determine areas of decreased fixation.

The radioisotope, of course, circulates in the vessels of the soft tissue parts surrounding the skeleton and may diffuse into them, creating a background which interferes with interpretation.

Results of bone scanning - Bone scanning was initially used to assess the viability of the femoral head immediately after fracture of the femoral neck in order to be able to predict necrosis, which so frequently follows these fractures, thereby, assisting in choice of method of treatment. Tucker[448] and Boyd et al.[61,62] were among the first to use this method, using radioactive phosphorous (P[32]) to detect a decrease uptake in the femoral head. However, the so-called primary non-traumatic ischemic necrosis of bone, when examined a long time after the onset of the circulatory problem, shows an increase in fixation. Bauer[40,42] was the first to demonstrate the importance of detecting localized increased uptake of Strontium[85] in diagnosis of the early stages of bone necrosis before radiologic evidence. He emphasized, however, that increased uptake was not at all specific for bone necrosis, as it is also seen in bone infections and metastasis.

Mechanism of increased uptake - Increased uptake is directly related to flow. Shim[412] showed that, when the circulation in the femoral head of the rabbit is stopped, the fixation of strontium is only 1.5% that of the normal femoral head. On the other hand, five minutes after ligation of the nutrient artery, the uptake is reduced by 50%.

Fixation is also directly related to bone accretion rate. According to Bauer[39], increased uptake is a sign of acceleration of the physiologic process of bone turnover and particularly the accretion rate, since strontium behaves within bone in the same manner as calcium. This hypothesis implies that, in bone necrosis (as in most metastases), the accretion rate would always be increased. It is well known that sclerotic lesions with trabecular thickening appear within or near the areas of long-standing ischemia. This bone sclerosis, which is not necrosis, behaves as if it were a defense reaction appearing relatively late. However, it is not often seen in the histological slides of core samples in Stage I of the disease.

According to some authors, the ionic exchange characterized in the first stage of incorporation of the isotope may be a simple, physical-chemical process of ionic equilibrium with exchangeable ions in the hydrated superficial shell which are not yet fixed into the matrix. This would explain how a completely dead bone devoid of circulation can trap radio-isotopes at significant rate[427].

Increased uptake and circulatory stasis - It would appear that there is a third mechanism which produces increased uptake of radionuclide. Vascular stasis is a constant and early phenomenon in bone necrosis[321]. We have demonstrated in our laboratories[187,188] that experimental venous stasis produces not only necrosis but also increases uptake of Strontium[85]. Also in the sympathetic reflex dystrophies, there are neither radiologic nor histologic signs of increased accretion but on the contrary, osteopenia is often intense. However, in these cases, increased uptake is the rule[362]. The common denominators between the two conditions, reflex sympathetic dystrophy and ischemic necrosis, is stasis, as we have shown[140,145].

NON-STANDARD METHODS OF ASSESSING BONE CIRCULATION

ARTERIOGRAPHY

Early workers emphasized the difficulty of visualizing the skeletal arteries in living man, particularly their intraosseous course. However, the work of the last twenty years has dispelled this idea.

At least three groups of workers have presented techniques which can be used in arteriography of the hip—Mossbichler in Sweden[326,327], Hipp in Germany[205], and Jung in France[239]. Since the work of Trueta[444,445], the anatomy and distribution of the arterial irrigation of the femoral head, both in the child and the adult, are now well known. In addition, new x-ray machines are better suited to selected angiography with rapidly taken serial films.

Technique

The principles of this technique are established and common to all arteriography. The mass of the injected dye must be sufficiently concentrated and, therefore, rapidly injected under pressure. A mid-thigh tourniquet is considered desirable by some authors. In order to opacify all of the arterial pathways to the hip, the level of injection should be at the common iliac artery or above it, since certain arteries to the hip (gluteal, ischiatic, and obturator) come from the internal iliac artery. However, in order to selectively visualize only the retinacular arteries, femoral or even selective catheterization of the medial circumflex artery can be carried out. The x-rays must be centered on the hip, using exposure technique for demonstrating bone. Serial x-rays are essential, since the speed of circulation may be decreased in pathological cases. Image intensification is also helpful. Both sides must be simultaneously injected if comparison with the normal, healthy side is to be utilized. To accomplish this, aortography, advocated by Jung, Wurtz, and Randrianorivo[239] is the procedure of choice. There are more problems, however, with this technique than with standard iliac or femoral arteriographies.

Our personal technique is as follows:

We use general anesthesia to avoid the discomfort and particularly movement of the patient, although the examination can be done under local anesthesia in older subjects. The catheter is inserted into the common femoral artery in the groin and then advanced to the common iliac or aorta. The same catheter can be used in the opposite direction to inject the posterior circumflex artery. A tourniquet is placed at mid-thigh: 10 to 20 ml of Vasurix 28 or Diodone 50% is injected with a power injector within two to three seconds. One film is taken every second for fifteen seconds.

Radiologic Anatomy of the Arteries to the Proximal Femur (Fig. 51)

The review article by Jung et al.[239] provides an excellent descriptive account. In the hip, there are six pathways with three main arterial pedicles which

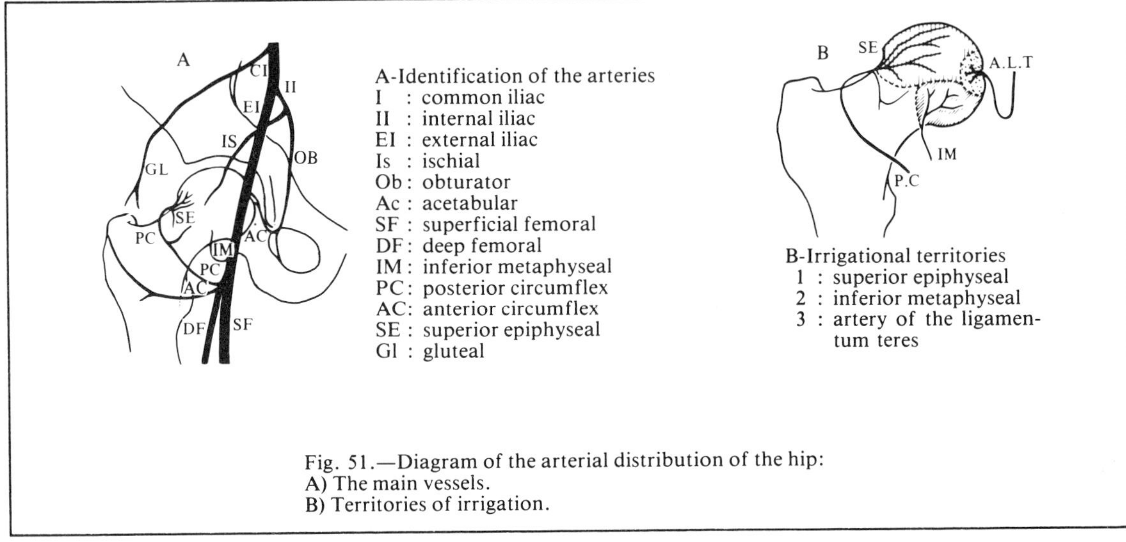

Fig. 51.—Diagram of the arterial distribution of the hip:
A) The main vessels.
B) Territories of irrigation.

must be analyzed. This analysis can only be done on serial films that allow the progression of the contrast medium up to the venous phase if one is to avoid false interpretation of thrombosis because of deficient filling. A good arteriography should allow all of the arteries of the proximal femur to be visualized (Fig. 52). Three arteries arise from the internal iliac artery: the superior gluteal artery descending vertically, the ischiatic artery descending obliquely, distally, and laterally, exiting the pelvis behind the head and neck of the femur along the axis of the neck and usually anastomosing with the posterior circumflex artery, and the acetabular artery or artery of the ligamentum teres, which is a branch of the obturator artery (80% of the cases) and which is not always present. Trueta[444] found it to be absent in 25% of adults.

Three arteries arise from the common femoral artery: the inferior metaphyseal artery traveling along the inferior border of the femoral neck penetrating the lower portion of the femoral head through two to four rami, the posterior or medial circumflex artery, and the anterior or lateral circumflex artery with an initial horizontal course from medial to lateral. The posterior circumflex artery is the most important artery of the femoral head and deserves special, detailed description. It arises from either the common femoral artery just before its division or from the profunda femora. There may be either a direct take-off from the femoral artery or a short common trunk with the anterior circumflex artery. Its initial course is proximal and lateral. If the inferior metaphyseal artery has not branched separately, it is given off at the inferior border of the femoral neck. The course then follows the intertrochanteric crest on the posterior surface of the femoral neck to reach the superior and lateral border of the neck. At this point the artery makes a 90° angle in the medial direction to follow the upper border of the femoral neck beneath the synovium. During this course, it gives off superior metaphyseal branches which descend vertically into the femoral neck. At the junction of the head and neck, the posterior circumflex artery branches into two to six superior epiphyseal arterioles that penetrate the femoral head. A good arteriography should show these arterioles inside the femoral head for a few millimeters.

From this description, we see that the proximal femur, including the femoral head, is irrigated by three main arterial pedicles. The medial pedicle, consisting of the ligamentum teres artery, irrigates the area around the fovea. The inferior pedicle, consisting of the inferior metaphyseal artery, irrigates the medial third of the metaphyseal part of the femoral head. The superior pedicle, which is the most important, arises from the posterior circumflex artery and irrigates the lateral two-thirds of the femoral head and most of the femoral neck.

MEASUREMENT OF CANCELLOUS BONE BLOOD FLOW

The principle consists of placing within the target tissue a defined quantity of radioactive marker and measuring the rate of decrease in radioactivity in the area of injection. The rate of decrease, which is an exponential function, is proportional to bone blood

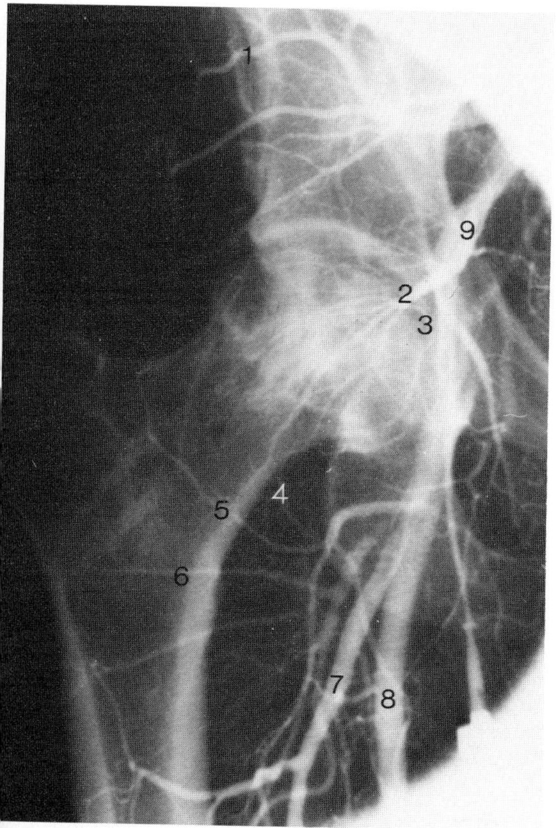

Fig.52.—Normal arteriography.
1 - gluteal a.
2 - ischial a.
3 - acetabular a.
4 - inferior metaphyseal a.
5 - posterior circumflex a.
6 - anterior circumflex a.
7 - deep femoral a.
8 - superficial femoral a.
9 - internal iliac a.

flow. By plotting the logarithm of the counts per minute of radioactivity against time in minutes, a straight line is obtained from which the following calculations can be made:

a. the time of 50% decrease in activity or T½;

b. the percentage of the radioactive material which is removed in one minute or slope of the line:

$$K = \frac{Log2}{T\frac{1}{2}}$$

c. the flow in ml/min/100 g tissue is then calculated by the formula 100 x λ x K, where λ is the coefficient of repartition of the marker between the blood and the marker tissue.

This method has been used by Petrakis[241] who used radioactive iodine to measure the bone blood flow in the sternal marrow of normal subjects and those suffering from various blood dyscrasias. He injected 0.1 to 1 ml of material in one or two minutes. At the end of injection, he removed the trocar and placed the counter over the sternum obtaining a single exponential curve. He found that K equals 7.37 and T½ equals 10 minutes on the average in normal subjects. One source of error may be the leaking out of injected material into the soft tissues between the injection and the measurement. This would lead to a second slower exponential curve. Najean and Clement[331] injected sodium chromate tagged with Cr^{51} into the sternal bone marrow of man and measured the radioactivity in the groin. The radioactivity measured is proportional to the disappearance of the marker from the injection site. Exact values cannot be calculated, but a bipolar curve is obtained. The first increase corresponds to the direct vascular entrance of the radioactive marker which measures medullary blood flow. The second slower curve corresponds to the diffusion of the radioactive marker from the non-circulating compartment to the circulating compartment that is not directly related to flow.

Hernborg[202] injected $Na\ I^{131}$ into the head and neck of the femur, monitoring radioactivity from the fifth to the sixteenth minute following.

We use the technique described by Semb[386] for the dog tibia. A curve of varying slope is obtained when counting over the metaphysis of the dog's tibia which has been injected with I^{131} labeled Iodoantipyrine. The initial steep slope lasts from two to ten minutes followed by one or two curves of more gentle slope that are, according to Semb, the result of iodoantipyrine degradation with the free iodine being released at a slower rate. Blood flow measured with this technique averaged 9 ml/100 gm/min. We have attempted to apply this method to man under local anesthesia by introducing a trocar horizontally, with the patient supine, in the distal part of the trochanter to reach the base of the femoral neck. IMP is measured and the pressure allowed to stabilize. A fine needle with a .01 ml volume is inserted into the trocar. A small quantity of the tracer solution (.20 to .30 ml) is followed by flushing 0.1 ml of isotonic saline. The valve is then closed to avoid reflux and the counter is placed anteriorly, directly over the tip of the needle. Since the counter is placed over the tip of the needle, it will be little affected by any residual radioactivity which might be left in the needle, and monitoring can begin with the injection. Two important points must be underlined. In order to avoid reflux, the system must be watertight. This is insured by a tight fit both between bone and the trocar and between the needle and the trocar. It is also important to inject as small a volume as possible in order to avoid disturbance in the local circulation which might produce pain and the vasomotor reactions which would influence local blood flow.

This technique gives us a single exponential curve, provided that a very small volume is injected (less than .5 ml). We believe that if a larger amount is injected, i.e., 1 or 2 ml, a steep, first slope occurs which represents a rapid decrease in radioactivity (Fig. 53), mainly due to the injection pressure more than to the action of the circulation.

Another important point concerns the choice of a tracer. Cancellous bone is a composite of very different tissues, including mineralized trabeculae, hematopoietic and fatty marrow. Iodine appears to be a good tracer because it permeates all of these tissues at the same rate with a mixing coefficient equal to 1. In about 15 patients, we have compared the results of the iodine injection with those of sodium pertechnetate injected and monitored during the same procedure. The results of these two measurements appear similar. If this is confirmed with further use, we will use the technitium for its more powerful radioactivity, shorter half life, and greater availability.

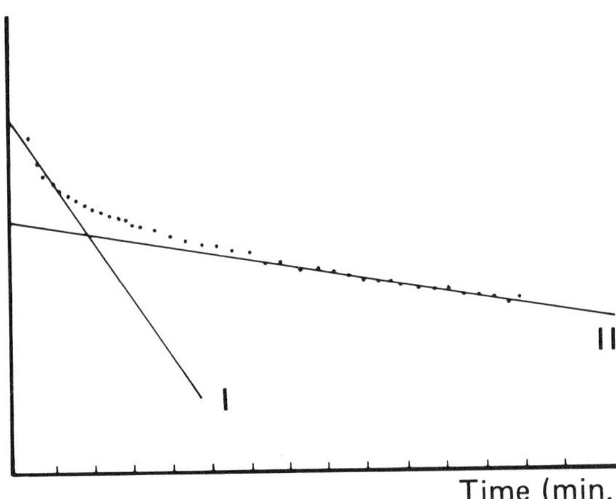

Fig. 53.—Measurement of blood flow in man by the study of the decreasing radioactivity curve after the injection of 0.5 ml of iodoantipyrine marked with iodine in the trochanteric region. The dotted line represents the logarithmic values of radioactivity in function of time in the trochanter after the injection of I^{131} antipyrine. This curve is formed by two exponential lines. The first slope is the fast exit of the radioisotope under the influence of the pressure injection. The second slope is a function of the bone blood flow.

OXYMETRY

The analysis of the partial pressure of oxygen from cancellous bone blood is theoretically an interesting parameter in the assessment of the circulatory status of a given bone. In fact, one way to measure ischemia is to search for the quantity of O_2 in any given region of a bone. Beginning with this fundamental concept, we have studied this aspect of the circulatory alteration of bone in a series of patients with the technique described below. A sample of blood is aspirated from the cancellous bone with a thick needle that has been inserted with a trocar obturator in place. We usually use the same needle with which the IMP measurements have been made, aspirating the blood after the pressure measurements but before injecting any substance, particularly physiologic saline. The region sampled is usually the intertrochanteric region approximately 2 cm in from the trochanteric surface and, therefore, at the base of the femoral neck. In this region, 2 to 5 ml of blood are easily aspirated. All of the precautions used when drawing arterial blood are used, including an airtight perfectly fitted syringe which has been heparinized in advance and a plugging of the tip of the syringe after completion of aspiration with immediate analysis for O_2, CO_2 and pH. Arterial blood gas and venous blood gases (from the femoral vein) are analyzed at the same time for comparison with the bone blood specimen. The "bone blood" comes from marrow vessels which have been opened by the needle. As we shall see in the section on analysis, the gas composition is between that of arterial and venous blood.

Unfortunately, we do not have enough samples from strictly normal subjects to give the normal values for these measurements in "bone blood". However, samples taken in the cases of early osteoarthritis at a distance from the osteoarthrosic lesion might be considered to represent normal values for this region. The most important parameter measured is oxygen saturation which measured 79.75% ± 3.9 in the 18 cases of osteoarthritis studied by us. Madrigal[294] studied the blood aspirated via transcutaneous puncture of the femoral head during surgical procedures under general anesthesia. In 40 normal hips, the median oxygen saturation was 96.6%. However, the absence of concomittant monitoring of arterial saturation level detracts somewhat from the value of these results.

INTRAOSSEOUS THERMOGRAPHY

Intraosseous temperature is a hemodynamic parameter which has been explored very little. The method described by Raynal and Levy[536] demonstrates that thermography is reliable and useful in the diagnosis of both post-traumatic and non-traumatic ischemic necrosis of the femoral head.

Technique

A fine thermistor probe is placed in contact with the bone marrow through the previously inserted trocar. The thermistor works on the principle of the Wheatstone bridge, allowing a sensitivity of measured temperature in the order of 0.1 degrees Centigrade (Fig. 54). For their recordings, these authors have calibrated the recorders so there is a deflection of 40 mm representing 4°C with the middle of the register corresponding to 37°C. The latter value is established by means of a phantom circuit which serves as a frame of reference for all measurements. The polyethylene tube may be sterilized either with ethylene gas or cold chemicals. The end of the trocar is connected to a pressure transducer, using a Statham P 23 DB transducer incorporated in a modular curve linearization machine of the Granjean-type to which an electromanometer is coupled. Very low flow was maintained in the system (3.5 ml/hr) to prevent clot formation. This allows studies to be carried out over a longer time. The damping of the pulse wave is dependent mainly on the nature of the catheter connected to the manometer. The more compliant the catheter, the greater the damping. A special set of stopcocks allows both the injection of fluid and the introduction of the thermisters.

Baseline marrow pressure is first recorded followed by the response to rapid injection of 5 ml of physiological saline. Both temperature and pressure can be recorded from the same location. In the thermometric tests, the tip of the probe must protrude 7 to 8 mm from the trocar to be certain that it is in contact with the cancellous bone. The probe must also be radiopaque in order to be able to use image intensification to control introduction. Several minutes are allowed to pass in order to allow the temperature to stabilize following introduction of the thermister.

Epidural anesthesia has been used which, from both an anesthetic and a circulatory point of view, provides a stabilized system. Once vasodilatation and analgesia have been established, they remain at a constant level. As long as the anesthesia does not produce change in arterial pressure, the circulation is established in ideal circumstances.

Results

In normal hips, thermographic values vary between 36.1 and 36.3°C. These marrow temperatures differ substantially from either rectal or esophageal temperatures. Hypothermia will decrease intramed-

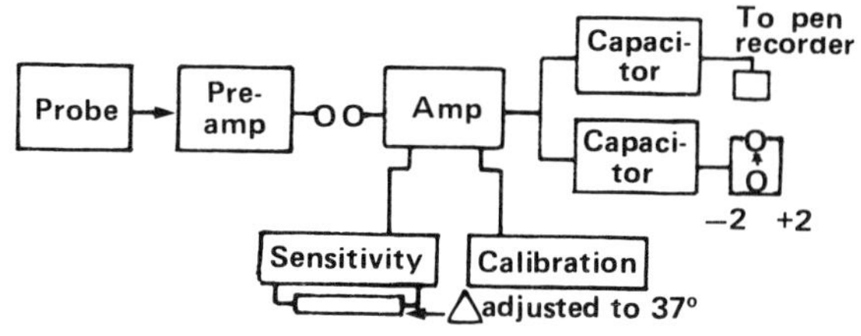

Fig. 54.—Diagram of the device used by Raynal and Levy for intraosseous thermometry of the hip.

ullary temperature and hyperthermia will increase it. However, this correlation between body temperature and bone temperature does not occur in advanced disease of bone.

SUMMARY—THE "FUNCTIONAL" INVESTIGATION OF THE INTRAOSSEOUS CIRCULATION

Radiography allows the study of the articular surface morphology, the integrity of the joint space, and the state of the bone texture, which reflects the functional remodeling of trabecular structures. It is the initial diagnostic test for all osteoarticular disorders. However, if it is negative, it should not be regarded as a certificate of normalcy. It reveals more what has taken place in bone than what is taking place at the actual time of the examination. For cartilage lesions, even greater changes need to occur before they are reflected in radiographic abnormalities. For this reason, the radiography must always be viewed with some suspicion since the early phase of the disease is radiologically silent.

The functional investigation of the intraosseous circulation can provide us with precise data on hemodynamic, histologic, biochemical, and metabolic parameters, giving us a true picture of the structures and, at the same time, of their functional capabilities. Most important, this investigation fills the radiologic gap for early diagnosis since it reflects the vascular component, projecting the diagnostician into the pre-radiologic phase of the disease and sometimes even into the preclinical phase[152].

The association of the two methods of investigation gives us both a morphologic and a functional picture of the two sectors of bone, trabecular and vascular, and, by doing so, provides a breadth and precision of diagnosis which has not previously been possible. For practical purposes, it is obvious that, except for very few cases, the functional investigation does not need all of the previously presented examinations. The triad of intramedullary pressure, phlebography, and biopsy constitute the essentials of the investigation and have been our routine procedure for many years. It can be even further simplified since when medullary hypertension exists, transosseous phlebography becomes superfluous. When the pressure value is abnormal, one can go straight to the biopsy which will bring with it the certainty of diagnosis (Fig. 55).

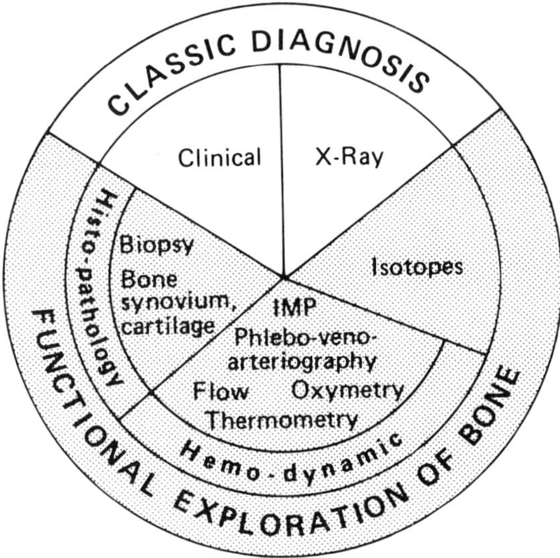

Fig. 55.—Diagrammatic summary of functional exploration of bone.

CHAPTER IV

NECROSIS OF THE FEMORAL HEAD

TERMINOLOGY

We have adopted the vague and general term necrosis of the femoral head, because all others appeared to us to be too restrictive, including osteochondritis dissecans[161,171,322,361], idiopathic, primitive, spontaneous, essential, aseptic, avascular, and ischemic necrosis. The latter term, ischemic necrosis, deserves to be rehabilitated because of the importance and the high frequency of ischemia in the process of necrosis.

CLASSIFICATION AND RADIOLOGICAL TYPES

The radiological picture is the most important criterion in any classification system because of its precision and objectivity. One should not infer, however, that a normal radiological picture signifies the absence of a lesion. As we shall see later, there exists both marrow and vascular pathology which can progress considerably without radiologic evidence. It is on this basis that there is such interest in the functional investigation as a means of early diagnosis. By using the two methods of evaluation, radiographic and "functional," we have been able to describe four successive phases in the evolution of bone necrosis, with the joint space being spared in the first three. At the same time we have been able to identify a special form of necrosis which is characterized by the early occurence of joint line narrowing which is quite similar to the evolution of osteoarthritis. This form of necrosis is osteo-chondral in type from the beginning, and we have labeled it "ischemic coxopathy."

OSSEOUS FORM

Stage I

This preradiologic stage (Fig. 56) is characterized by the absence of radiologic signs and the presence of a stiff and painful hip, usually with some limitation of movement. Nonetheless, there are some cases which are quite silent from a clinical point of view, particularly in renal transplants who reach an advanced stage without having had symptoms. Under most circumstances, when x-rays have been available from the very beginning of the symptomatic period, the silent radiologic phase is evident. We have labeled this Stage I instead of Stage O because hemodynamic, isotopic, and histopathologic signs already exist and make the diagnosis possible in spite of the absence of radiologic signs. This phase is predictable, but too often it is forgotten that pure bone necrosis is not radiologically visible. To be convinced of that, one needs simply to have a radiograph of an old skeleton, even a prehistoric one (Fig. 56A). In this phase, of course, there are no changes in the epiphyseal outline nor the joint space. The bony trabeculae may be strictly normal or present a very discrete homogeneous or spotty osteoporosis that even in retrospect is nonspecific and without any apparent pathologic significance. Only functional investigation can document this phase wherein early diagnosis is essential for therapeutic reasons[11,13,40,42,151,182].

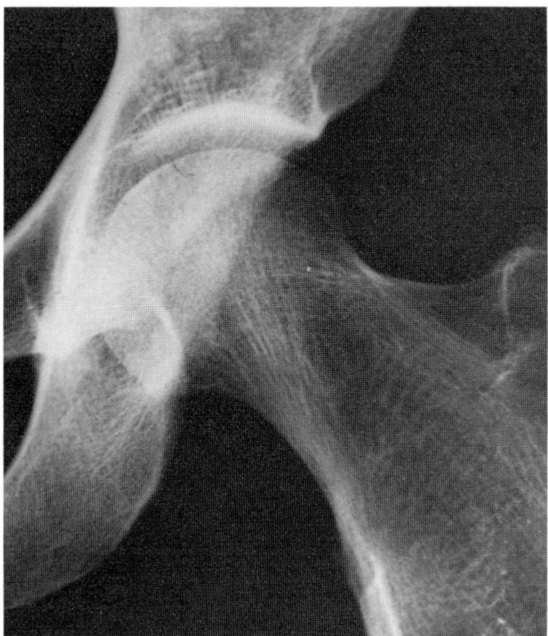

A: X-rays of a person dead for over a century, showing all the appearances of a normal hip.

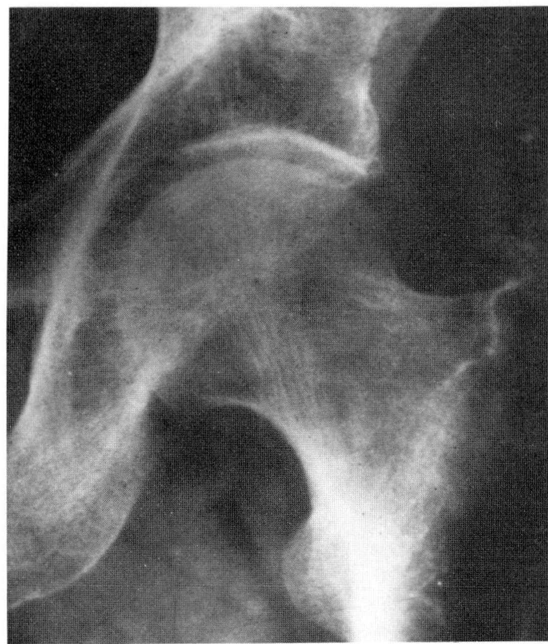

A': X-rays of a femoral head necrosis of the left hip in a patient affected with Stage I necrosis of the right hip.The necrotic nature of this lesion was eventually proven by core biopsy.

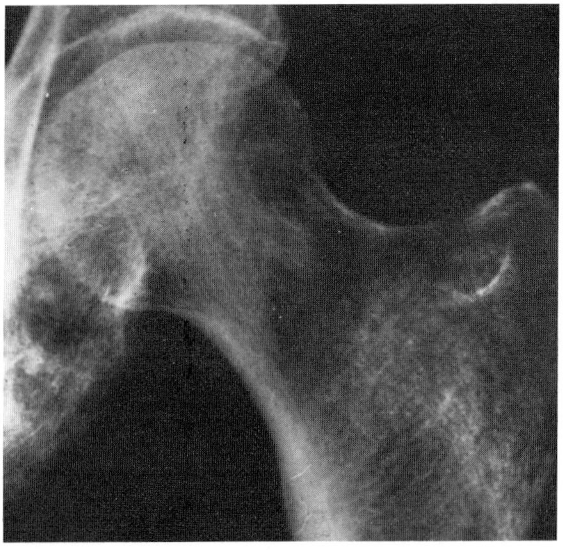

B

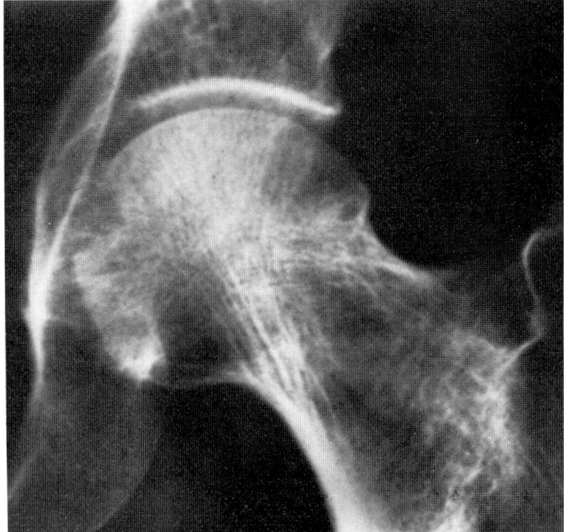

B'

B,B': Two cases of Stage I necrosis with almost normal x-rays.
B: Slight flattening above the fovea and a small superolateral cyst at the junction of the head and neck; the weight-bearing trabeculae are blurred in this bone which shows subtle osteoporosis.
B': Small superolateral cyst at the junction of the head and neck; the weight-bearing trabeculae are blurred in this bone which shows subtle osteoporosis.

Fig.56.—X-rays of cases at Stage I compared with "normal hips."

Illustrative Case 1.(Fig. 57) - Mr. CIE . . ., a 55-year-old administrative secretary, was seen for the first time on December 28, 1966, after two months of pain in the right lower extremity. He was treated initially and unsuccessfully as sciatica. Constant, severe, disabling pain, initially felt in the groin and buttock and radiating towards the knee, was felt suddenly after prolonged walking. On physical examination, passive flexion of the right hip was normal, but abduction and internal rotation were restricted and painful. AP and lateral radiographs of the right hip were entirely within normal limits. Functional investigation of the hip showed a normal baseline pressure; but with the stress test the pain was reproduced, and the pressure rose to 40 mm Hg. Intramedullary venography revealed a complete lack of drainage with contrast medium refluxing the length of the diaphysis. Core biopsy showed marrow and trabecular necrosis of considerable severity and extent. Following decompression, the pain disappeared, and the recovery has been maintained for the past 12 years.

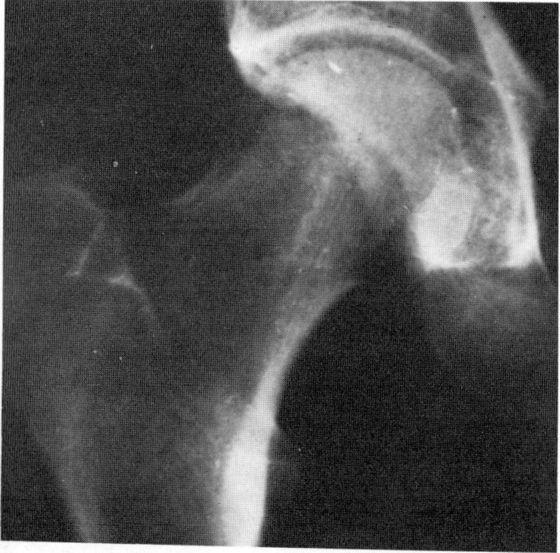

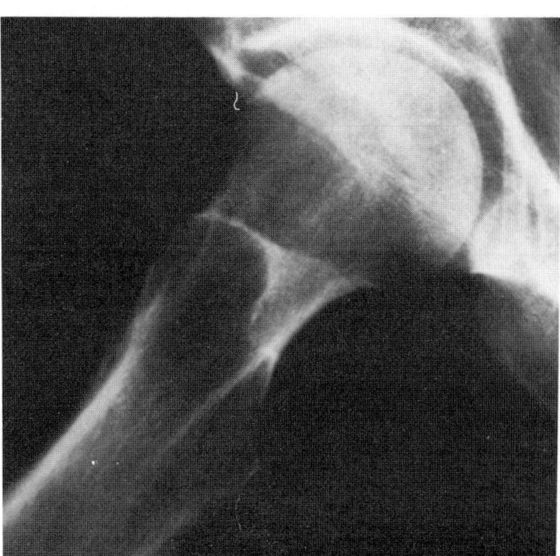

A　　　　　　　　　　　　　　　　A'

A, A': AP and lateral views of the right hip (no appreciable changes in spite of severe pain and limitation of motion).

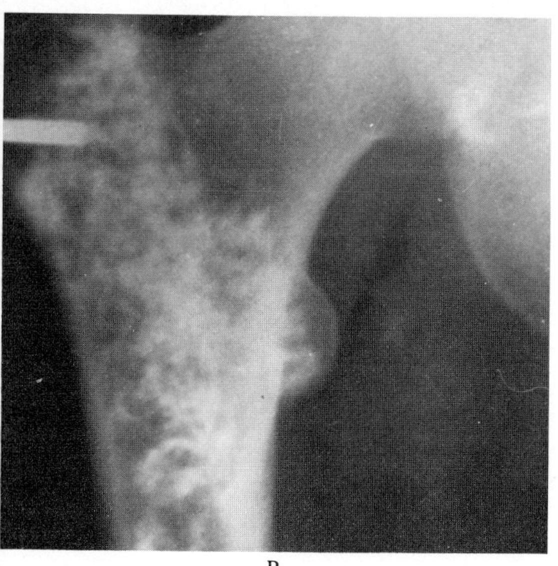

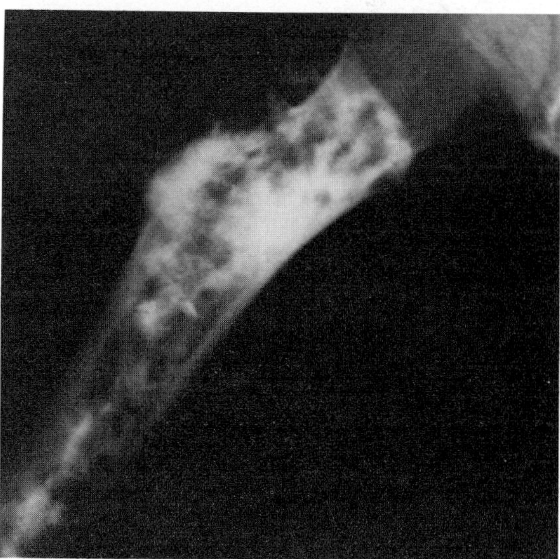

B　　　　　　　　　　　　　　　　B'

B': Pertrochanteric phlebography: total absence of efferents (even the circumflex is absent), considerable reflux down to the knee and stasis lasting several hours.

Fig.57.—Case 1

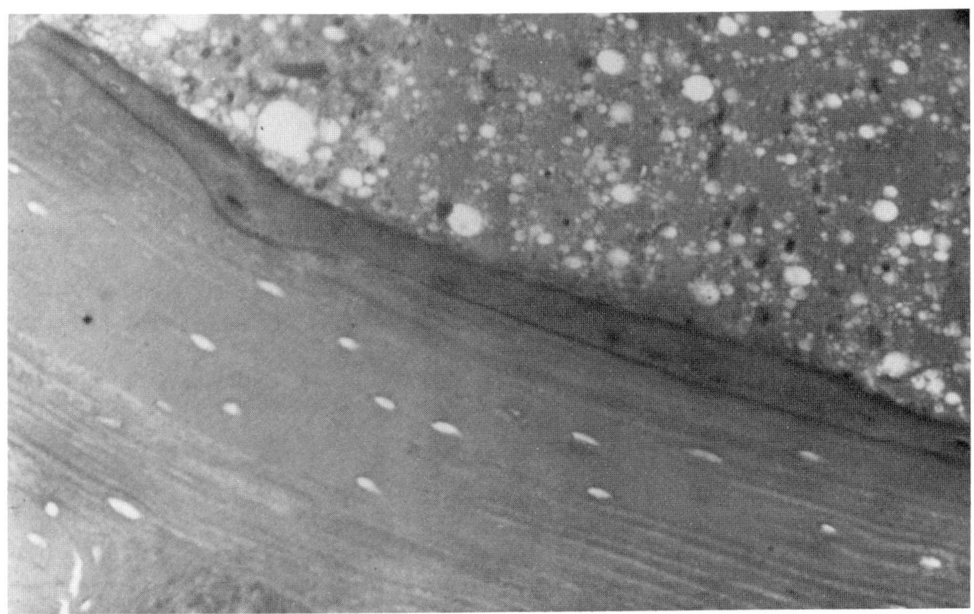

C: Total marrow and trabecular necrosis.

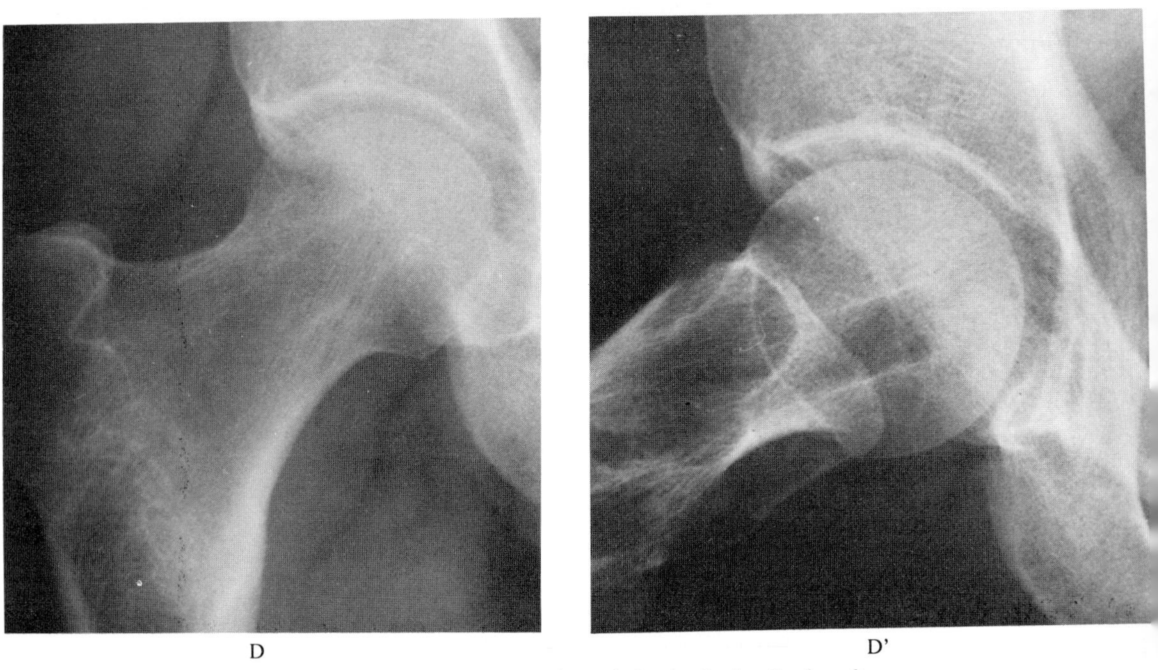

D   D'

D, D': Nine years later, normal x-rays. Complete symptomatic remission beginning the day after sugery.

Fig. 57.—continued.

Stage II (Fig. 58)

This phase is characterized by the radiologic appearance of evidence of bone remodeling but still without any changes in the overall shape of the head or the joint space. Three types of bone reactions can be distinguished: the osteoporotic type and the mixed or sclerotic-cystic type.

The osteoporotic type may present in several ways. The first way is diffuse and marked with regional overlapping involving the acetabulum and blurring the epiphyseal contour but with maintenance of the joint space. It looks very similar to a post-traumatic osteoporosis. In occasional cases, this may be temporary and may recede after a few months.

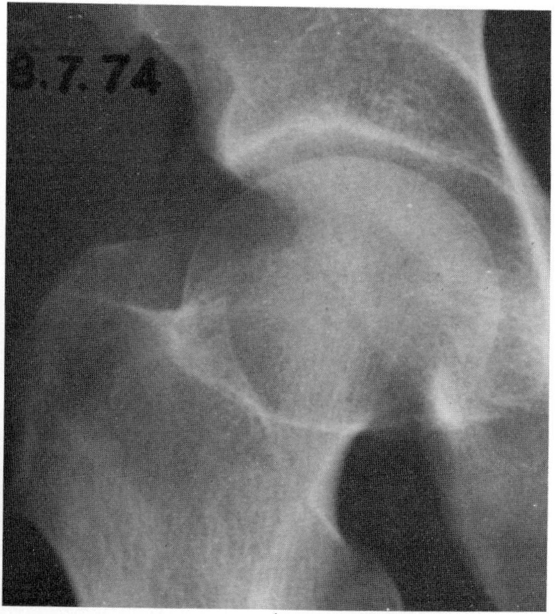
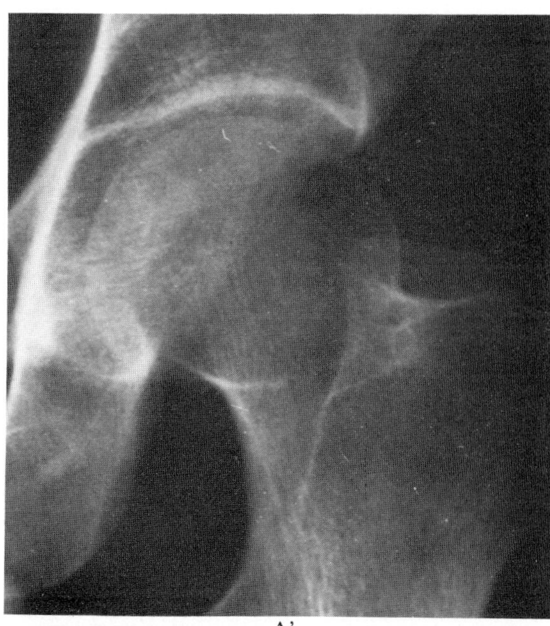

A   A'

A, A': In A' diffuse osteoporosis when compared with the opposite normal hip A.

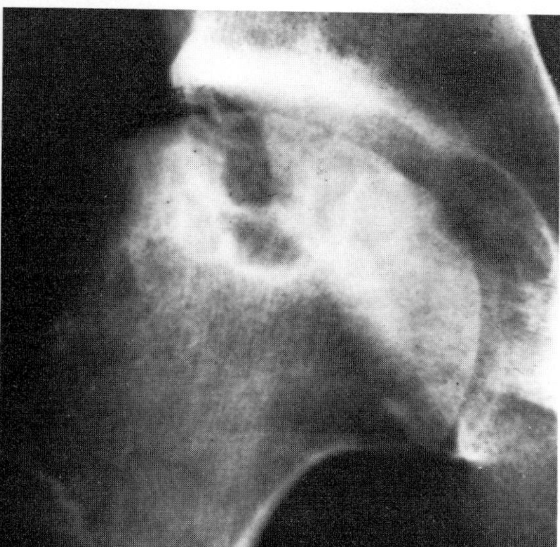
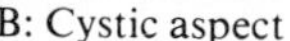

B: Cystic aspect

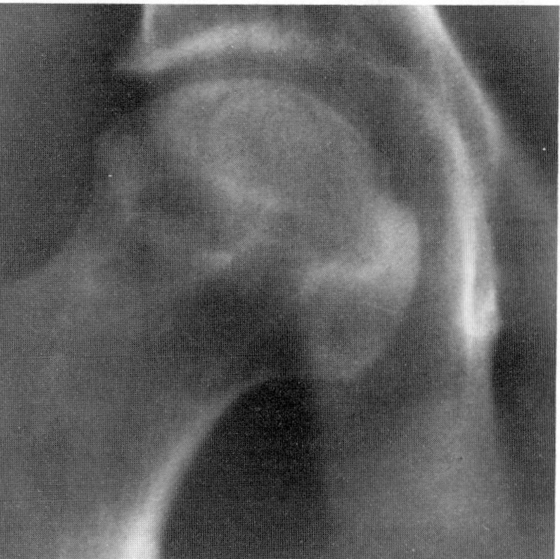

B': Clear subchondral crescent sign as an egg shell, representing a transitional stage before sequestration.

Fig.58.—Main different radiological aspects of Stage II.

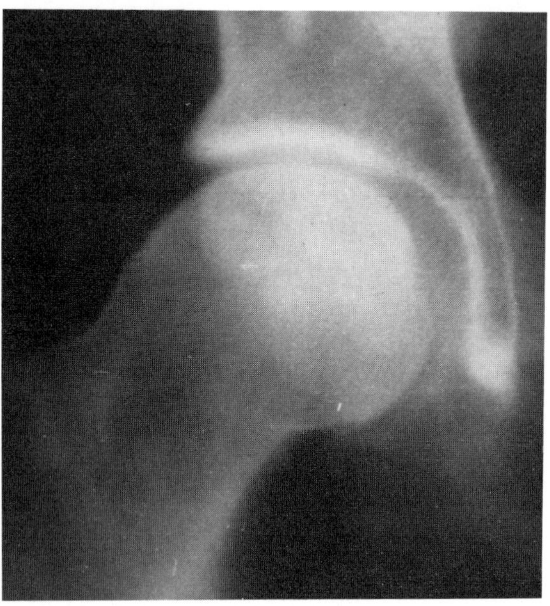

C

C: Homogenous sclerosis of two-thirds of the femoral head.

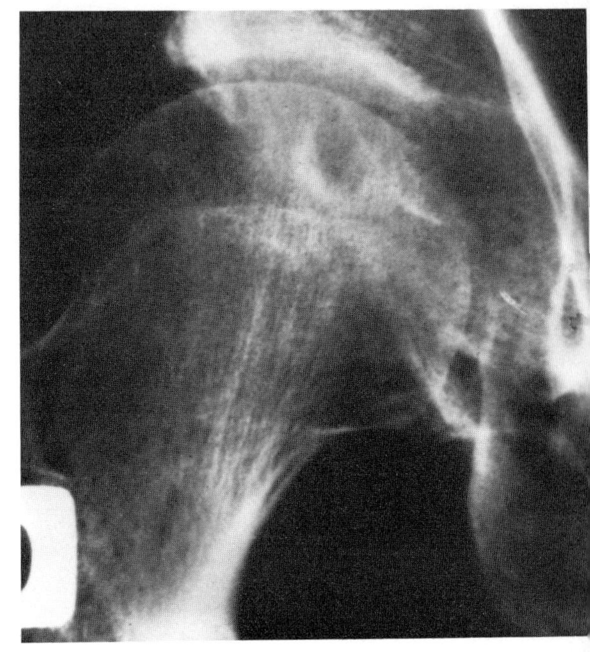

C': Sclero-cystic type on the weight-bearing cone.

Illustrative Case 2 (Fig. 59). - Mr. ESC..., a 37-year-old baker, was examined for the first time in December, 1965. The patient complained of pain for only a few days located in the left groin, radiating to the calf. It began suddenly after strenuous effort while loading a car and was aggravated by cough. Physical examination of the left hip revealed a good range of movement although it reproduced his pain. X-rays showed diffuse osteoporosis of the femoral head with slight superomedial narrowing. There were no signs of inflammation, but the uric acid was elevated (7.2 mg). Since the patient had a history of tuberculosis in 1949, he was suspected of beginning with tuberculosis of the hip. Functional investigation of the left hip revealed an abnormal trochanteric intramedullary pressure following injection of physiologic saline (43 mm Hg), and the venogram was definitely pathological with stasis and diaphyseal reflux. In March, 1966, the patient underwent open biopsy, synovial membrane and bone, in order to rule out synovial tuberculosis. The synovial membrane was completely normal. However, the bone specimen showed marrow lesions and trabecular necrosis that was extensive but with signs of revascularization and repair. Following the decompression, the patient became asymptomatic and resumed full activity. However, eight years later in 1974, he returned with the same signs in the opposite hip: groin pain, moderate limitation of movement, and diffuse demineralization. The core depression confirmed the necrosis and rendered the patient asymptomatic which he has been for the past four years.

The microcystic, osteoporotic type, in contrast to diffuse osteoporosis in the head, may present with one or more cysts in various positions. These may be at the upper border between the head and the neck and appear as a string of small cysts in the immediate, subcondral region or occassionally appear considerably removed from the joint surface near the center of the head. They have a very different appearance from osteoarthrosic cysts.

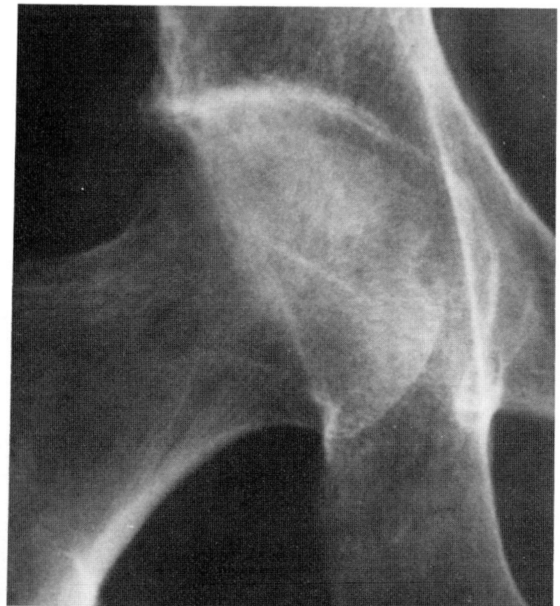

A: The right hip in March 1972; diffuse osteoporosis with blurring of the outlines and slight superomedial joint narrowing. Cyst with sclerotic margin in the femoral neck.

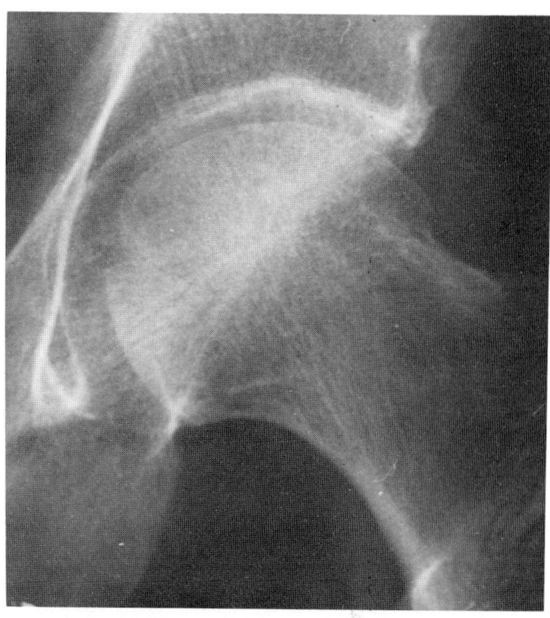

A': The left hip in 1972, healed for the last six years; she had exhibited the same type of osteoporosis.

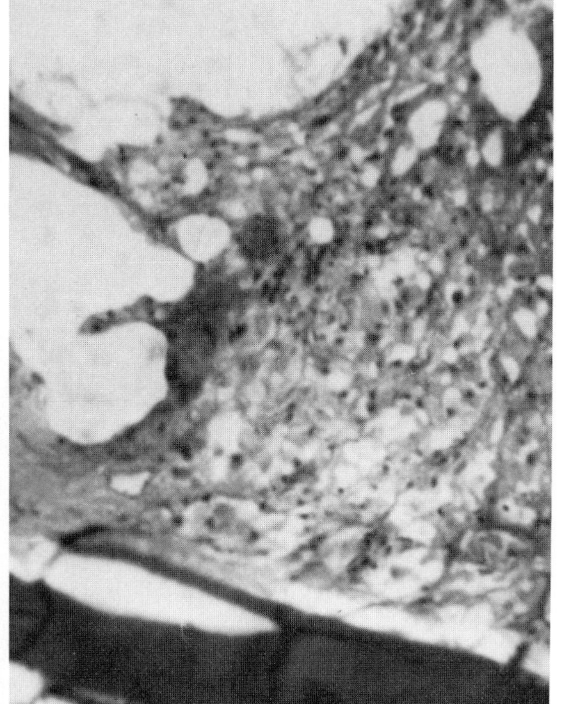

B: Marrow necrosis with disintegration of the lipocytes and pseudocytes.

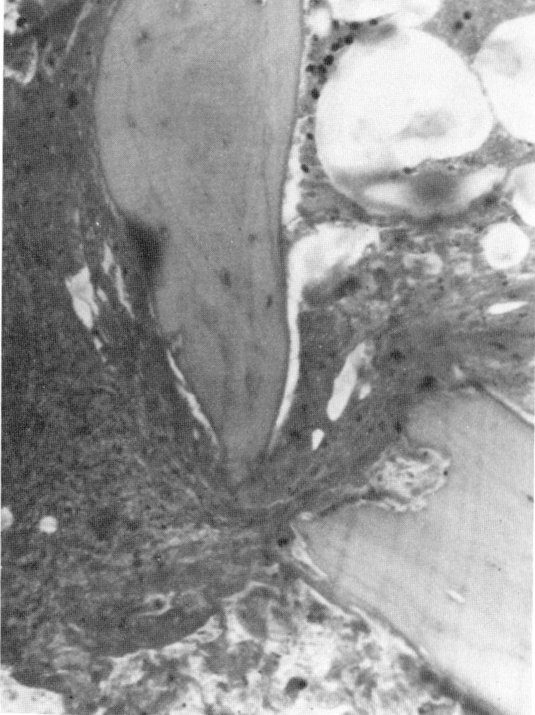

B': Hemorrhagic necrosis of the marrow.

Fig.59.—Case 2—Osteoporotic type.

Illustrative Case 3 (Fig. 60). - Mr. CAD . . ., a 37-year-old farmer, was seen initially in 1965 with a 20-month history of moderate, left groin pain on weight-bearing. The hip demonstrated significant painful limitation of movement (flexion to only 100°). The x-ray showed a large cyst with well-defined margins situated laterally and proximally to the fovea. The superior pole of the femoral head had a normal outline. Intraosseous venography (10-12-65) showed considerable stasis at ten minutes and moderate diaphyseal reflux. Core biopsy (1-21-66) demonstrated extensive marrow lesions of necrosis and fibrosis. At follow-up ten years later, the patient is asymptomatic and has resumed normal activity, although the movement is somewhat more restricted than the contralateral side (flexion, 110°). X-ray taken in 1975 shows some sclerosis within the head with very slight narrowing of the joint space. The cyst is no longer visible.

The sclerosing type of ischemic necrosis of the femoral head is characterized by homogeneous and uniform sclerosis which extends more or less over the entire head, occasionally with a spotty appearance. Such cases usually have a better prognosis than the other types of Stage II.

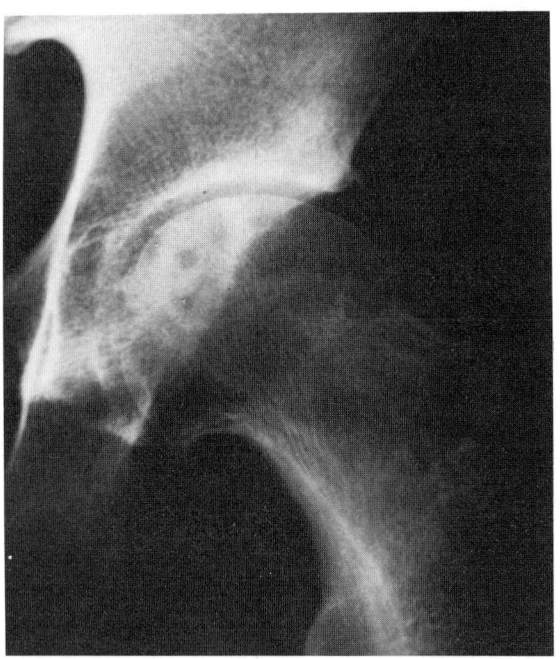

A: X-rays of the left hip taken in November 1965; cyst formation aspect, intact joint line.

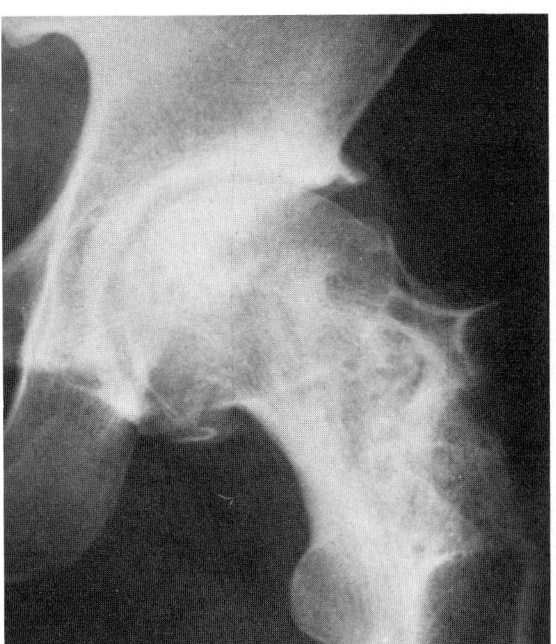

A': X-rays taken nine years after core decompression: sclerosing changes in the head and neck. Clinical healing in spite of slight superolateral joint line narrowing.

Fig.60.—Case 3

Illustrative Case 4 (Fig. 61). - Mr. BAR..., a 36-year-old salesman, presented in 1965 with a three-year history of left groin pain radiating to the knee. He had previously been treated for arthritis and sciatica without improvement. At the time of presentation, the pain was constant, present at night, and interfered with sleep. The hip showed painful limitation of movement in all directions. X-rays demonstrated homogeneous sclerosis affecting the whole head. On February 11, 1965, a functional investigation was carried out. Baseline IMP was normal. During this period, the stress test was not being carried out. However, phlebography demonstrated marked stasis with diaphyseal reflux down to the knee. The core biopsy demonstrated extensive necrosis. Following the decompression, the patient was asymptomatic for five years following which symptoms began to appear after exercise. At that time, flexion was 100°, abduction 50°, internal rotation 20°, and external rotation 40°. In November,

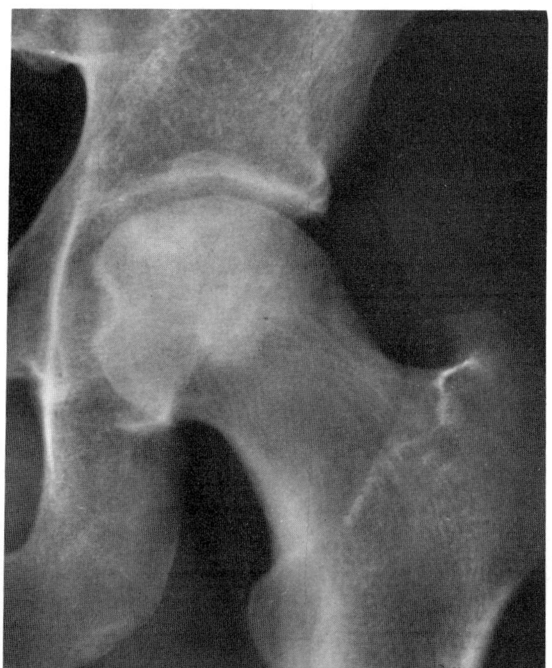

A: Pre-operative x-rays.

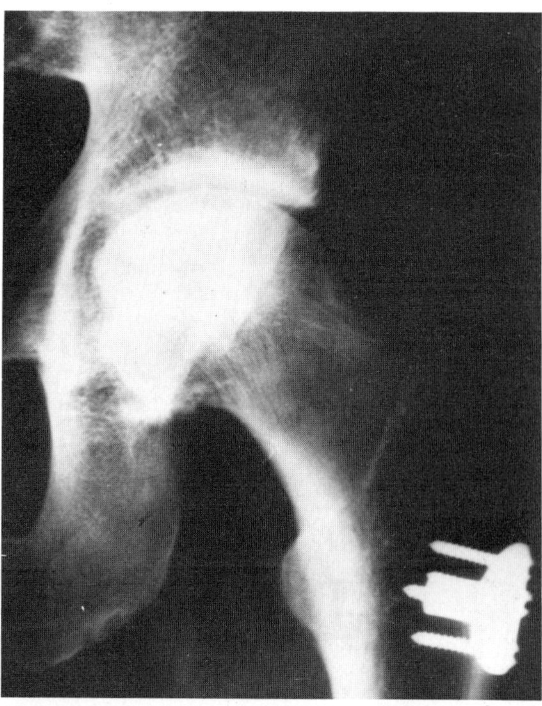

A': Post-operative x-rays 1965: Sclerosis of the whole femoral head, the joint line slightly narrowed. In this film, the metallic cylinder, first used in an attempt to keep the channel open, is seen.

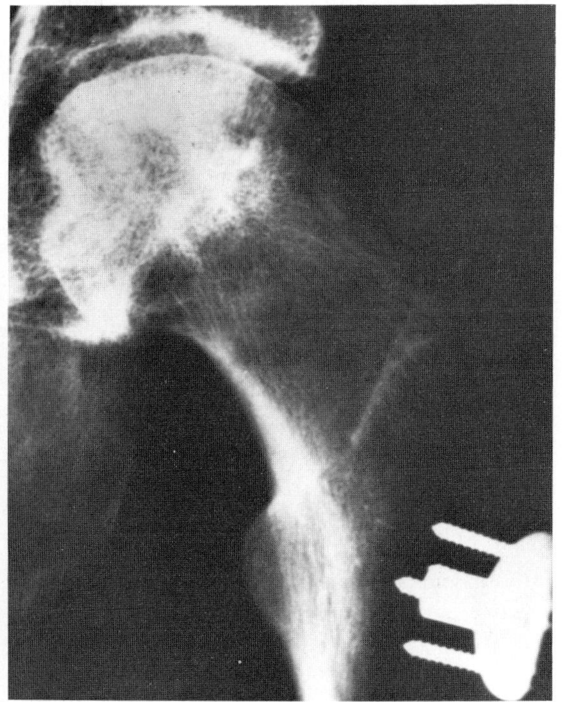

B: Film taken one year later: the bone texture is clearer and the joint line seems normal.

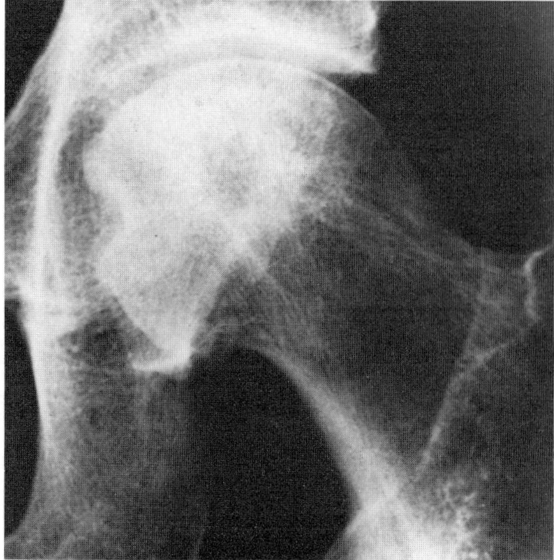

C: Film taken eight years later (and three years after a second forage, performed in 1970 when pain had reappeared). For the last ten years, remission has been practically complete without interference with work.

Fig.61.—Case 4—Sclerosing type.

1969, the ring was removed, and a new decompression was carried out. Histological analysis showed marked changes of the fibrous type and practically no necrosis. The patient was immediately relieved of his symptoms, and at latest follow-up ten years after the initial decompression, he was still working as a salesman with a painless hip which showed minimal restriction of movement.

We could also include in this category the type described by DeSeze[397] in which a linear sclerotic line appears at the junction of the head and neck. The sclerocystic type is more common than the preceding classification and characterized by mixed areas of increased density, alternating with radiolucent areas.

All types of both Stage I and Stage II have the integrity of both the joint space and the outline of the head. Because the gross anatomical morphology of the proximal femur is undisturbed, we have labeled this uncomplicated or simple necrosis. The appearance of the crescent sign is a forerunner of the trabecular sequestrum and represents a transitional phase between Stage II and Stage III[390,394]. Stages III and IV, on the other hand, are characterized by the advent of morphological and irreversible complications, consisting of either collapse of the epiphyseal shell (Stage III) or narrowing of the joint space (Stage IV). The advent of these changes results in progressive deterioriation of the joint as a functional entity.

Stage III (Fig. 62)

This stage is characterized by disruption in the continuity of the epiphysis. Partial collapse or flattening of the roof might not even be visible in the AP projection. For this reason, a lateral view and tomograms are important before determining the stage of the disease.

The previous partial collapse which is limited to the anterolateral portion may be combined with a more medial portion of the head, representing the inner border of the weight-bearing aspect of the acetabulum. The two sections represent the limits of the sequestrum which corresponds topographically to the pressure area of the femoral head. This is a functional topography and not an anatomical one, contrary to what has been asserted by some authors who believe that the shape of the sequestrum corresponds to the territory of the superior epiphyseal artery.

The sequestrum begins to fragment and impact into the femoral head, flattening the superior margin and giving a false appearance of an increased joint space. Loss of sphericity of the head is an important sign of complicated necrosis as it represents cancellous bone compression. This can be seen in the

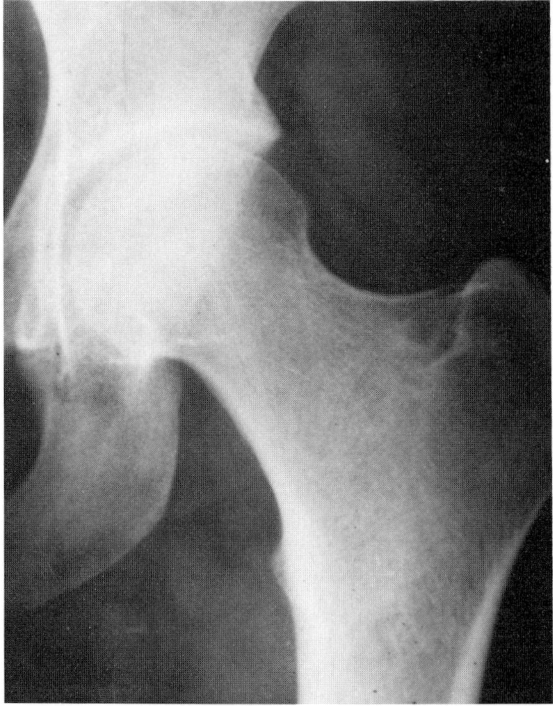

A

A,A': AP view, normal; lateral step-off sign seen on lateral view (A').

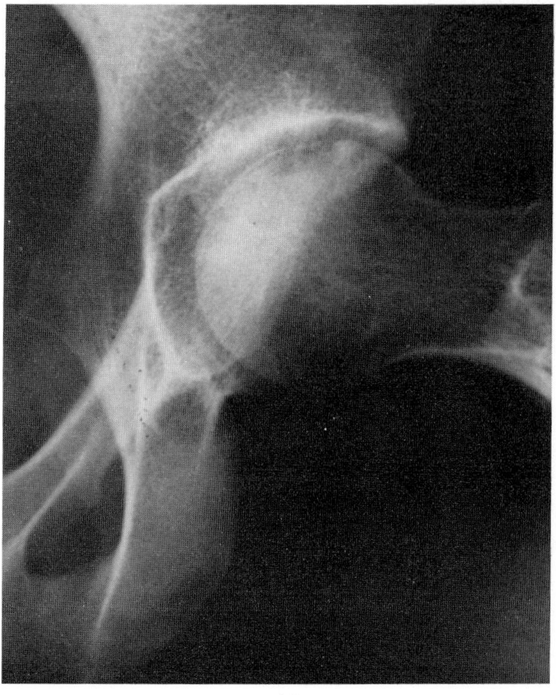

A'

Fig.62.—The main radiographic varieties of Stage III.

lamellar compression in the crescent sign or in the typical conical collapse. There is, however, a variety of lesser collapse in which there is only small segmentary interruption of the sphericity of the head without any separation of bone in the area. The significance of this can be debated, since it is occasionally observed in clinically normal hips. Conversely, a rapid collapse without sequestrum formation also exists; and, from a radiologic point of view, it resembles the rapidly destructive osteoarthrosis reported by some authors [100,193,274].

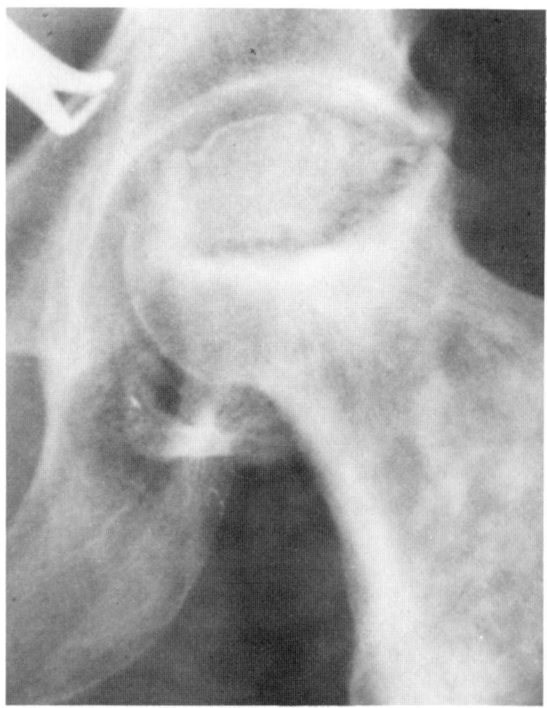

C: Medial and lateral subchondral infraction with collapse of the sequestrum and arcuate sclerosis.

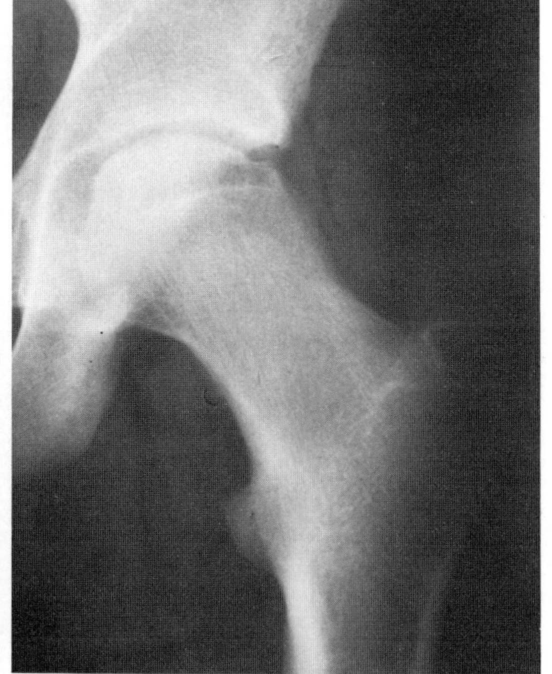

B: Subchondral step-off at the lateral margin of the head.

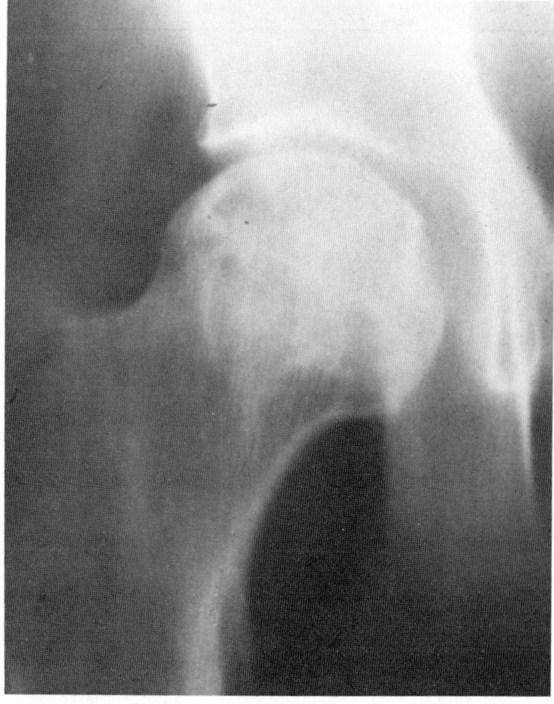

B': Indentation at the medial margin of the weight-bearing cone.

Fig. 62.—continued.

Illustrative Case 5 (Fig. 63) - Mr. MON..., a 42-year-old cook, was examined for the first time in 3-29-67 with a history of moderate right inguinal pain of three months duration, beginning while carrying a heavy load. Movement of the hip was full with exception of lateral rotation which was limited and painful. X-ray revealed sclerocystic changes with flattening of the head in the region on the right side. The left side was normal. Trochanteric IMP on the right was 30 mm Hg. Pertrochanteric phlebography showed stasis and diaphyseal reflux. Core biopsy (4-6-67) confirmed the necrosis and relieved the patient of his symptoms for a two-year period during which he returned to work. In September, 1967, the patient began to have similar symptoms in his left hip but refused a core biopsy. The pain reappeared on the right side in April, 1969, and x-rays revealed complicated necrosis of both hips, more severe on the left. He was seen again in April, 1973, when he still continued to work as a cook but with considerable difficulty. Both hips demonstrated marked, painful restriction of movement. Included among the etiologic factors in this case were obesity, chronic alcoholism, blood lipid abnormalities, and chronic arterial and venous circulatory problems.

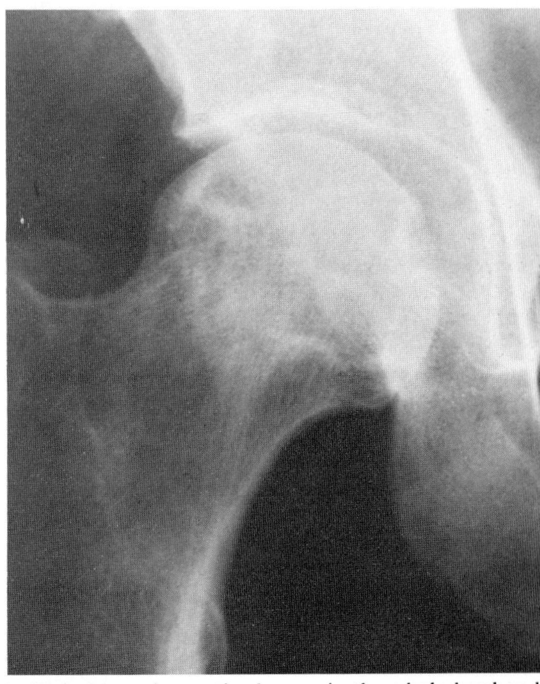

A: Right hip: sclerocystic changes in the whole head and flattening above the fovea core biopsy in 1967 confirmed the necrosis.

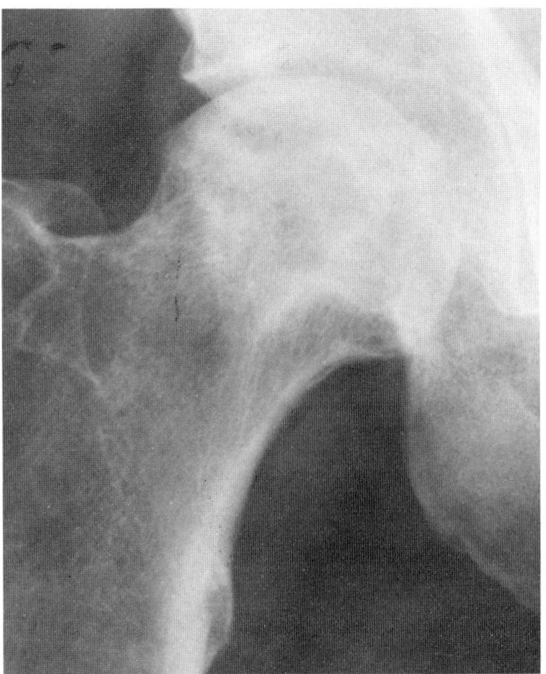

A': Right hip: two years after the core. During this time he continued working, but the pain had reappeared.

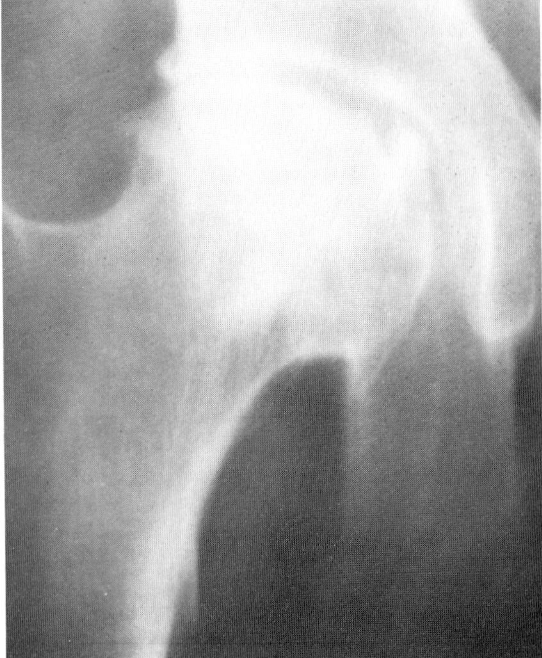

A'': Right hip: three years post core. The sclerosis has increased, and there is subchondral infraction medially and superior flattening.

Fig.63.—Case 5

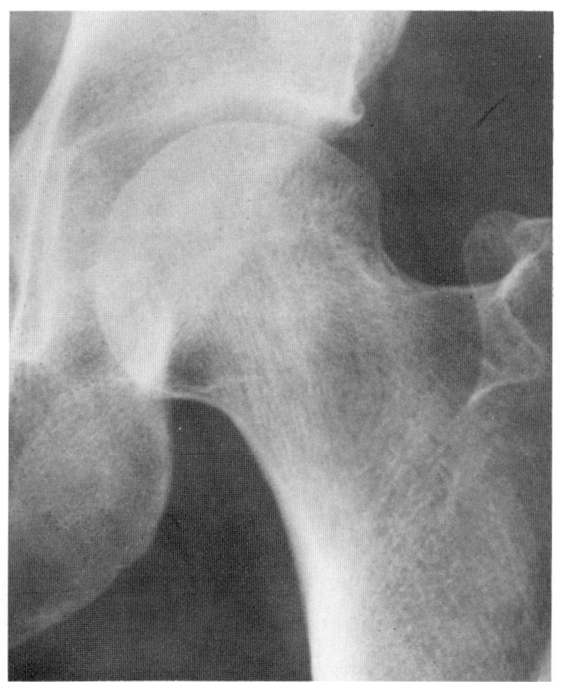

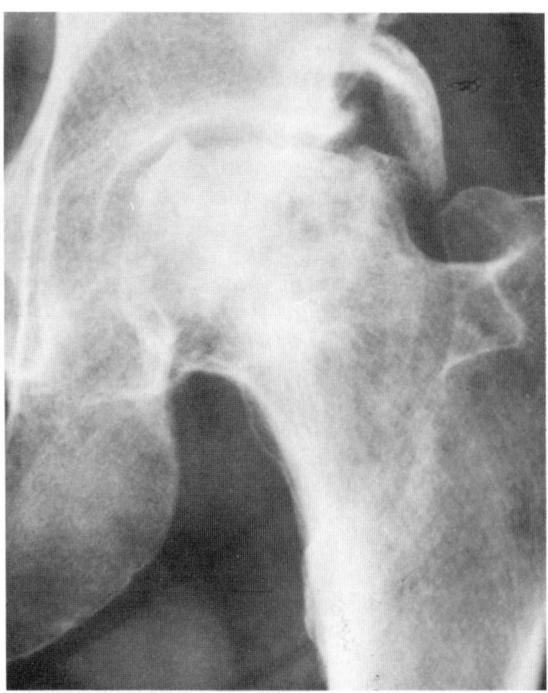

B: Left hip: in 1967, during a recurrence of right hip symptoms. Normal appearance in spite of the pain. The patient refuses the forage.

B': Left hip: two years later, bipolar irregularities with collapse of the sequestrum and peri-articular ossification.

Fig. 63.—continued.

Illustrative Case 6 (Fig. 64) - Mr. CLA..., a 52-year-old farmer, was first seen by us in May, 1971, with a ten-month history of moderate groin and knee pain. Since March, 1968, he had been treated with Prednisone equivalent, 15 to 30 mg/day for pulmonary sarcoidosis. On physical exam, the right hip showed slight but definite limitation of movement. X-rays of the pelvis showed abnormal, non-homogeneous densities in both femoral heads, leading to a likely diagnosis of cortisone induced

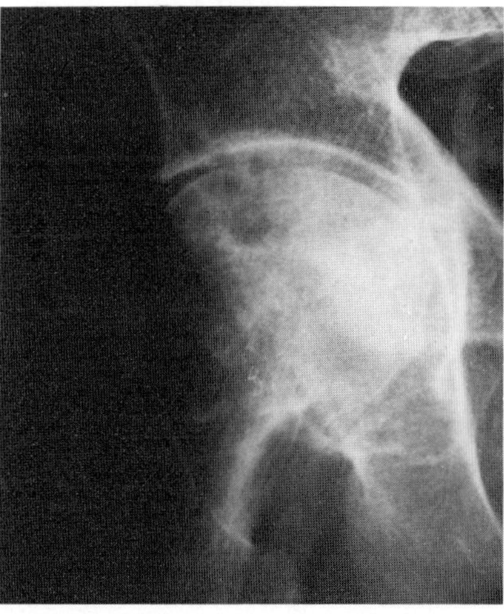

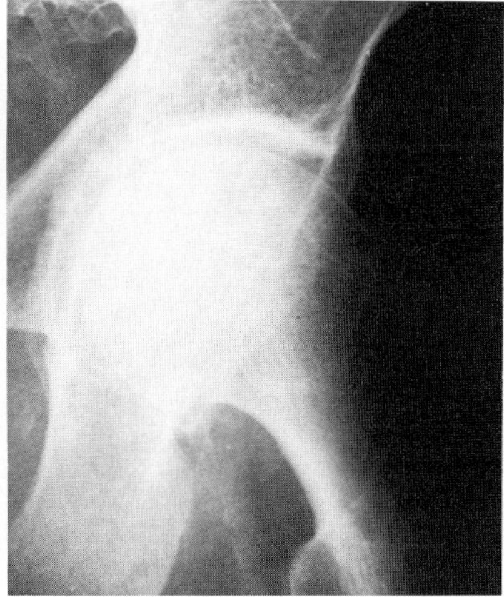

A: Bilateral necroses of the hips: on the right with sclerocystic changes and lateral, subchondral infraction; on the left, homogeneous sclerosis.

Fig.64.—Case 6

bilateral femoral head necrosis. In spite of protected weight-bearing, the left hip also became painful in August, 1971. By October, 1971, the right hip lesion had become more severe. At the time of functional investigation, IMP measurements were normal in the greater trochanter (18 mm Hg in the right, 15 mm Hg in the left) but high in the head (50 mm Hg on the right and 55 mm Hg on the left after stress test). The core biopsy specimens revealed obvious necrotic lesions with important reactive lesions (marrow fibrosis, mixed bone resorption, and sclerosis). This patient did not have any blood lipid abnormalities, but alkaline phosphatase and calcium were abnormally elevated. He also had vertebral osteoporosis and compression fractures. At his March, 1975, follow-up, he had resumed work. His left hip had good range of movement and was painless, although the right hip remained painful with limitation of movement and evidence of radiographic progression. When last seen in 1977, there was no change in his clinical situation.

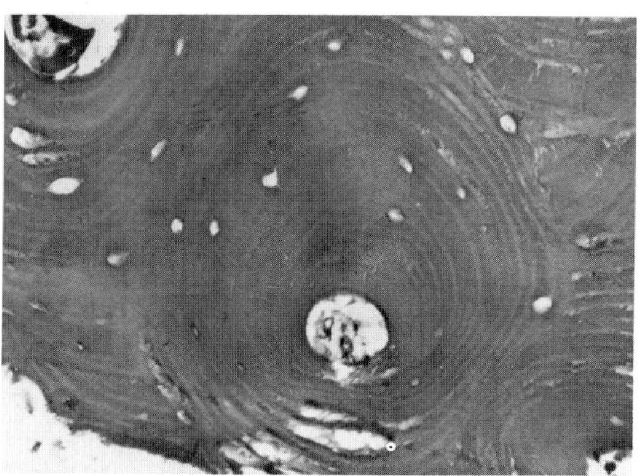

Fig.64B: Trabecular necrosis

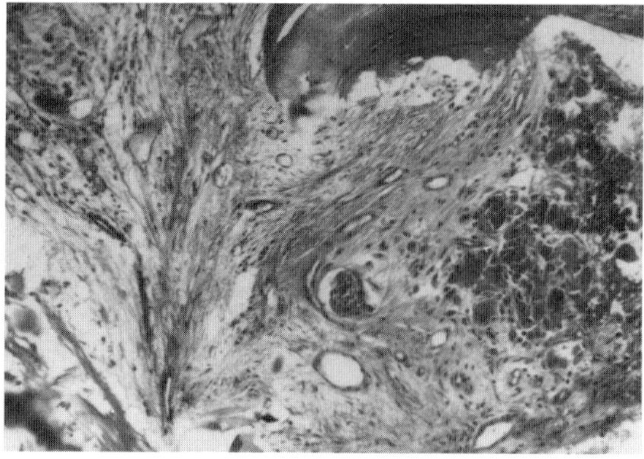

Fig.64C: Hemorrhagic area surrounded by fibrosis.

Stage IV (Fig. 65)

The last phase in the evolution of femoral head necrosis is characterized by a progressive secondary deterioration of the cartilage revealed by late joint space narrowing and the establishment of typical osteoarthrosic changes. The acetabular roof becomes deformed to accommodate the flattened deformity of the head, transforming the spherical joint into a cylindrical one that preserves flexion to a large degree but results in almost total loss of abduction and rotation.

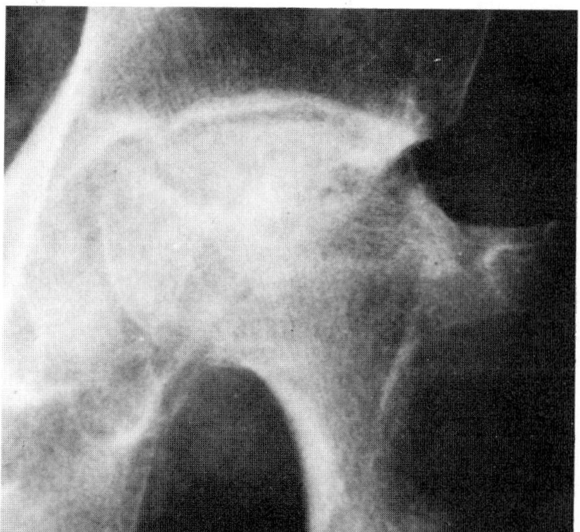

A: Flattened head with collapse of the sequestrum and global narrowing of the joint space.

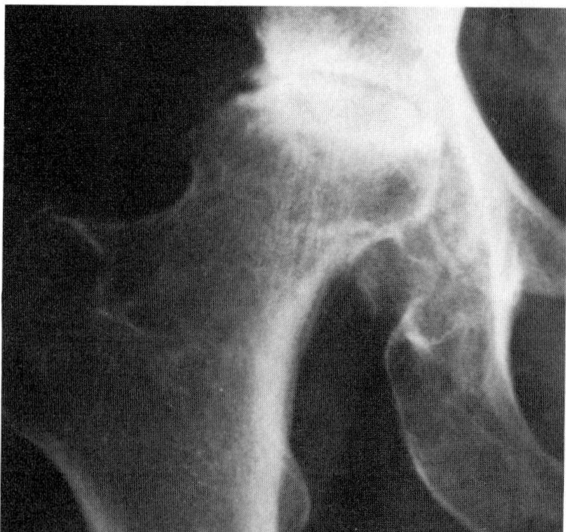

B: Flattened head produced by progressive wear; sclerosis with global narrowing and irregularity of the joint space.

Fig.65.—Radiologic features of Stage IV

Illustrative Case 7 (Fig. 66) - Mrs. HU..., a 37-year-old housewife, was seen initially in January, 1966, with a four-year history of right, groin pain. The pains had started rather suddenly after pregnancy in which she delivered twins and during which she experienced severe edema of both lower extremities. Clinical examination revealed definite limitation of both hips, although the left hip was pain free. The initial x-rays which had been taken in 1962 were available for review and showed, on the right side, poorly limited, subchondral lucencies in the superomedial zone with radiodensity on the opposing acetabular surface. On functional evaluation, January 14, 1966, the venography showed marked stasis and diaphyseal reflux on the right and definite abnormalities on the left. The core biopsy on the right confirmed the presence of extensive medullary necrosis. Surgery improved the patient, but the lesion progressed quickly to Stage IV on the right (Fig. 67) as well as on the left, non-operated side. In spite of the advanced radiologic appearance, the patient had reasonable function and was able to ambulate without assistance when seen in 1979.

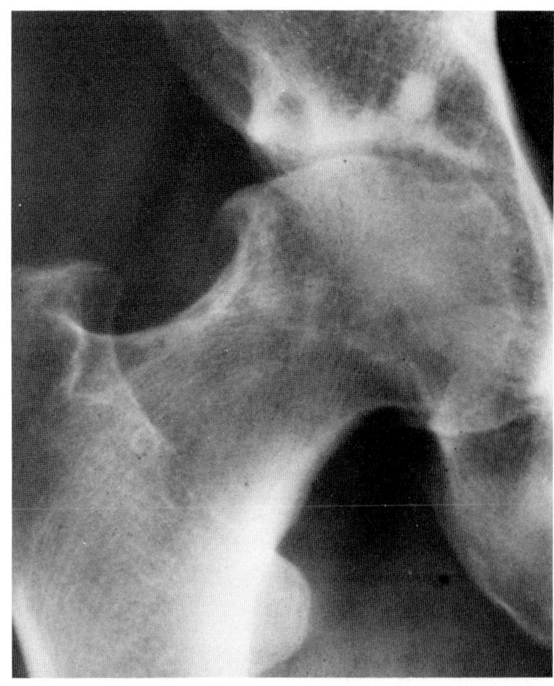

B: Right hip (January 1966): collapse of the superior pole of the femoral head with subchondral infraction. Superolateral joint-line narrowing with marginal osteophytes. Acetabular changes have also progressed.

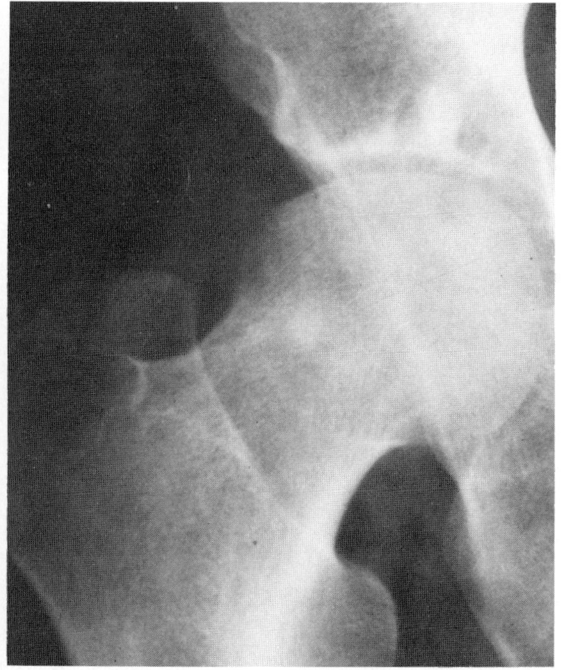

A: Right hip (June 1962): subtle sclerocystic changes within the femoral head which is slightly out of round; sclerosis along the margin of the acetabulum.

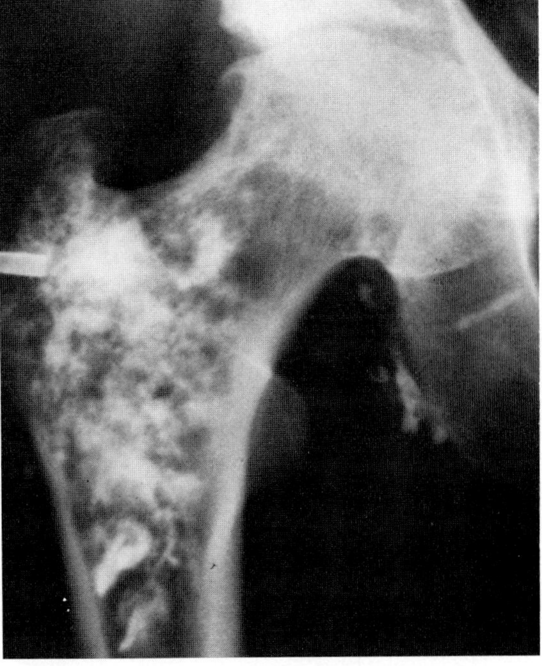

C: Right hip (January 1966): very abnormal pertrochanteric phlebography (absence of efferents; marked reflux and stasis).

Fig.66.—Case 7 (Stage IV)

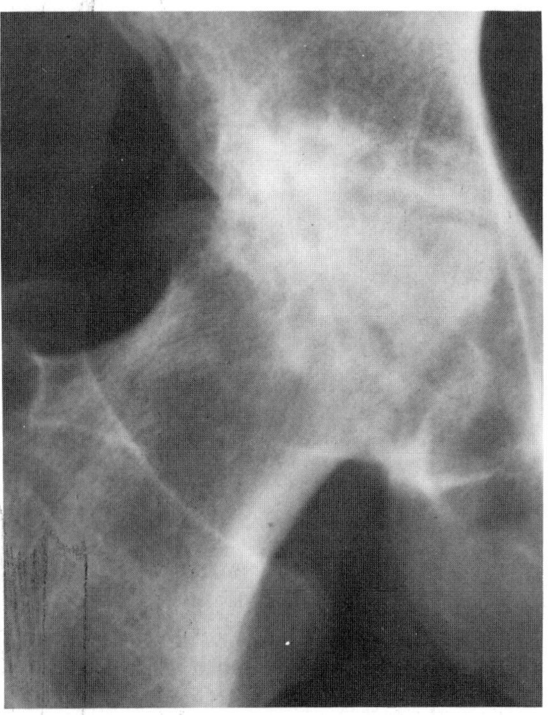

Fig.67.—Right hip (November 1966): complete collapse of the whole superior pole of the femoral head and sclerocystic mirror image of the acetabulum. The joint has become cylindrically shaped with joint-line narrowing.

The characteristics of the four stages of femoral head ischemic necrosis are outlined in Table VIII. Although this classification system has been primarily developed for the femoral head, which is the most common site of involvement of bone necrosis, it is applicable to bone necrosis in general where an epiphysis and, eventually, an articulation is involved. It is particularly useful for ischemic necroses of the knee and shoulder, the next two most common sites of involvement.

OSTEOCHONDRAL TYPE: ISCHEMIC COXOPATHY

(Fig. 68 and 69)

Besides the classical type which we have just described, it is necessary to describe an osteochondral-type of necrosis which is characterized by early narrowing of the joint space. This joint space involvement begins with the onset of the disease, whereas, in the classical osseous form such involvement occurs only in the terminal stage. It is for this reason that we propose to label this form ischemic coxopathy[148]. This is a peculiar process and somewhat surprising at first since its radiological presentation is similar to either early coxarthrosis or rheumatoid synovitis. The bone necrosis hides behind a mask of non-specific bone changes and is interpreted as a secondary reaction to the arthrosis. The necrotic component of the condition becomes

TABLE VIII

RADIOLOGIC CLASSIFICATION OF ISCHEMIC NECROSIS OF THE FEMORAL HEAD
I. OSSEOUS FORM: CLASSIC "NECROSIS"

	Stages	*Jointline*	*Femoral Head Contour*	*Trabeculae*	*Diagnosis by X-Ray*	*Diagnosis by Functional Exploration of Bone*
Simple Necrosis	I	N	N	N or very slight osteoporosis	Impossible	Hemodynamic-probable
	II	N	N	Osteoporosis mixed sclerosis/porosis	Probable	Histopathological certain
Necrosis Complicated by Collapse	III	N	Flattened subchondral infraction collapse	Sequestrum formation	Certain	Confirmation
	IV	Narrowed	Collapsed	Destruction of superior pole	Very difficult between arthrosis, flammatory arthritis, and necrosis	Hemodynamic insufficient combined biopsy necessary

N = Normal

evident in some cases with the terminal evolution towards sequestrum formation which is more typical of necrosis. The two forms of osteonecrosis, the osseous type and the osteochondral type, through different processes come to a common end-stage: complete destruction of the joint. Without initial x-rays, it is impossible to reconstitute the sequence of the degenerative lesion. The differences between the osseous and osteochondral types, however, remain somewhat schematic and artificial because we have observed in a few cases that the sequestrum formation and the joint narrowing develop simultaneously. Moreover, radiologic preservation of the joint space is no presumption of the integrity of the articular cartilage which may be severely affected with advanced lesions detected by arthrography and confirmed by histology. According to Patterson et al.[337], the sparing of the articular cartilage is not necessarily characteristic of necrosis, as he has observed moderate narrowing of the joint space in 23% of the cases and marked or disappearing joint line in 8% of the cases. In the remaining 69% of the cases, the narrowing was "discrete or absent." Most authors, like Patterson, accept the possibility of a concurrent joint narrowing without considering its nosologic significance. We have seen some examples of ischemic coxopathy which can evolve like an arthrosis for several years only to show late sequestrum formation followed by collapse.

We have collected 42 hips in 36 patients as examples of ischemic coxopathy according to three criteria: well-centered, non-dysplastic hips from a radiologic point of view, no evidence of synovitis seen either in the laboratory or in histology at the time of synovial biopsy, and no evidence of trauma. All of these cases fall within the traditional category of primary osteoarthrosis of the hip and are always diagnosed as such if the functional exploration is not used. This method, therefore, allows us to define an important new category of pathology. A review of the essential characteristics of this series will allow us to outline a diagnostic profile.

In the 36 patients that we have seen with ischemic coxopathy, there is slight female predominance (20:16) as well as right-sided predominance. Thirteen cases were bilateral. Twelve patients experienced sudden onset of symptoms, while 15 patients complained of night pain as well. Restriction of movement was usually moderate and seemed to effect mostly extension and internal and external rotation. Flexion and abduction were often decreased but not to an important degree. The x-rays exhibit a variable location of the joint line narrowing with 5 cases superolaterally; 10 cases superomedially; 7 cases

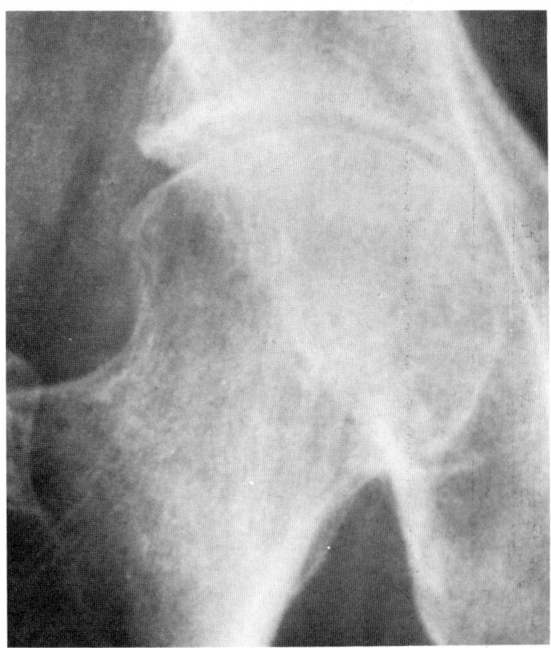

Fig.68.—Radiologic features of the osteochondral type or ischemic coxopathy. Beginning of ischemic coxopathy with superomedial joint-line narrowing and bone formation in the inferior border of the femoral neck.

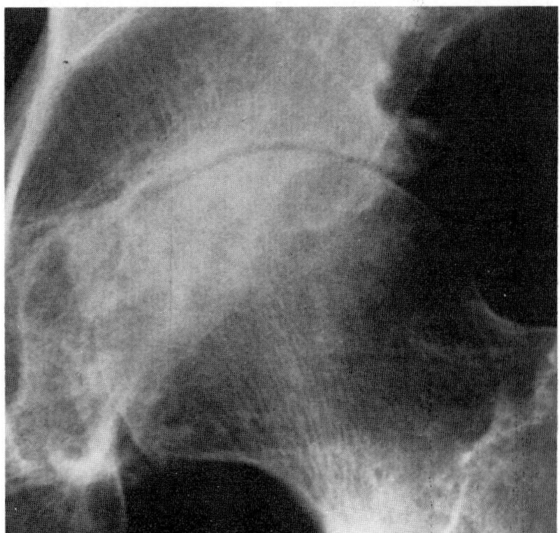

Fig.69.—Advanced ischemic coxopathy with smooth, global joint-space narrowing. Sclerocystic changes in the femoral head with subtle marginal osteophytes.

superiorly; and 20 cases showing symmetrical joint-line diminution. The changes in bone texture are more frequently toward increased density with pure sclerosis in 16 cases, mixed sclerocystic changes in 17 cases, cystic alone changes in three cases, and non-specific changes in three cases.

Intramedullary pressure investigations were carried out on 38 hips. Twenty-six cases showed an increased baseline pressure of more than 30 mm Hg as measured at the level of the greater trochanter. In 25 instances, marrow pressure was measured within the head and in 20 of those cases, the baseline pressure was elevated. In 11 cases with normal intertrochanteric intramedullary pressures, the "stress" test was positive in the greater trochanter in six cases, and at the level of the femoral head in four cases. In the only case with both normal trochanteric and femoral head pressures and a negative saline test in the head, the pressure curve in the head showed complete absence of the osseous pulse which constitutes a sign of severe ischemia. We can, therefore, say that abnormalities have been found on functional investigation of all cases.

Intraosseous venography was carried out in 20 cases and revealed stasis in 19 cases. Core biopsy was carried out in 42 cases and classified according to the histologic classification system explained in Chapter VI. Six cases were of Type 1; 25 cases were of Type 2. Type 2 seems to be the most typical for ischemic coxopathy. Ten cases exhibited Type 3 changes, of which one had signs of repair (Type 4). Only one case did not show necrosis. In that case, the histology showed only typical arthrotic changes in spite of an intramedullary pressure of 50 mm Hg. It is interesting to note that the contralateral hip showed a typical histologic appearance of necrosis.

These findings lead us to two conclusions. Firstly, there does appear to be a significant ischemic element in the development of some cases of hip pathology which is different from the pure osseous form of necrosis. Ten cases showed Type 3 changes with complete, uniform, and extensive necrosis of the whole bone marrow, a picture totally incompatible with a diagnosis of simple osteoarthrosis. Secondly, the findings emphasize the importance of bone marrow necrosis (25 cases of Type 2 lesions) as an intermediate, and probably constant, transition between ischemia and trabecular necrosis.

It is likely that these ischemic lesions exist before radiologic abnormalities are seen, and we have been able to demonstrate this in one case. The joint space narrowing can be either symmetrical or eccentric from the beginning. When eccentric, it is usually superomedially but then may extend to involve other portions of the joint. There is a tendency toward progressive disappearance of the joint space, occasionally proceeding to destruction of the superior pole which is typical in destructive arthroses of the hip.

Conclusion - This concept of ischemic coxopathy rests on the association of a cartilaginous, radiologically evident lesion coupled with diffuse necrotic bone and bone marrow lesions seen on the histological specimens. This association brings up the crucial problems of diagnosis and pathophysiology which will be discussed in Chapter VI on differential diagnosis.

Illustrative Case 8 (Fig. 70). - Mrs. SCH..., a 54-year-old midwife, presented to our clinic in January, 1974, with a two-year history of right knee pain which had started suddenly and quickly involved the groin and thigh. The symptoms became continuous, severe, and associated with night pain. Physical examination in January, 1974, revealed painful limitation of movement with flexion to only 95°. Range of movement on the opposite side was normal. X-rays showed a subfoveal cystic lesion of the right femoral head. Although the joint line appeared to be of normal width, arthrography showed considerable thinning of the articular cartilage on both the femoral head and the acetabulum in the superior pole. On the left side, there was definite joint line narrowing superolaterally, although on that side the patient was asymptomatic. Trochanteric IMP was elevated on both sides (42 mm Hg on the right, 45 mm Hg on the left). Combined biopsy of the right hip showed normal synovium, degenerated articular cartilage, and necrotic intracapital bone. In July, 1974, the patient no longer had pain in the right hip but presented with a few days history of pain in the left hip. Core biopsy on the left hip revealed necrosis as well. Possible etiologic factors for consideration include an eight day course of Cortisone in 1973 for asthma, increased beta lipoproteinemia (29%), and venous insufficiency of the lower extremity. This observation is a typical one in that on the right side there was a Stage II osteonecrosis of the cystic-type (normal head contour, normal joint line but with histologic evidence of cartilage damage). On the left side, there was a clear ischemic coxopathy which was suspected in the preclinical stage because of the joint space narrowing and the increased pressure, which was later confirmed by biopsy at the time of presentation with symptoms.

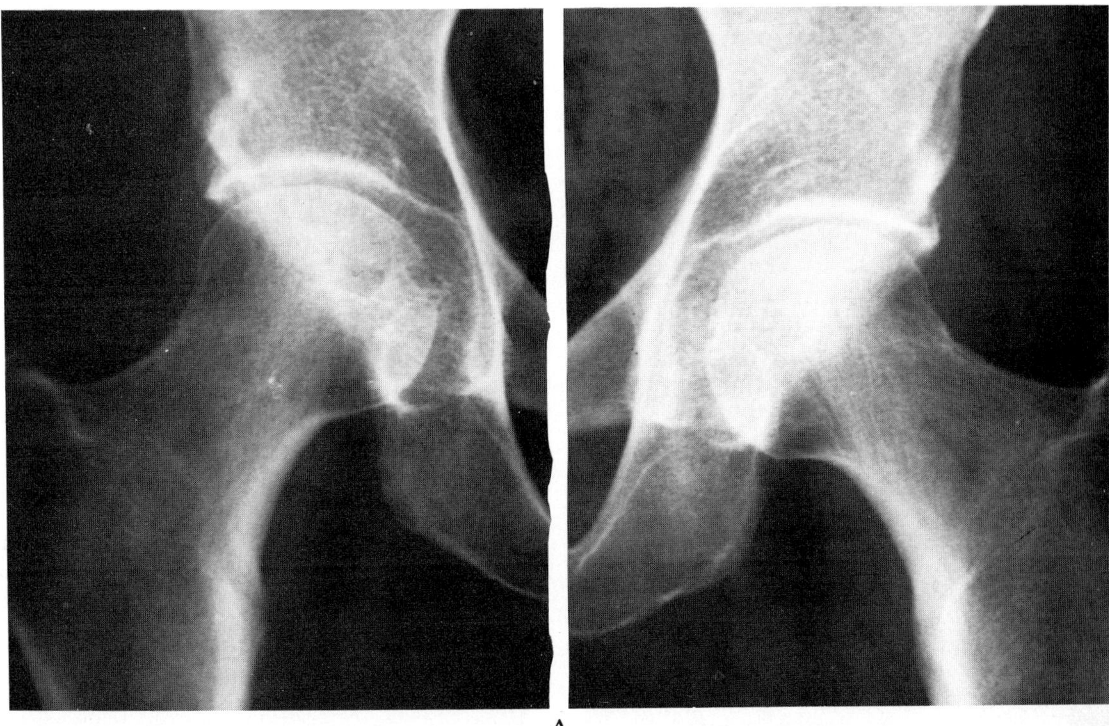

A

On the right side, subtle sclerosis and suggestion of a medial cyst (A). Good preservation of the joint-line confirmed by tomograms (A') but the contrast arthrography (A'') demonstrates a thinning of the articular cartilage, particularly on the acetabular side. The necrosis was confirmed by biopsy (February 1974). On the left side, the joint space is relatively narrowed in relation to the right side, comparing the tomograms (B with that of the right side (A'). At that time it was painless, but the necrosis was confirmed two years later by a core biopsy carried out because of the onset of severe pain. The right hip had remained painless since the core decompression.

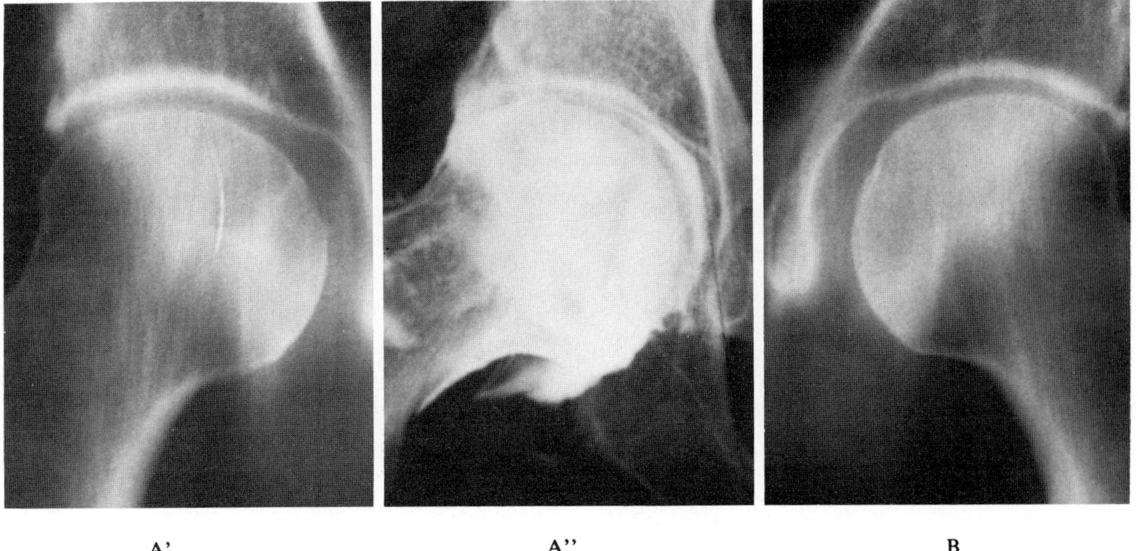

A'A''B

Fig.70.—Case 8.

Illustrative Case 9 (Fig. 71). - Mr. LAF..., a 53-year-old bricklayer, presented in March, 1974, with a three-year history of right hip pain. The patient had been unable to work for the nine months prior to his initial presentation. Physical examination showed painful limitation of movement (100° flexion). X-rays showed bilateral lesions, right side more developed than the left, with concentric joint line narrowing and sclerosis in the head. The inter-trochanteric IMP was elevated on the right (48 mm Hg). Intraosseous venography showed definite intramedullary stasis within the femoral head. The biopsy showed both medullary and trabecular necrosis extending into the head and femoral neck. Possible etiologic considerations include clinically evident gout appearing in 1970, eight injections of long-acting Cortisone in the right shoulder and neck in 1972, and increased pre-beta lipoproteinemia (20%).

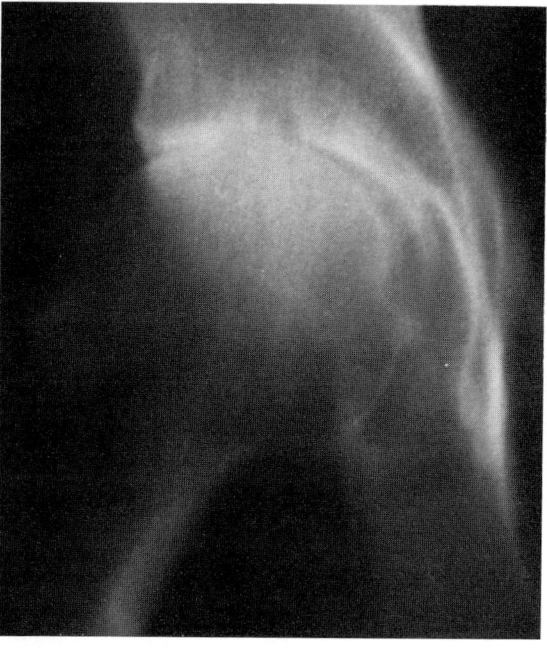

A: Tomogram of the right hip, showing severe superior joint-line narrowing.

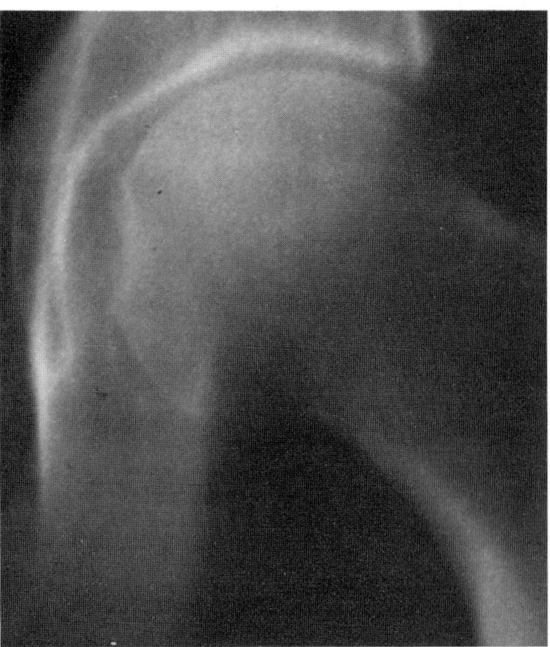

A': Tomogram of the left hip with joint narrowing, mainly superomedially.

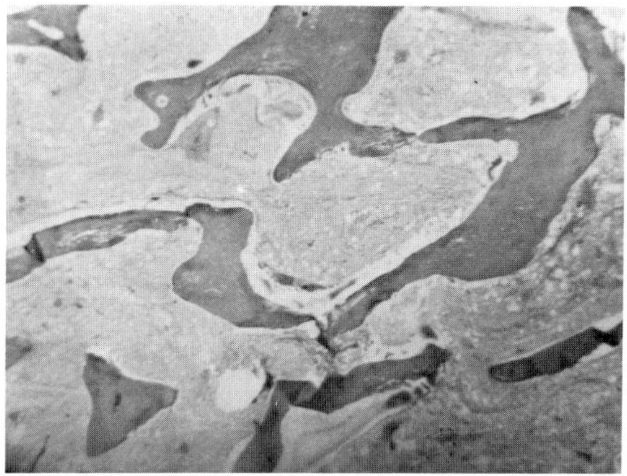

B: Complete marrow necrosis.

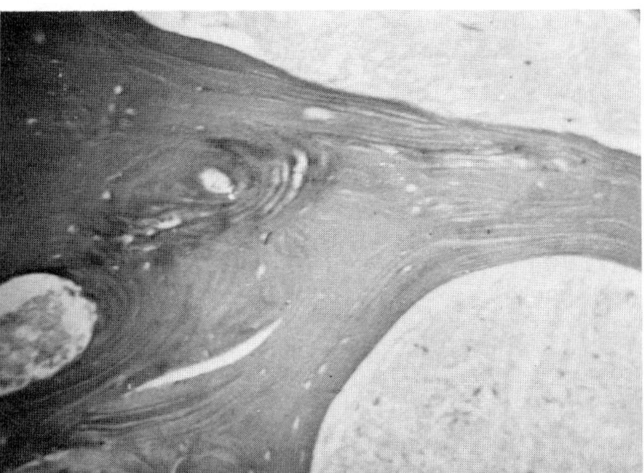

B': Trabecular necrosis surrounded by necrotic marrow.

Fig.71—Case 9

Illustrative Case 10 (Fig. 72) - Mrs. LAF..., a 52-year-old housewife, was examined for the first time in October, 1967, with a four-year history of bilateral groin pain which had recently increased in severity, considerably restricting her ambulation. The hips showed moderate painful limitation of movement (flexion 115°) and were radiologically abnormal. On the left more than on the opposite side, there was superior narrowing of the joint line with marginal osteophytes, subchondral cysts, and a picture suggesting a sequestrum formation. On the right side, the joint line was relatively intact but the superior aspect of the head was flattened with extensive sclerocystic changes. The patient had been diagnosed as having osteoarthrosis. However, intraosseous venography showed definite stasis, more pronounced on the left than on the right. Bilateral core biopsies showed diffuse medullary necrosis on the right and extensive medullary and trabecular necrosis on the left. The patient, therefore, demonstrated ischemic coxopathy. With the core decompression, the pain subsided considerably. The patient was followed up in 1970 and again in 1974, at which time she had painless range of movement, led a normal, active life, and was able to walk three to four kilometers a day. The lesions remained unchanged on the right although on the left, there was considerable improvement in both the radiologic appearance of the head and the joint line (Fig. 72B).

Nonetheless, in 1977, the symptoms reappeared associated with a significant change in the radiologic appearance. Increased symptoms led to total hip replacement on the left in December, 1977, and on the right in October, 1978.

Table IX summarizes the findings in the different stages of evolution of this disease entity.

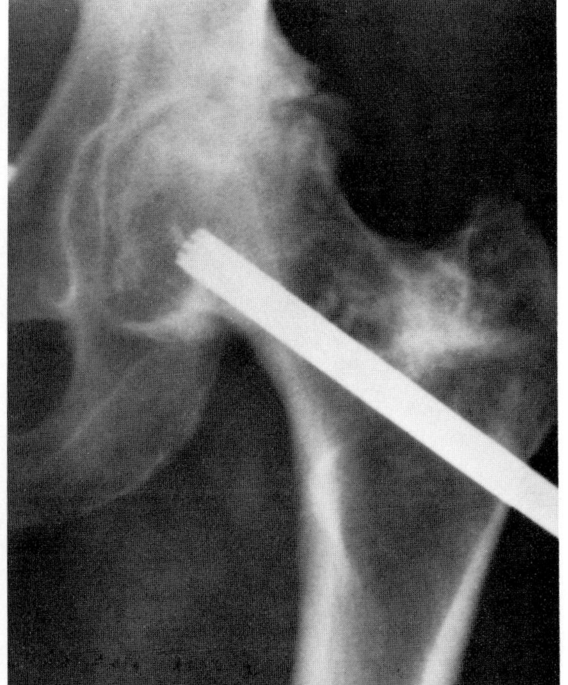

A: Intra-operative x-rays during core decompression. The joint-line is non-existent superiorly with sclerotic changes on both sides of the joint, simulating a sequestrum in the head.

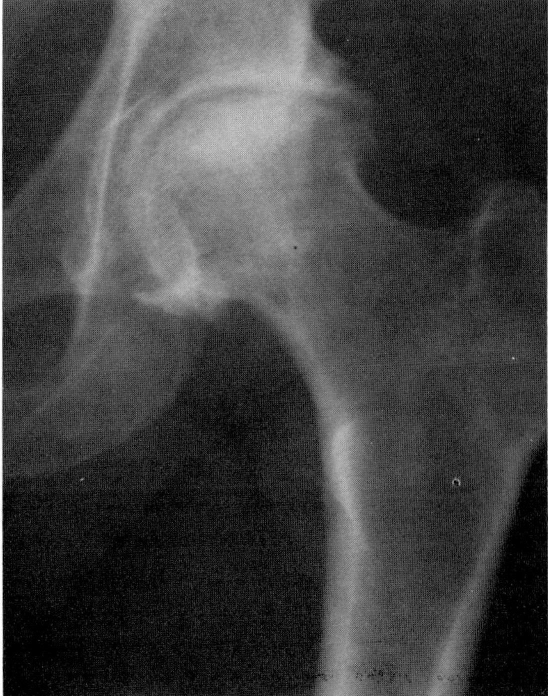

B: Radiological aspect two years after the forage; the joint line is partially constituted.

Fig. 72.—Case 10

TABLE IX

RADIOLOGICAL CLASSIFICATION OF THE FEMORAL HEAD NECROSES
IL Osteochondral Form: ischemic coxopathy

Stage	Joint Line	Head Contour	Trabeculae	Diagnosis by X-ray	Diagnosis by Functional Exploration
Earliest onset	Normal	Normal	Normal or slight porosis	Impossible	Hemodynamic: probable histologic:certain
Established	Narrowed Localized or diffuse Slight-complete	Normal	Decalcification Disorganization	Very difficult between: —arthrosis	Combined biopsy:
End—stage	Complete disappearance	Flattened	Wedge-shaped sclerosis Increased density	—inflammation —necrosis	Synovium/ bone: certain

CHAPTER V

THE SYNDROME OF BONE ISCHEMIA

INTRODUCTION

Before we began applying our method of functional investigation to all disorders of the hip, we mainly concentrated on osteonecrosis in which the radiologic diagnosis was apparent. From this we arrived at the conclusion that all cases had certain factors in common which we shall describe under the term, the "ischemic syndrome." We have chosen this particular term because it describes the diminution in circulation which we find in most cases. Total arrest of circulation leads to massive and irreversible necrosis. However, on the other hand, a decrease in blood flow and slowing of the circulation leads to signs of chronic ischemia which is characterized by a mixture of necrotic lesions and evidence of reconstitution of bone. Although our initial concepts were formulated by applying these methods of functional evaluation to radiologically-evident osteonecrosis, we have only found reinforcement of the ideas in the findings in the earlier stages (Stages I and II). We believe that these findings tie together all stages of bone ischemia which justify the description of an ischemic syndrome. The ischemic syndrome is composed of a series of signs, each of them revealing, in turn, a different aspect of the same circulatory problem. The only type of necrosis which might be an exception to these would be a direct cytotoxic process as can be caused by radiotherapy. Even in such cases, our experience has shown that the functional investigation may be positive, indicating that a circulatory disturbance could be concomitant with or secondary to the cytotoxic death. This syndrome can be described and understood in terms of six areas of investigation: clinical, radiologic, hemodynamic, isotopic, histopathologic, and metabolic.

CLINICAL SIGNS

Although the clinical findings are only presumptive, they should lead us to include the possibility of ischemia in the differential diagnosis.

PAIN

The pain is characteristically associated with bone ischemia is deep and usually not precisely localized. It was of sudden onset in 50% of our cases. Pain does not always coincide with the beginning of the disease, since x-rays sometimes already demonstrate the formation of a sequestrum, and one might believe that the pain represents the occurence of a subchondral fracture. It is this aspect of pain which most likely brought about the name of "coronary artery disease of the hip[87]," since it resembles an infarction. The intensity of the pain is quite variable, and we have rated it according to a code (see Table XXXIII). Night pain which wakes the patient is less common (24.5%). Night pain is also encountered in inflammatory hip disease. The mechanism is not well understood although among the hypotheses are included the concept of increased venous stasis at night and diurnal hormonal variation can be mentioned.

The distribution of the pain is not characteristic for ischemia since, like most hip pain, it radiates to the groin (63%), sometimes to the trochanteric region, and occasionally to the buttock, simulating sciatica. In a few cases associated with osteoporosis, trochanteric pressure can produce discomfort. Thirty-five percent of the cases demonstrated pseudoradicular radiation of the pain extending anteriorly and medially down to the level of the knee and occasionally to the upper third of the tibia. Occasionally, increase in pain with coughing or sneezing was present. It is well to be aware of this so as not to attribute this finding to be pathognomically true radicular pain. Sudden compression of the abdominal wall and thorax increases both synovial fluid pressure as well as venous pressure in the trunk, the latter having its effect on intramedullary pressure.

Patients may also experience a type of claudication. The circulatory demands are increased by exercise, increasing the ischemia, which suddenly increases the pain, forcing the patient to stop the exercise. The pain then improves with rest. In this way, it is very similar to the claudication of chronic, peripheral vascular disease and also must be differentiated from claudication of spinal or venous origin. Peripheral vasomotor disturbances may also be associated with the painful syndrome, including edema, pallor or cyanosis, and coldness and numbness. These are undoubtedly due to an associated reflex circulatory disturbance with manifestations, including the whole extremity down to the foot. However, it is also possible to observe segmental vasomotor problems. In one patient, we were able to record a 3°C drop in skin temperature on the side of the necrosis, affecting only the upper two-thirds of the thigh.

LIMITATION OF MOVEMENT

As with other hip disorders, a generalized restriction of movement may be present or the motion may be restricted in only some directions and not others. Internal rotation and abduction are particularly affected. Careful examination is necessary to detect these limitations. There is no particular type of stiffness for the ischemic syndrome, but demonstration of limitation of hip motion is usually sufficient to identify the hip joint as the source of the symptoms. It is particularly useful when the restriction of movement is associated with a normal x-ray, since such restriction could not otherwise be explained. The only other explanation for the painful limitation of movement in the face of a completely normal hip x-ray would be an adhesive capsulitis of which we have encountered several cases in the course of the combined synovial/bone biopsy. Degree of limitation is also measured by a standard numerical guide.

RADIOLOGICAL SIGNS

For a long time in the past, only the appearance of the sequestrum in the weight-bearing area of the femoral head has been recognized as the pathognomic picture of death and separation of a bone fragment. This is the basis for the concept of an osteochondritis dissecans. The radiologic picture of necrosis following femoral neck fractures showed more or less intensive and extensive development of sclerosis. Although this picture is not pathognomonic, it is of considerable value because of the context in which it develops. Aside from posttraumatic cases, this type of sclerosis is also seen in 50% of the cases of chronic ischemia. However, two important points must be emphasized. First and foremost, this is only a suggestive and not a pathognomonic sign as it can also be found in Paget's Disease or in metastatic bone disease. The similarity of the appearance with medullary infarction is, however, very suggestive. Secondly, the radiologic appearance is not produced by the necrosis but rather the process of reconstruction and repair of the ischemic and/or necrotic bone. Another radiologic lesion which should suggest the diagnosis of bone necrosis is a fairly large and well-defined cystic lesion located outside the weight-bearing zone. The functional investigation has allowed us to confirm that radiologic appearances are associated with the ischemic syndrome, since we have encountered this form in 25% of our cases.

The functional investigation used systemically has allowed us to relate the ischemia and necrosis to two radiologic aspects which have not been mentioned in classic descriptions. The first is an osteoporotic appearance characterized by a homogeneous, regional osteoporosis or a spotty multifocal osteoporosis, sometimes extending to include the acetabulum. The second finding is one of segmental or global jointline narrowing without the usual radiologic changes associated with arthrosis (see Ischemic Coxopathy, Chapter IV).

Finally, the normal x-ray is completely compatible with a diagnosis of the ischemic syndrome, in fact, it is even one more reason to think of it. The normal x-ray corresponds to the preradiologic or Stage I of the ischemia which has been confirmed from many points of view, etiologic, clinical, and experimental. This fundamental concept which has now been adequately demonstrated should be sufficient to alter our diagnostic approach to articular pathology.

Periosteal new bone formation has been reported by several authors[3,241,296,299], although mainly on the lower femoral metaphysis and diaphysis. It has also been described, however, at the lower border of the femoral neck, where it cannot be called periosteal but rather subsynovial. Some authors have reported it in arthrosis and others in necrosis. This new bone formation has been interpreted as a bone reaction to the increase in mechanical stresses occurring on the femoral neck[299]. However, other factors can also be argued, including the transmission of increased in-

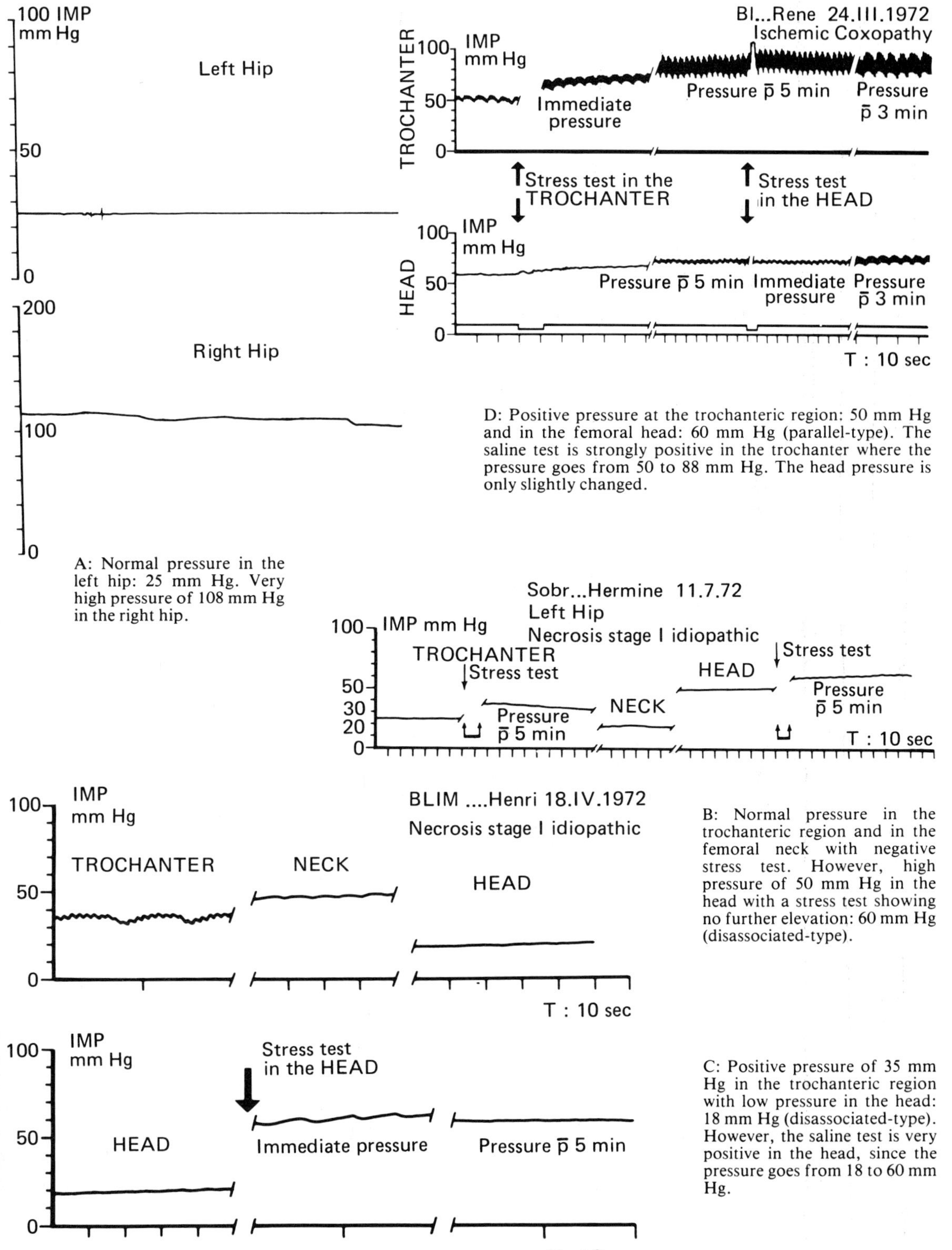

A: Normal pressure in the left hip: 25 mm Hg. Very high pressure of 108 mm Hg in the right hip.

D: Positive pressure at the trochanteric region: 50 mm Hg and in the femoral head: 60 mm Hg (parallel-type). The saline test is strongly positive in the trochanter where the pressure goes from 50 to 88 mm Hg. The head pressure is only slightly changed.

B: Normal pressure in the trochanteric region and in the femoral neck with negative stress test. However, high pressure of 50 mm Hg in the head with a stress test showing no further elevation: 60 mm Hg (disassociated-type).

C: Positive pressure of 35 mm Hg in the trochanteric region with low pressure in the head: 18 mm Hg (disassociated-type). However, the saline test is very positive in the head, since the pressure goes from 18 to 60 mm Hg.

Fig.73.—Examples of intramedullary pressure recordings.

tramedullary pressures to the foramina of the cortex and a response to the compensatory increase in vascularization in the area surrounding the ischemia.

HEMODYNAMIC SIGNS[11,21]

INTRAMEDULLARY PRESSURE (Fig. 73)

For several years, we have measured pressure only in the intertrochanteric region of the proximal femur. Baseline intramedullary pressure was more than 30 mm Hg in 72% of the cases. The highest baseline pressure that we have recorded is 100 mm Hg. These statistics are significant in themselves. They are, however, rare cases where in acute ischemia the medullary pressure is abnormally low, being less than 10 mm Hg[317]. We have also observed such a low baseline pressure in a case of Gaucher's Disease.

THE STRESS TEST

The next step in the functional evaluation is to provoke increased intramedullary pressure by injecting 5 ml of normal saline. We began by doing this in a systematic fashion in 1968. The pain associated with this intramedullary injection is very precise and usually reproduces the patient's symptoms. Even under general anesthesia, there may be a withdrawal phenomenon of the lower extremity. Resistance to injection is a rough guide but accurately portrays the compromise of the bone marrow vascular bed and its difficulty in accepting and dispersing an injected saline load. Under normal circumstances, this is remarkably easy. In bone necrosis, it is sometimes not even possible to inject 5 ml of saline. The stress test may not be necessary when the baseline pressure is already significantly positive, but it is of great interest in those cases where the baseline pressure is normal or borderline, since it allows us to uncover more minor or latent problems. In such cases, its abnormality is of great help in contributing to the diagnosis.

We have occasionally seen a fall in intramedullary pressure with the stress test, even in some cases that were clearly pathologic. This mainly occured when the baseline pressure was very high. It is possible that the injection of fluid may have opened a drainage pathway, thus producing better evacuation for the localized region under evaluation.

When limiting the IMP evaluation to the trochanteric region, we occasionally had the feeling that we were missing some cases of bone ischemia and considered that the intertrochanteric circulation might remain unaffected, even in the face of an epiphyseal circulatory disorder, at least in the early

stages. We, therefore, compared intramedullary pressure values measured both in the trochanteric region and in the femoral head in a series of 60 patients, of which 25 were for arthrosis and 35 for necrosis. This study revealed that in 40 cases the values were raised in both the trochanteric and the femoral head regions. In these cases, the baseline IMP was usually increased. However, in three of 15 cases of arthrosis and three of 25 cases of necrosis, the abnormalities only occurred through the stress test. In the remaining 20 cases, there was a dissociation of the IMP values in the trochanteric and the femoral head regions (10 arthroses, 10 necroses). In nine cases, it was increased in the trochanteric region and lower in the femoral head (4 arthroses, 5 necroses). In 11 cases, it was normal or mildly elevated in the trochanteric region and high in the femoral head (6 arthroses, 5 necroses).

The finding of 20 cases (33.3%) with dissociation of the findings in the femoral head and intertrochanteric region would seem to argue for always taking the IMP in the femoral head. However, this impression is not as strong if one considers that this dissociation with an increased pressure in the trochanteric region would have been considered pathological even in the absence of alterations in the head pressure. There were only three necroses and five arthroses with normal pressures at the level of the greater trochanter with high femoral head pressure. Even in these eight cases, one should take into account that the stress test was not always done.

In spite of its somewhat simplistic appearance, the finding of increased IMP has proven to be an excellent diagnostic test, particularly in the hip with painful limitation of motion but without x-ray changes. This test has allowed us to identify ischemic necrosis at Stage I. It seemed logical that all hips should pass through such a stage but, before this, there had never been demonstrable proof. Intertrochanteric, intramedullary pressures are of great diagnostic value even in the cases where the lesion is located in the femoral head. In our experience with 100 cases, the baseline pressure was positive in 72% of the cases. The stress test increased the positive results to 85%. Of the remaining 15%, 10% will also be positive when the pressure is taken in the femoral head. The remaining cases seem to be paradoxical forms of osteonecrosis without elevated pressure.

Intramedullary venography (Fig. 74)[15,168] - The abnormalities demonstrated by intramedullary venography are often quite dramatic and suggest some derangement of venous drainage of the bone. The picture suggests engorgement of intramedullary vessels and a blockage to evacuation of blood from the bone. The absence of one or several efferent ex-

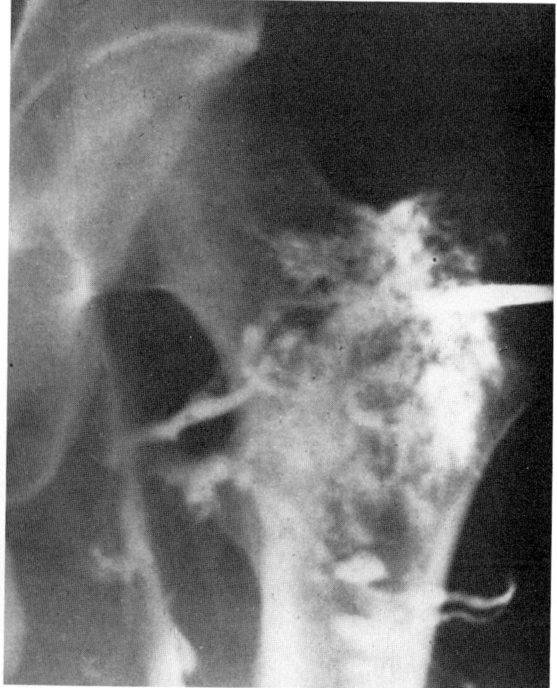

A: Pertrochanteric venography. Absence of the ischiatic vein.

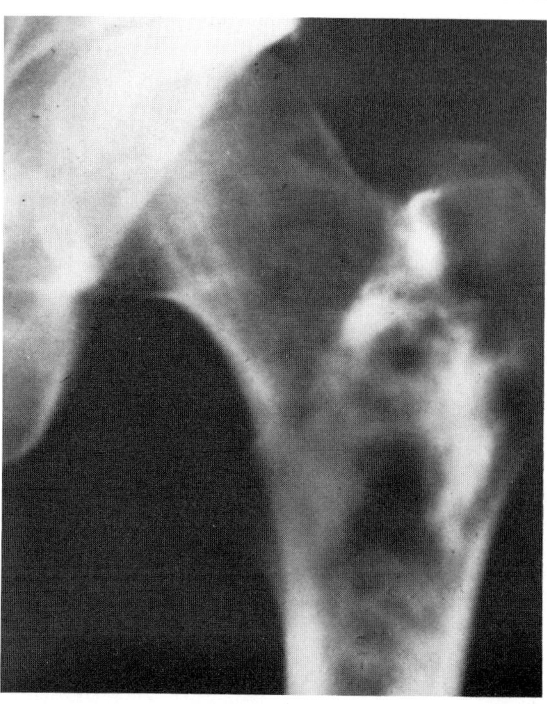

A': Metaphyseal-diaphyseal stasis 12 hours after the venography.

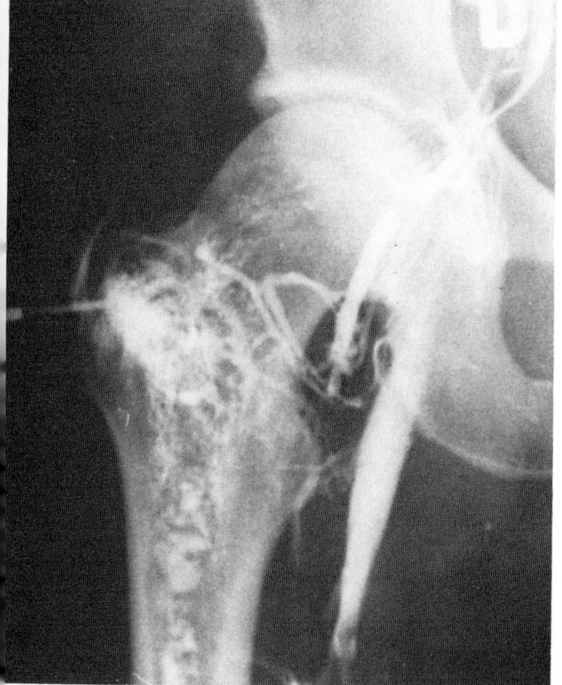

B

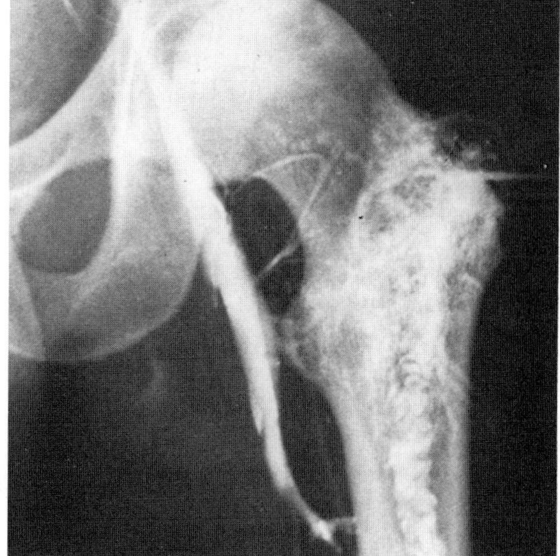

B'

B & B': Bilateral pertrochanteric venography in a sclerotic type of necrosis at Stage II. Diaphyseal reflux in both femurs.

Fig. 74.—Osteoporotic type of femoral head necrosis at Stage I.

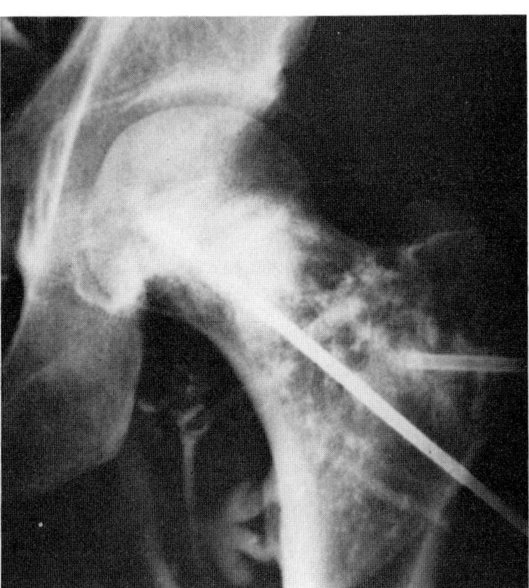

Fig.74C: Venography of the femoral head, showing absence of obturator and ischial veins, metaphyseal reflux and pooling within the neck.

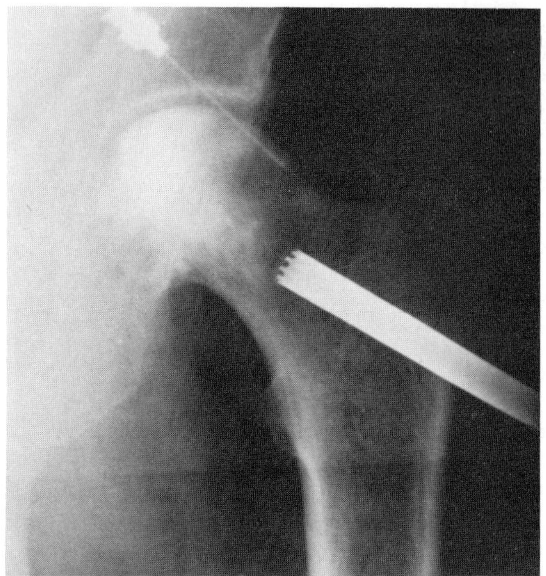

Fig.74C': Osteoporotic type with sudden onset of necrosis at Stage I in which diagnosis of tuberculosis had been entertained because of past history (sed. rate = 33). Intramedullary pressure: 20 mm Hg in the greater trochanter. Stress test: 47 mm Hg. Intra-capital stasis, 20 minutes after venography. Double biopsy: normal synovium. Diffuse eosinophilic reticular bone necrosis. Complete healing at five-year follow-up.

traosseous veins may be significant, particularly if one of the main efferent veins such as the circumflex or the ischial is the missing one. It is not uncommon that only one efferent, particularly the anterior circumflex, is seen although we have occasionally encountered nonvisualization of all the metaphyseal veins including the circumflex. In these cases, the contrast medium refluxes into the diaphysis and is slowly eliminated through the nutrient vein (Fig. 57B and 57B'). Even the visualization of all metaphyseal veins is no guarantee of good drainage, since the flow may be impaired, as seen when the five-minute film shows significant intramedullary stasis.

Diaphyseal reflux is very characteristic of the impairment of the metaphyseal drainage system. The contrast medium refluxes into the medullary canal and the main central venous sinus of the diaphysis is visualized with its irregular, serpentine shape down towards the distal metaphysis. Occasionally, one even sees epiphyseal reflux although, for hemodynamic reasons, it is very uncommon.

Intraosseous stasis may be demonstrated in two forms. In the first instance, persistance of the intraosseous dye for longer than five minutes is abnormal. We have seen this evident for more than several hours and sometimes even 24 hours following the injection of the dye. Secondly, the usually reticular appearance of the intraosseous dye may take on a globular-blotted appearance, usually implying stasis.

The painful reaction to the injection which we reported with the saline test is even more marked with contrast medium, probably due to the increased osmolality of the contrast material. The intramedullary pressure is also generally increased significantly more than with the saline stress test, although one can also occasionally see this in the normal. The painful nature of intramedullary venography is such to justify either strong, systemic analgesia or general anesthesia.

The extraosseous venous channels may show both functional and morphologic abnormalities which are best seen on cineradiography. These irregularities and distortions of the vascular walls are observed as distensions with abnormal sinusoids, reflux produced by incompetent valves, and prolonged visualization of a dye in a main venous trunk. Occasionally, non-visualization of the femoral vein suggests blockage by a thrombus. All of the above abnormalities suggest the sequelae of phlebitis which has usually not been clinically obvious. It is, however, not uncommon to see significant intraosseous circulatory derangement with no abnormality in the extrinsic veins. We believe that this can be explained by blockage of the cortical foramina under the influence of medullary hypertension or by thrombosis of the periosteal veins as suggested by Burkhardt[80].

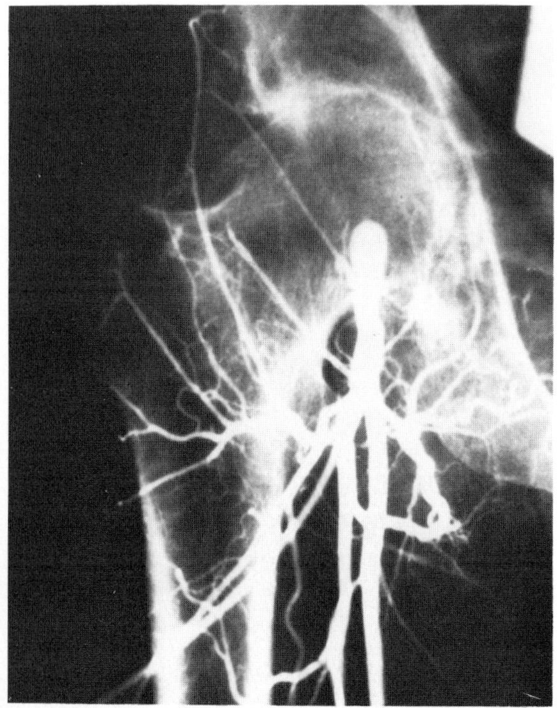

A: After a first injection, there is no visualization of the termination of the posterior circumflex in its retro-cervical segment. One could wrongly conclude that it was blocked.

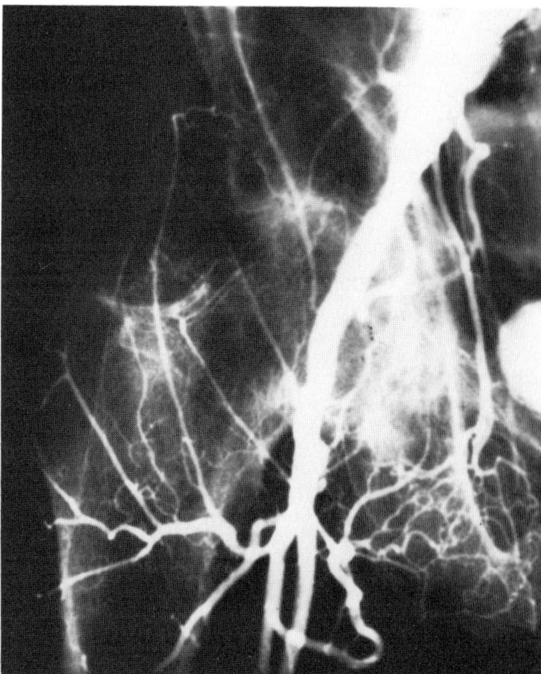

B: After a second injection, the posterior circumflex and its epiphyseal branches completely filled.

Fig.75.

Selective arteriography of the hip - The technique has been already reviewed, but it is important to remember that it is optimal to visualize both sides simultaneously, either by aortography so as to include the large pelvic vessels or bilateral femoral catheterization with retrograde injection. The opacification of the major proximal arterial trunks permits identification of lesions of either the vessel walls or areas of stenosis but sometimes even total obliteration. Diffuse narrowing of the entire arterial tree with poor filling of the secondary branches has been seen in four of our patients, suggesting the diagnosis of Buerger's Disease[464].

The second type of information, more specific but more difficult to obtain, is given by the filling of the epiphyseal-metaphyseal arteries of the femoral head, arising, as indicated in the chapter on normal exploration from four main pedicles: a.) the ischiatic artery perfusing the acetabulum and anastomosing in the back of the neck with the posterior circumflex artery, b.) the obturator artery and its acetabular branch, from which usually springs the artery of the ligamentum teres, c.) the inferior metaphyseal artery penetrating the inferior medial third of the femoral head, and d.) the superior epiphyseal pedicle, constituting the termination of the posterior circumflex artery through several branches.

The study of these vessels is difficult because of their small caliber, the natural density of the bone, and the lack of experience of most radiologists. Finally, technical deficiencies (insufficient injection rate or volume of the contrast medium) may be responsible for the lack of filling. Of course, it is essential to study all films or else a false conclusion of obliteration could be reached (Fig. 75). Our personal experience, based on about 30 cases, is still small, but we have been able to visualize, in some of these cases, unquestionable lesions of the posterior circumflex artery, contributing at least in part to the occurrence of ischemia and necrosis (Fig. 76 and 77).

Hipp[205] first used arteriography to confirm the role of traumatic rupture (or of compression followed by thrombosis) of the post-circumflex artery or of its branches in the occurrence of post-traumatic necrosis of the femoral head. Mussbichler[328] demonstrated obliteration of the posterior branch of the circumflex artery in one case and filling delay in 13 cases in a series of 21 instances of necrosis of the femoral head following femoral neck fracture. The visualization delay of the posterior circumflex in its retrocervical course was the most typical finding in this type of necrosis.

The role of arterial lesion in non-traumatic cases of osteonecrosis of the femoral head has not yet been

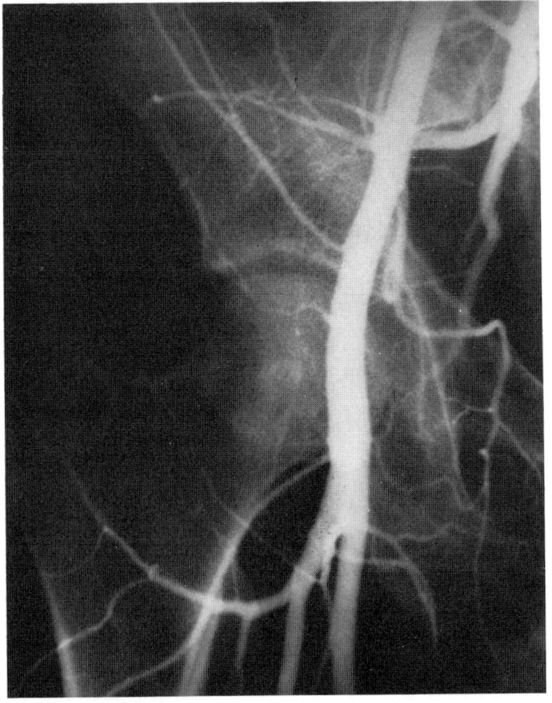

Fig.76.—Example of a thin posterior circumflex artery blocked at the level of the superior margin of the neck in a necrosis at Stage II-III.

conclusively demonstrated. Hipp[205] often found, in such cases, hypoplasia either of the posterior circumflex, of its epiphyseal branches, or of lesions of this artery with occasional evidence of a complete block. He does not hesitate to interpret these findings as confirming Chandler's concept of "coronary disease of the hip." Jung, Kehr, and Hamid[240] published similar observations in non-traumatic ischemic necrosis at each stage of the disease, including the preradiologic stage (Stage I with histologic confirmation). They have also demonstrated similar lesions in Perthes' Disease and in slipped capital femoral epiphysis. It must be remembered that arteriography demonstrates flow. Diminution in flow could result from obstruction further down the vascular tree. Therefore, non-visualization of a given artery does not necessarily indicate that the lesion lies within the artery itself. The classic example of this is non-visualization of the anterior tibial artery in the anterior compartment syndrome. Decompression of the compartment immediately results in visualization of the artery. We believe that there are, unquestionably, some necroses which result from circumflex artery lesions. However, the overall importance of this lesion for the general field of necrosis of the femoral head remains to be determined.

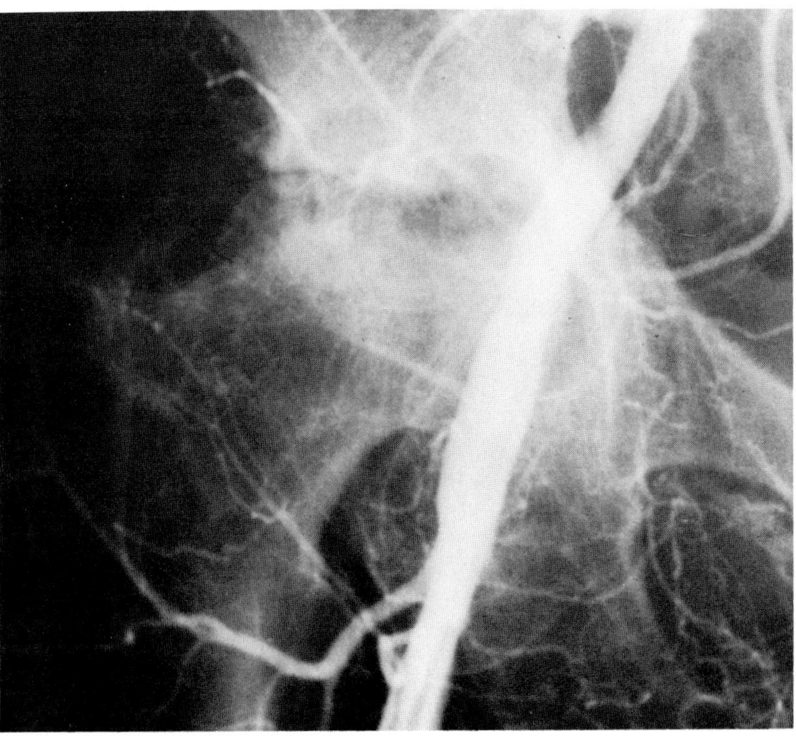

Fig.77.—Example of thin and irregular posterior circumflex in the upper third of its retro-cervical course in a necrosis at Stage IV. Patient has atherosclerosis.

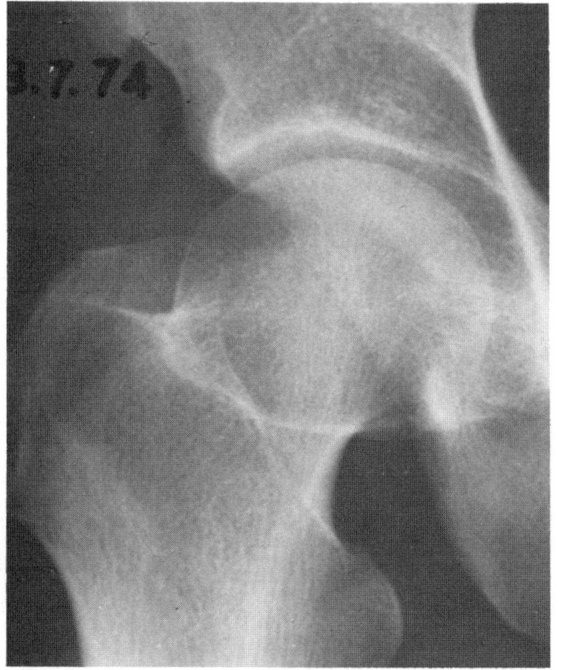
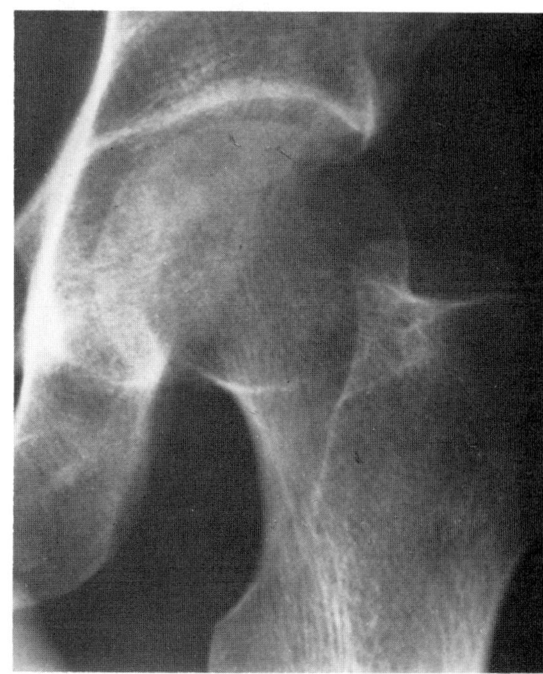

Fig.78.—Osteoporotic type of left hip necrosis diagnosed by biopsy, showing increased uptake of Technetium99m-labeled pyrophosphate in the left hip.

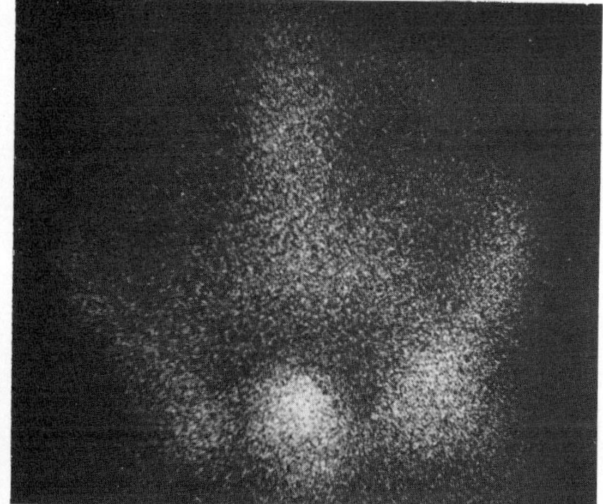

RADIOISOTOPIC SIGNS

Since Bauer's pioneering work[41] using radio-isotope scintimetry, many authors have used this as a method in diagnosing bone necrosis[182,192,270]. Gilet et al.[182] used Strontium[87] in 20 patients presenting with clinical signs compatible with osteonecrosis but with no x-ray changes. The patients were followed up for at least six months. The 13 patients who demonstrated increased uptake of the radionuclide underwent radiologic changes which confirmed the necrosis in all cases. The seven patients who did not show increased uptake neither persisted in symptoms nor had x-ray changes. In our own experience[192], 11 patients suspected of osteonecrosis of the femoral head in the preradiologic stage had core biopsy carried out after initially positive bone scans. Bone marrow necrosis was confirmed in 10 of the 11 cases (Fig. 78). In the eleventh case, the bone lesions were compatible with the diagnosis of reflex sympathetic dystrophy. When radiologic lesions were advanced, increased uptake was always marked. However, as Bauer has shown (Fig. 79), such increased uptake can be shown in osteoarthrosis and in inflammatory hip disease. Increased uptake, then, is nonspecific. Nonetheless, Crutchlow[104], using Strontium[85] in 189 hips (105 patients with 75 arthroses and 48 typical necroses radiologically), commented that Stage IV osteonecroses characteristically showed greater uptake than arthrosis. He concluded that these findings allowed one to differentiate between the end stages of osteoarthrosis which were apparently "primary" and those which were secondary to necrosis. The greatest value of the increased radionuclide uptake in ischemic bone is in the setting of a painful hip with limited movement but normal x-rays. Gaucher et al.[178] have confirmed this in a recent study of bone necrosis in patients with renal transplants.

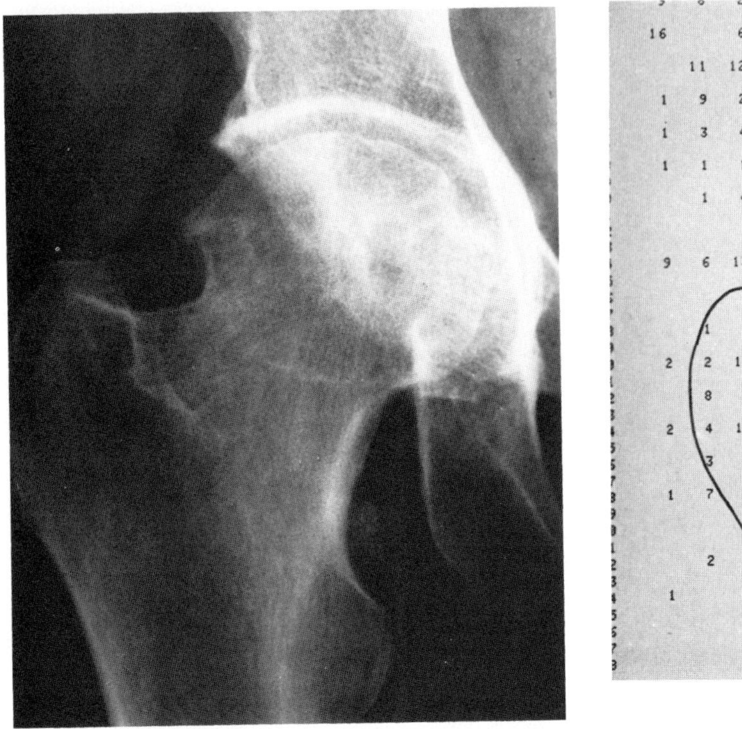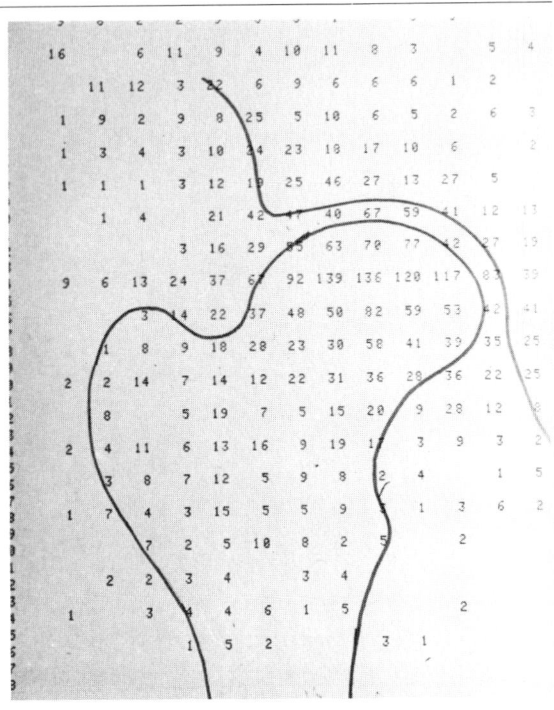

Fig. 79.—Scintimetry with Strontium [85m] (G. Bauer's technique) in a Stage III necrosis. Notice the regional diffuse character of the increased uptake (film given by Professor G. Bauer).

HISTOPATHOLOGICAL SIGNS

EXPERIMENTAL BACKGROUND

The experimental work of Rutishauser et al.[378] has greatly contributed to the recognition of the spectrum of histologic changes associated with bone and bone marrow ischemia. A summary of his findings will serve as a backdrop for our experience with the tissue removed at core biopsy from patients with non-traumatic bone necrosis (Fig. 80). Although there are numerous histopathologic studies on human femoral head necrosis, these are virtually all concerned with advanced cases of necrosis with the femoral heads being taken at arthroplasty. Although these specimens are interesting for comparison with the radiologic and hemodynamic signs of Stage III of the disease, they are too advanced to be of any help in understanding the early pathophysiology.

Rutishauser, Rohner, and Held[378] produced both arteriolar- and venous-initiated ischemia in an experimental model. The arteriolar ischemia was produced by injecting carbon particles of approximately 30 microns in diameter into the nutrient artery of the rabbit femur. The particles produced obliteration of the precapillary arterioles. Post-capillary obstruction was accomplished by injection of thrombin into the

bone marrow itself. The lesions observed were identical in both types of ischemia. It is interesting to note that both types of ischemia produced reversible histologic lesions, although the bone required longer to recover from the venous thrombosis type of ischemia. By comprehensive examination of the tissue, the authors were able to rank histologic findings with degree of ischemia. The first change described was labeled as plasmostasis. An eosinophilic material was evident between the bone marrow cells. The authors felt that this was plasma within the interstitial sinusoids. It would, however, be difficult to distinguish this from interstitial extravascular edema. The first cellular evidence of ischemia is the disappearance of hematopoietic tissue which requires high oxygen saturation levels in order to proliferate. Reticular proliferation is also an early event. The interstitial spaces fill with reticulum cells and collagen fibers. A loose, fibrous tissue appears similar to that occurring in other areas of the body under circumstances of chronic edema. The lipocytes first show atrophy, then disappearance of nuclei and cell walls, and finally breakdown of the cytoplasm. This fat necrosis leads to phagocytosis of the debris by mononuclear macrophages or foam cells. Trabecular necrosis is the last event preceded by osteo-

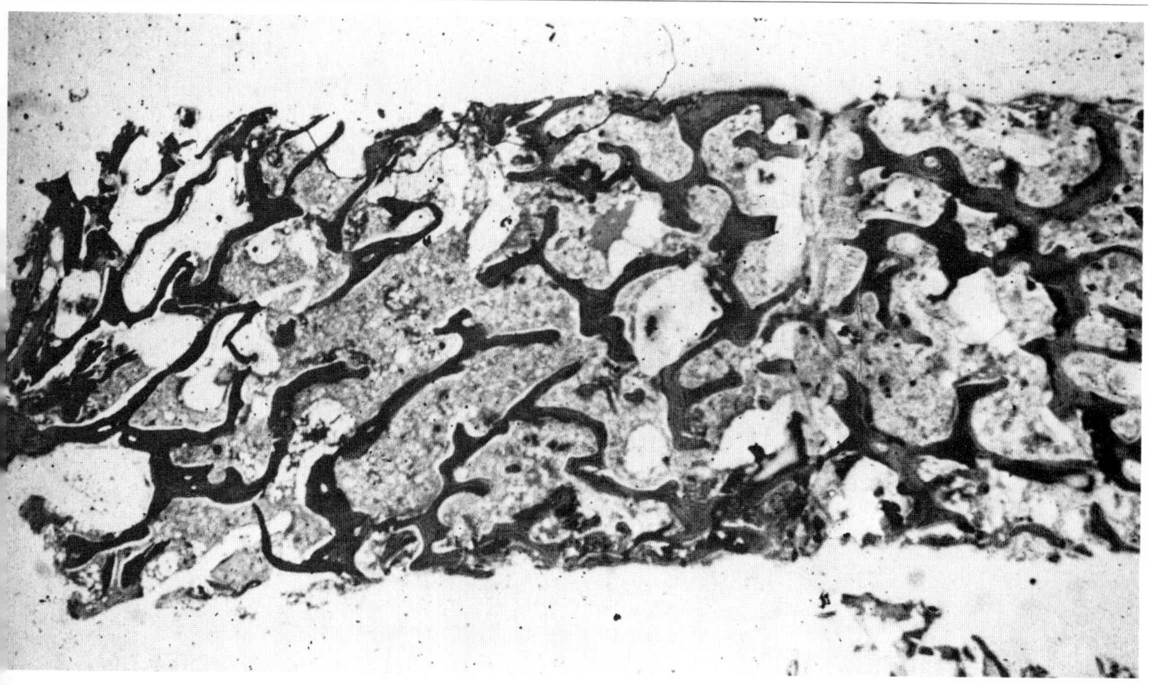

Fig. 80.—Photomicrograph of the core specimen from a patient with cortisone-induced necrosis. The eosinophilic reticular medullary necrosis is already quite visible in most of the bone marrow spaces.

ytic osteolysis. Finally, the nuclei show pyknosis and then disappear. Bone turnover occurs early in the ischemia with histologic evidence of increased osteoblastic and osteoclastic activity. The trabeculae frequently show increased thickness and increased numbers of cement lines, explaining the radiologic appearance of increased radiodensity. In the same specimen, one can see normal looking trabeculae and other areas showing bone marrow and/or bone trabecular necrosis. Rutishauser believes that the histologic lesion observed is dependent both on the degree of ischemia and on the reaction of the tissue to the unfavorable circulatory environment. Evidence of repair may be slight or complete with partial fatty or fibrous tissue replacement of the hematopoietic tissue. Necrotic lesions in this model could be observed up to five months after the precipitating episode.

HUMAN BIOPSY MATERIAL

Our data consists of over 200 specimens taken at the time of core decompression [9,17,22]. We have many cases of advanced necrosis at the Stage III level, but the most interesting specimens come from radiologically intact femoral heads. These 80 cases have allowed us to define the preradiologic stage (Stage I) of bone necrosis.

Bone Marrow Lesions In Stage I And II

Prenecrotic vascular changes - These involve, primarily, ischemic or prenecrotic "vascular" abnormalities. The cellular elements are separated by lightly colored, gray-blue (H & E stain) amorphous material adapted to the bone marrow cell outline. Rutishauser[378] believed this to be the blood plasma in the sinusoidal network, although it would be difficult to differentiate this from an extrasinusoidal exudate (Fig. 81). Another finding at this same stage is sinusoidal congestion or interstitial hemorrhage. The lipocytes are separated by an accumulation of red blood cells which form a network limited by the lipocytes themselves (Fig. 82). Normally, the morphology of the red cells is easily distinguished. Occasionally the outlines are indistinct, and there are some signs of old hemorrhage with red cell necrosis and hemosiderin pigment. There may be some reticular or mesenchymal proliferation with mesenchymal cells and reticular fibers appearing in areas of interstitial edema. Later, the fibers become more numerous and the cells take on a fibroblastic appearance, resembling young "edematous" fibrous tissue[402] (Fig. 83).

Necrosis of the fatty marrow - Much as in Rutishauser's model, the nuclei of the lipocytes disappear. Since these nuclei are generally at the

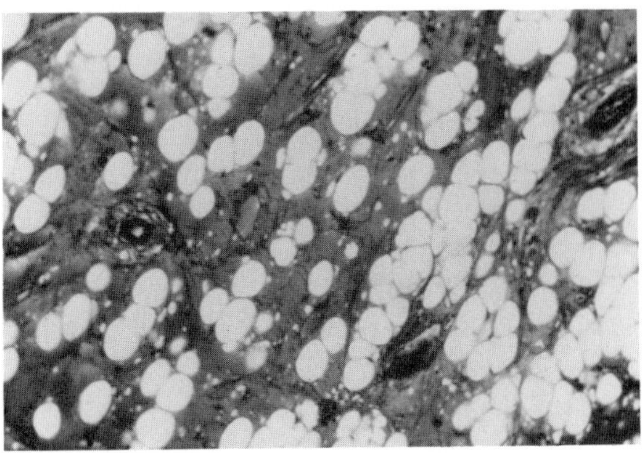

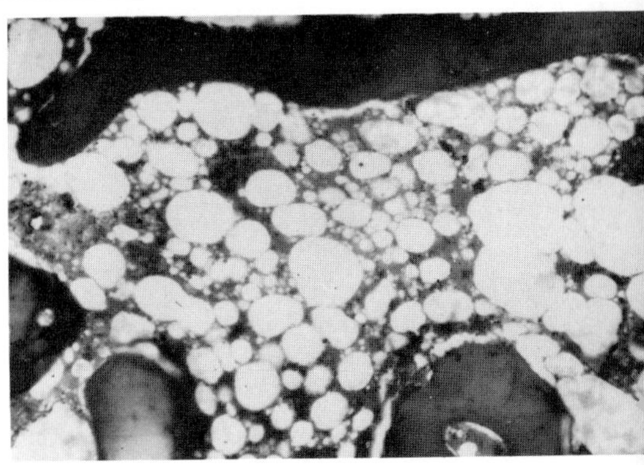

A: Area of stasis separating the lipocytes on the right side of the marrow space.

B: Separation of the lipocytes.

Fig.81.

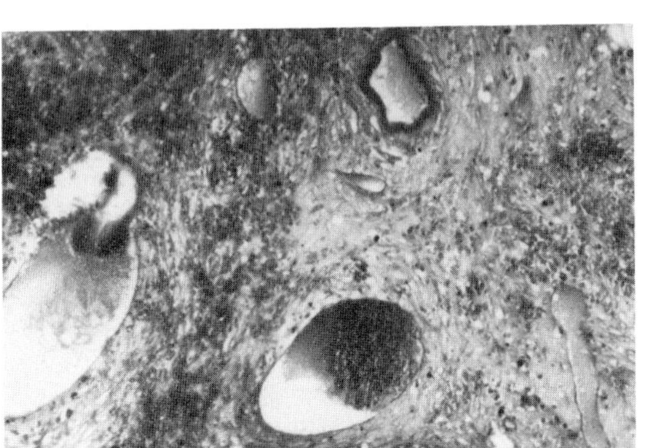

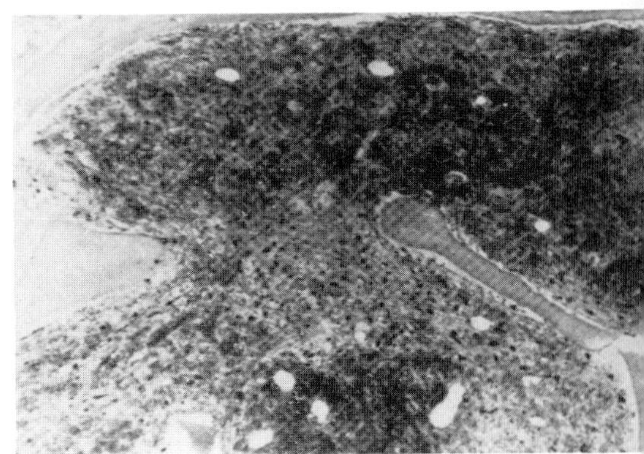

Fig.82.—Multiple hemorrhagic foci infiltrating the bone marrow.

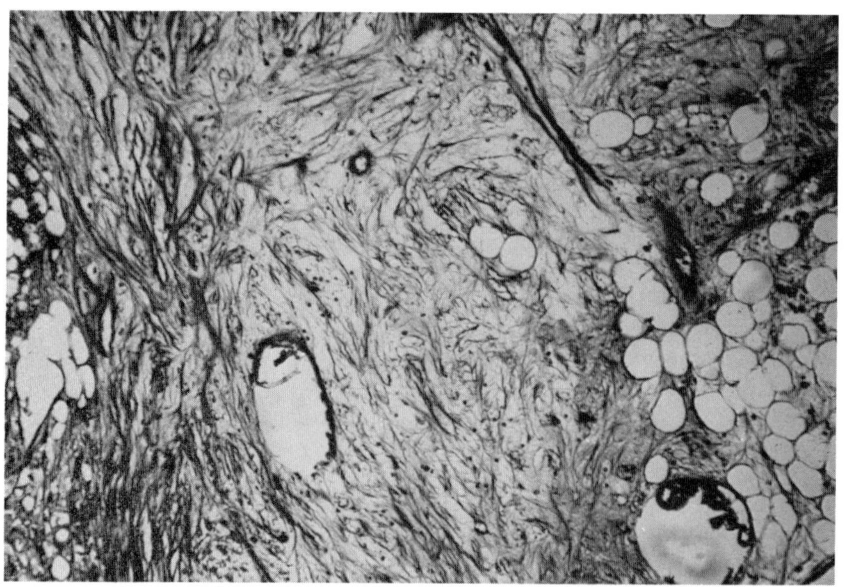

Fig.83.—Reticular p⟩liferation.

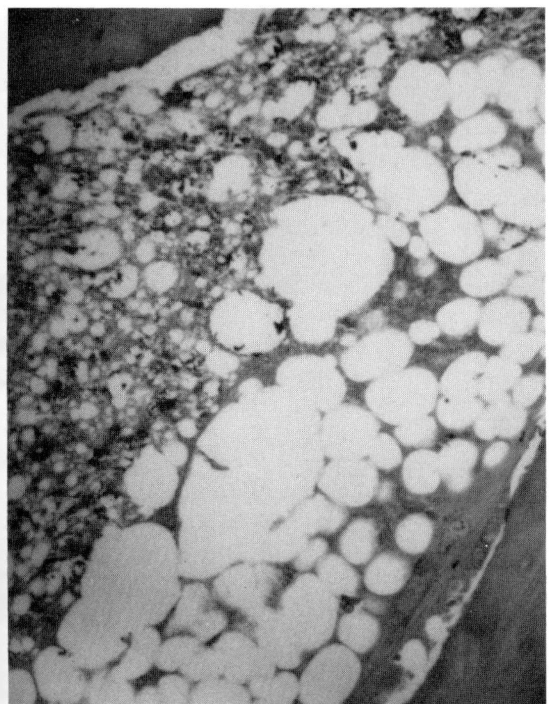

A: The left half of the medullary space is filled by an area of eosinophilic reticular necrosis.

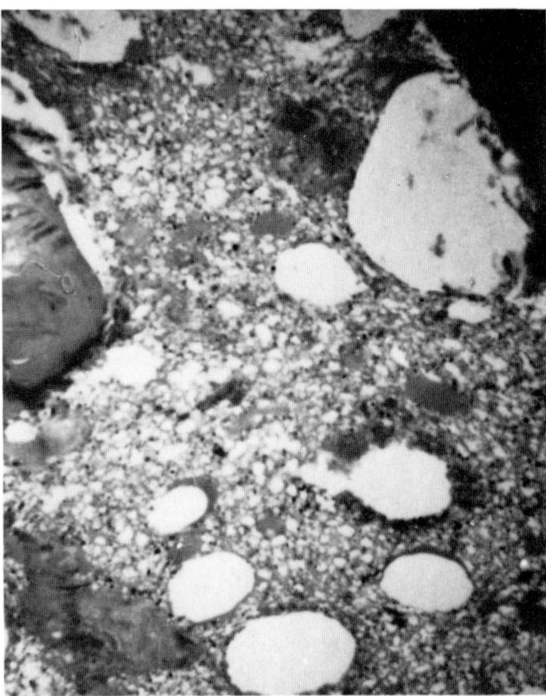

B: The diffuse eosinophilic reticular necrosis.

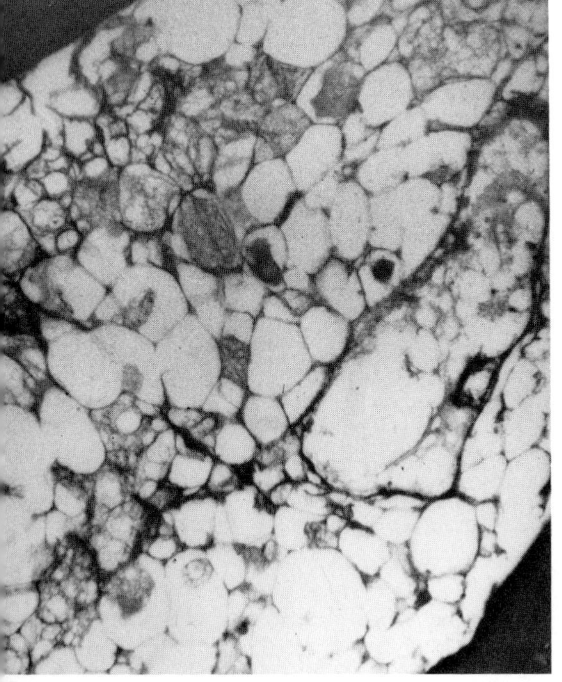

C: Foci of eosinophilic reticular necrosis in a case of cortisone-induced necrosis.

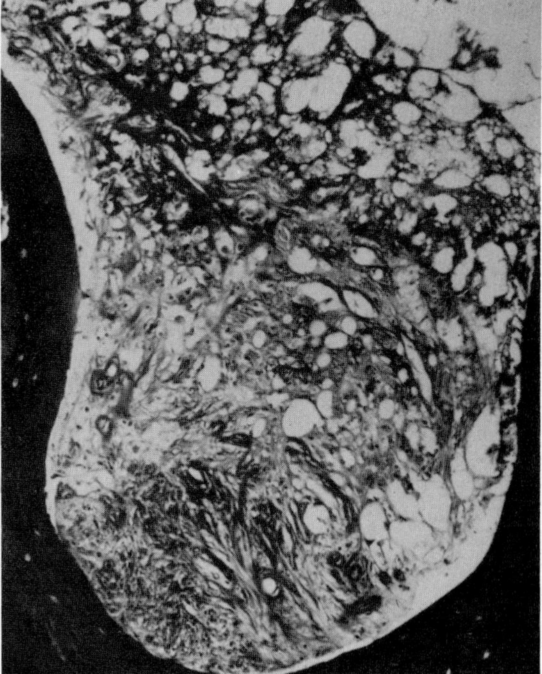

D: In the upper part, eosinophilic reticular necrosis with thick walls. In the lower part, medullary fibrosis (patient with gout and INFH).

Fig.84.

periphery of the cell and are not always well visualized, their absence as the singular, cellular sign cannot be used for establishment of the diagnosis. However, at a more advanced stage, the lipocytes rupture, and evidence of phagocytosis of the lipid debris is evident. Simple rupture of the thin cellular walls of the lipocytes alone may be an artifact of the processing of the specimens. However, fragmentation of the lipocytes associated with an acidophilic fibrinoid network is a very frequent finding associated with necrosis (Fig. 84). We proposed the term of eosinophilic reticular necrosis of the fatty marrow. The lipocytes are no longer true cells but only fragments of lipid droplets within the macrophages. These foam cells are round or polyhedral with small, dark, homogenous nuclei centrally located in a lightly stained, granular cytoplasm. These are usually grouped in clusters. Similar histologic findings are often found in steatonecrosis (Fig. 85). Another finding affecting the fatty marrow is the rupture of lipocytes producing large, empty, round cavities on the standard sections. These cavities, however, are well outlined by a thin wall and occasionally have a ring of histiocytes justifying the interpretation of liquefaction necrosis. Mazabraud[305] has also confirmed these findings in the early lesions of osteonecrosis.

Necrosis of the hematopoietic marrow - This is less frequently seen in our biopsy specimens because the hematopoietic tissue is not particularly abundant either in the regions biopsied or at the age of our patients. It is also possible that the ischemia first induces arrest of myelocytic proliferation and a simple disappearance of the hematopoietic tissue. However, necrosis of the hematopoietic tissue is sometimes observed, giving a much denser appearance than the fatty marrow necrosis. This can be recognized by an array of a variety of cellular structures with blurred cellular outlines and pyknotic, fragmented nuclei. This gives a more homogeneous appearance which is predominantly acidophilic. A second aspect of red marrow necrosis presents with cellular structures that can no longer be recognized, showing granular acidophilic nuclei with a thinner basophilic debris. We have labeled this granular necrosis. Finally, a more advanced form consists of a dense accumulation of acidophilic material in which fragments of collagen fibers can be recognized. It is difficult to tell whether this represents necrotic hematopoietic tissue or reactive connective tissue which has also necrosed because of persistance or worsening of the ischemia (Fig. 86).

Evidence of post-necrotic marrow regeneration - Complete regeneration of bone marrow tissue after

necrosis seems to be a possibility in the animal. Perhaps this is also true in man although, to our knowledge, it has never been documented. On the other hand, one often sees ischemic areas side-by-side with necrotic foci, areas of fibrous or fibrovascular proliferation with areas of bone formation. This "replacement" fibrosis is often quite dense, rich in fibers and poor in cells. Sherman[402] called it "inactive dense fibrosis." It more or less fills the marrow spaces and is often adjacent to an area of marrow necrosis (Fig. 87). It is not known whether this fibrosis is an intermediate stage between the necrosis and regeneration or whether it does indeed constitute a definitive scar which is inactive and incapable of being replaced by normal marrow tissue. Although marrow fibrosis is often seen in both ischemic and necrotic bone, it is neither constant nor characteristic. These are very common lesions which are seen in almost all pathologic bone conditions, for example, around metastatic foci.

Vascular lesions of bone marrow - These have not been properly evaluated by the histopathologist for several reasons. They are often preoccupied with the mineralized tissue. Also, the quality of the marrow tissue in the slides is often poor, making interpretation difficult. However, sinusoidal distension, thickening of the arteriolar walls, and arteriolar thrombosis are frequently observed (Fig. 87B). A microangiographic study in ischemia of the femoral head has been done by Collard and Collard[95], showed important atherosclerotic lesions predominantly in the posterior circumflex artery with changes in the appearance of the intraosseous branches of that artery.

Trabecular Lesions In Stage I And II

These lesions are neither as obvious nor as frequently observed as marrow lesions. Total necrosis is rarely seen in all of the trabeculae within the biopsy specimen. Usually only some trabeculae show evidence of bone death, and the bone and bone marrow lesions are usually contiguous (Fig. 88). The most obvious sign of trabecular death is the presence of empty lacunae, i.e., the disappearance of the nuclei. When all of the lacunae are empty, the necrosis is apparent. These dead trabeculae show fissures which develop selectively along cement lines. The trabeculae which appear necrotic as such seem to fragment more easily at the time of sectioning. This phenomenon is associated, in our experience, with advanced trabecular necrosis, suggesting that they are secondary to the necrosis, not pre-existing the necrosis, and a cause of the necrosis as has been suggested by some. Occasionally, completely necrotic trabeculae show notches which probably represent resorption lacunae but in which no osteoclasts are

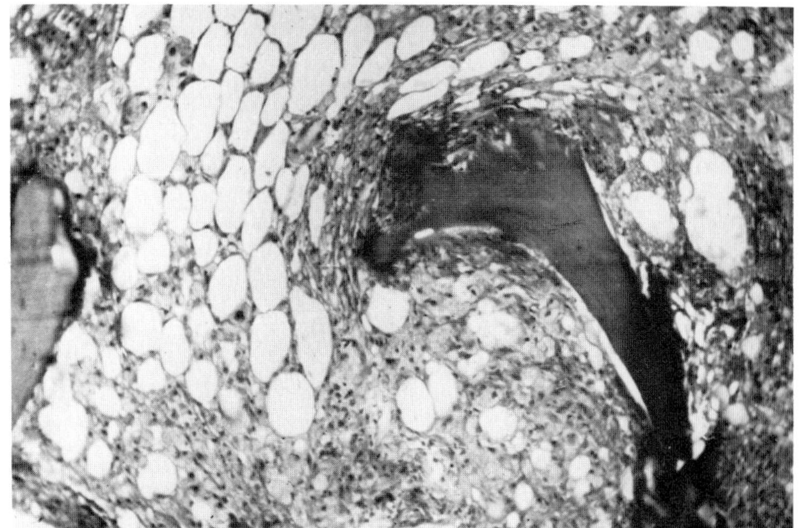

Fig.85.—Foci of foam cells or lipophages (fat necrosis).

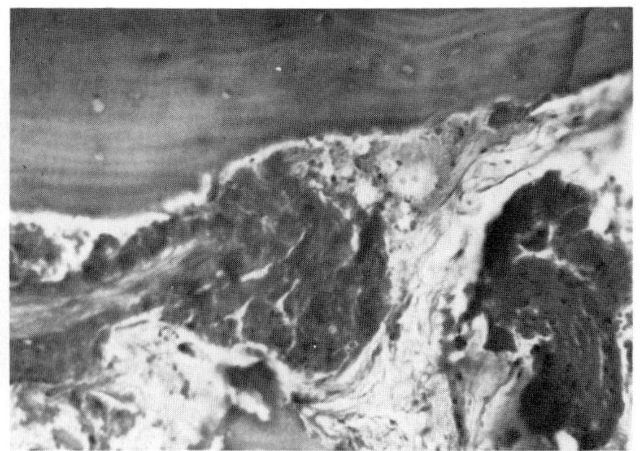

Fig.86.—Granular necrosis in clumps.

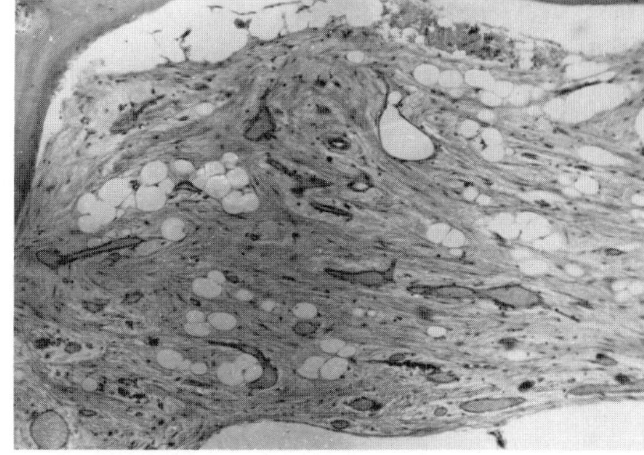

Fig.87a.—Fairly dense medullary fibrosis.

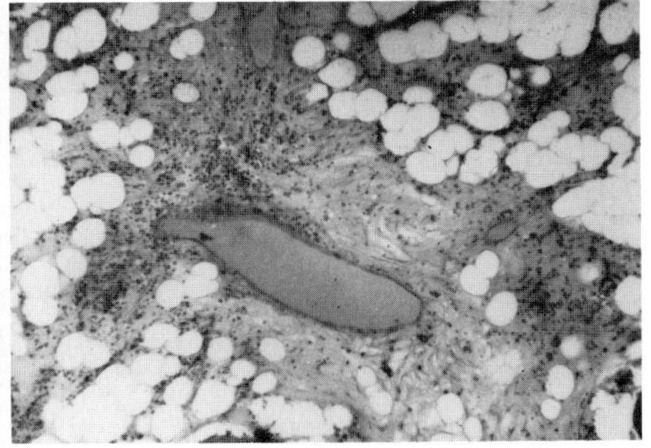

A: Sinusoid distension.

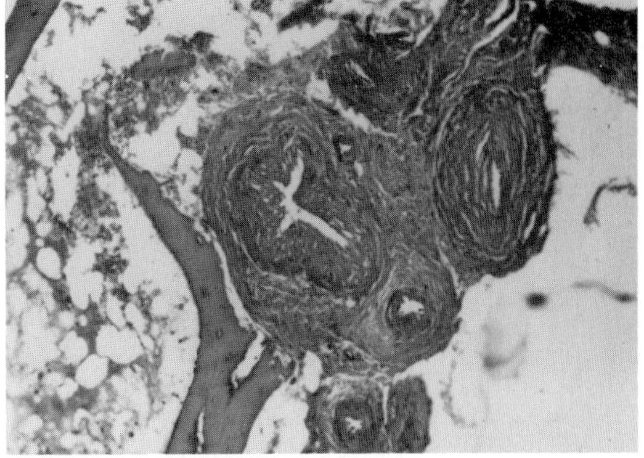

B: Arteriolar wall thickening.

Fig.87b.

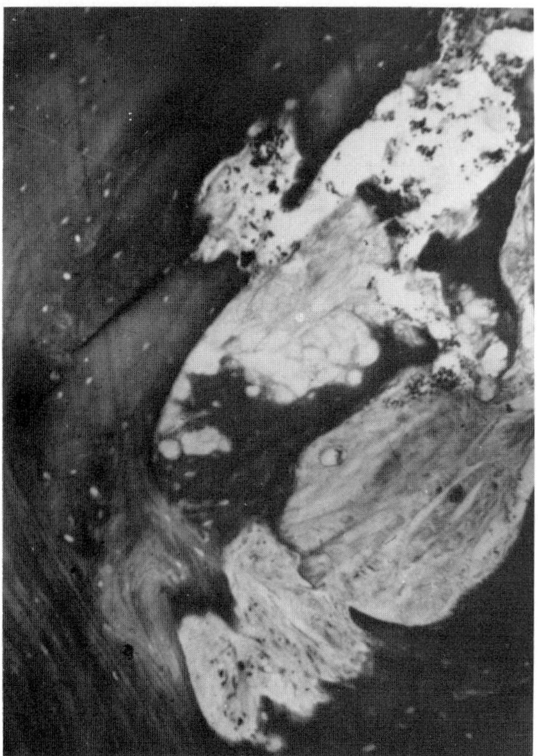

A: Total necrosis of the bone trabeculae, even those more recently formed, with foci of osteoclasts.

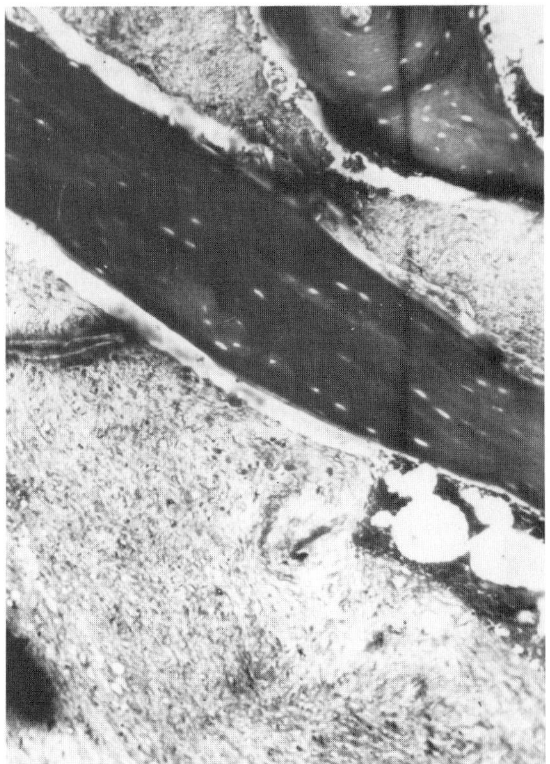

B: Usual aspect of a complete necrosis of the cancellous trabeculae in a case of necrosis at Stage I.

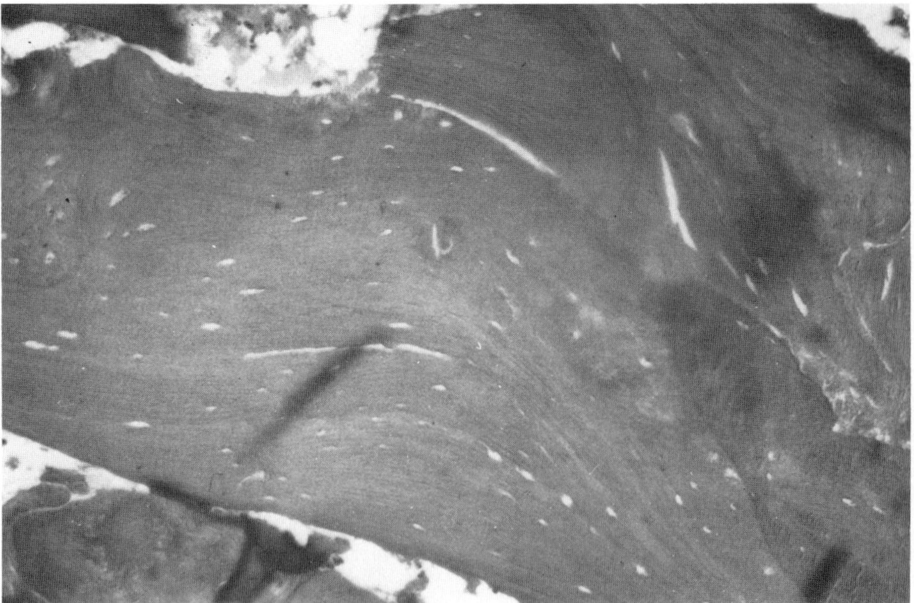

C: Total necrosis.

Fig. 88.

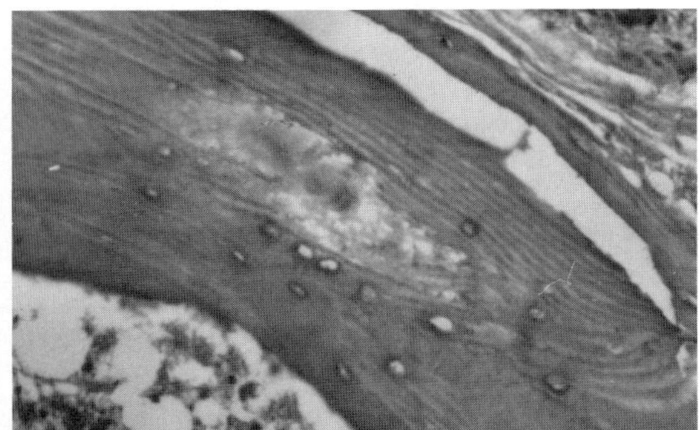

Fig.89.—Enlargement of the lacunae (osteocytic osteolysis).

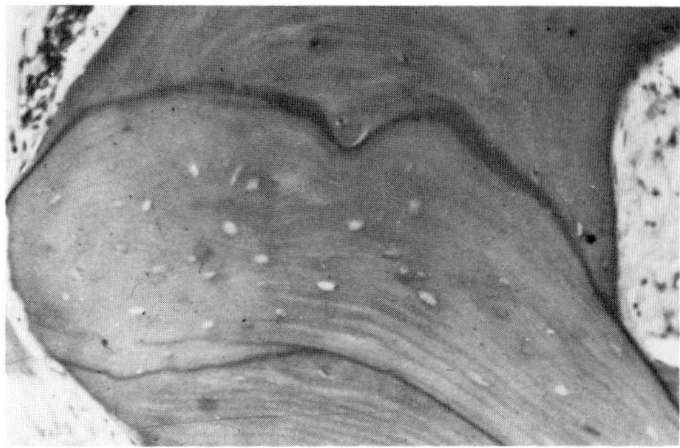

A: Total necrosis of an old trabecula between two living trabeculae.

seen. It is probable that partial or complete resorption of dead trabeculae can occur, and focal areas of decreased bone density are frequently evident. However, it is also probably true that the mechanism for resorption is not by normal physiologic osteoclastic resorption, a fact which has already been suggested by Coutelier[102].

Partial trabecular necrosis is more difficult to diagnose on standard H & E preparations. The only sign is emptiness of some of the lacunae. As is well known, completely normal trabeculae may have some empty lacunae. Here, it is a question of quantity. We consider that a trabecula is necrotic when the number of empty lacunae reaches at least 50%. In fact, one should study osteocyte viability, since a dead cell may be present in the lacuna and give the appearance of viability.

According to Duriez and Cauchoix[129], the slow death of an osteocyte may be characterized by enlargement of the lacuna through periosteocytic osteolysis (Fig. 89). However, this phenomenon is characteristic of not only osteocytic death, being an important and usual sign in hyperparathyroidism. Jowsey has also observed this in biopsies of normal subjects[236]. Laurent[267] did not observe these changes in the seven cases of necrosis he studied.

Bone reconstruction is frequently observed on the surface of dead trabeculae which frequently become surrounded by the new bone. The presence of an osteoid seam with large numbers of osteoblasts, irregularly distributed on a clearly dead trabecula, is a very interesting observation which emphasizes the reaction of bone tissue stressed by chronic but incomplete ischemia, probably changing both in time and in space (Fig. 90). It is difficult to accommodate this data within the concept of creeping substitution, since one commonly sees successive layers of bone being laid down on the trabeculae with the newer layers also dying. In any case, it is not known if this

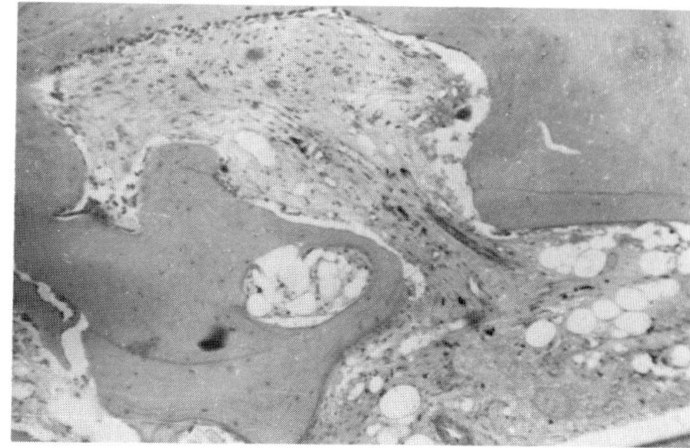

B: Reconstruction process with increased osteoblast activity.

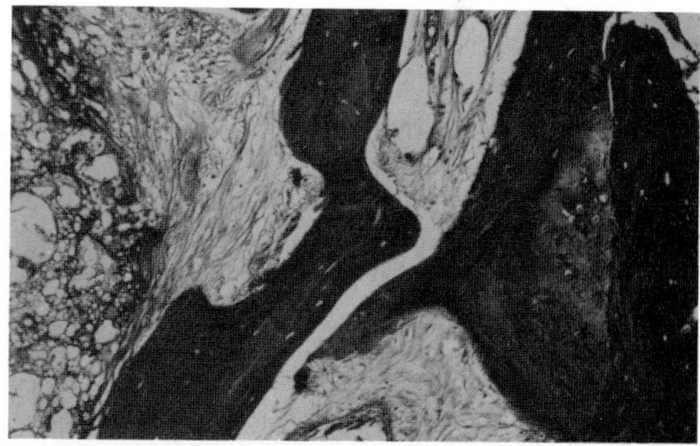

C: Typical example of the classic necrosis. From left to right can be seen:
-an area of eosinophilic reticular necrosis.
-an area of fibrosis.
-a dead bone trabecula.
-and a newly formed trabecula next to a dead one.

Fig.90.

type of necrosis may heal by total resorption of the dead trabecula and replacement by new, live trabeculae.

Advanced Lesions In Stage III And IV

Our experiences are based on both core biopsy specimens and complete femoral heads removed at the time of hip arthroplasty (Fig. 91). The description of Merle D'Aubigné, Mazabraud, and Cahen[309] is an excellent one which we will summarize in part although our experience differs in one point — the status of the cancellous bone underneath the osteosclerotic area. The radiologic picture, which is quite typical of the collapsed sequestrum, has three distinct segments as viewed from top to bottom. Superiorly, the articular cartilage with a small portion of subchondral bone is separated from the rest of the femoral head and overlies a segment which is impacting into the remainder of the head. Beneath this is a zone of variable radiodensity which is collapsing into the head. Inferiorly, this sequestrum is separated by a dense sclerotic margin which is generally in the form of an arc, concave superiorly. The surgeon removing such a femoral head can easily demonstrate the collapse of the weight-bearing zone, generally forming a circular area on the anterolateral segment of the head and in which the articular cartilage can be manually depressed. The cartilage itself, overlying this area, is generally without sheen and slightly discolored.

On a coronal section, the articular cartilage and the thin layer of dense subchondral bone firmly adherent to it are typical of the advanced cases. The subchondral bone is separated from the underlying, supporting cancellous bone by a fracture line. This explains the mobility of the osteocartilaginous cover which is easy to remove from the remainder of the sequestrum. The quality and viability of this cartilage are variable. Sometimes it is thick, apparently normal cartilage while at other times the surface is replaced with a layer of fibrous tissue, and the chondrocytes are more or less altered. Chondrocyte abnormalities are even more obvious in electron microscopic studies (Fig. 100). Cartilage lesions of the arthrosic type can also be seen as reported by Laurent[267].

The sequestrum itself, that is the zone of cancellous bone underlying the separated articular cartilage, is completely dead. The trabeculae, however, are of irregular thickness, indicating that significant changes had taken place preceding death. They are totally devoid of osteocytes and are sometimes fractured. The marrow spaces are filled with necrotic debris in which no cellular structure can be recognized (Fig. 91).

The living base of the sequestrum is generally formed by two superimposed areas, one mainly fibrous and the other mainly osseous. The fibrous

Fig.91.—Photomicrograph of a femoral head necrosis at Stage III. Notice:
-the subchondral defect,
-the dense triangular sequestrum,
-the sclerotic osseous border and the subjacent medullary lesions.

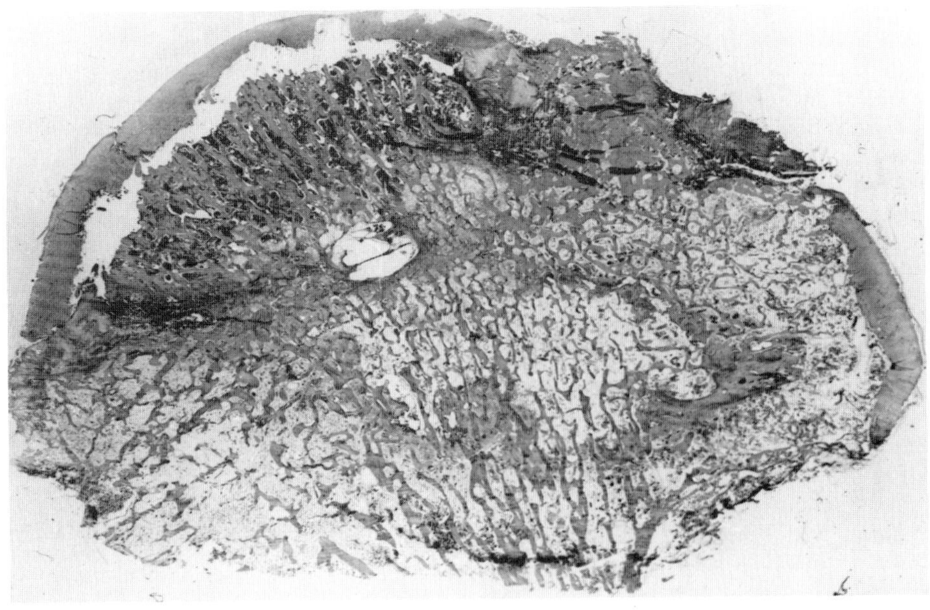

area is often rich in vessels and may show cartilage metaplasia. The bony layer consists of thick, osteosclerotic, irregular trabeculae with superficial layers all showing signs of viability and the recent new bone formation, while the deeper zones are sometimes dead. The marrow spaces are filled with connective, vascular tissue. Osteoblasts and osteoclasts are abundant. The borders of the sequestrum are not always clearly demarcated. The fibrous area may be incomplete, with living trabeculae of the bony base being in continuity with the dead of the sequestrum. Beneath the demarcation of the sequestrum in the lower part of the femoral head and upper femoral neck, we have observed, in many cases, both marrow and trabecular lesions that give evidence of widespread circulatory problems. The fatty marrow is partially atrophied and in a state of eosinophilic reticular necrosis. Reticular fibrosis and interstitial edema are often seen in adjacent areas. The trabeculae are thin and irregular (Fig. 92). These observations agree with those of Jacqueline and Rutishauser[221].

Classification And Evolution Of The Histologic Lesions

It is obviously not possible to observe in man the evolution of bone lesions of ischemic origin, such as one can do in the rabbit. Moreover, human pathology is much more complex than those of the experimental ischemia, particularly because one is usually dealing with chronic incomplete ischemia in which truly ischemic lesions, secondary reactive lesions, and reconstruction phenomenon may be both sequential and simultaneous, depending upon time and area. Through our experience with core biopsies, we have learned that these lesions may be quite different from one area to another within the specimen. However, this has not always been true, and, in the majority of cases, there was a type of lesion which was quite uniform throughout the whole biopsy specimen. We have proposed a classification of four types of histologic change which are summarized in Table X[22,130].

In Type 1, the predominant lesions are clearly prenecrotic and confined to bone marrow, although, occasionally, one sees both foam cells and small areas of eosinophilic reticular necrosis of the fatty marrow. The most common lesion is the interstitial edema or plasmostasis, according to Rutishauser[378]. In Type 2, the most characteristic finding in our preradiologic cases is that all the medullary spaces are filled with necrotic tissue, resulting in eosi-

TABLE X

HISTOPATHOLOGIC LESIONS IN INFH

Type	Bone Marrow Lesions	Trabecular Lesions
1	Plasmostasis, reticular proliferation, hemorrhage, accumulation of foam cells	0
2	Necrosis of fatty marrow	0
3	Medullary necrosis	necrosis
4	Necrosis and fibrosis	necrosis and reconsitution

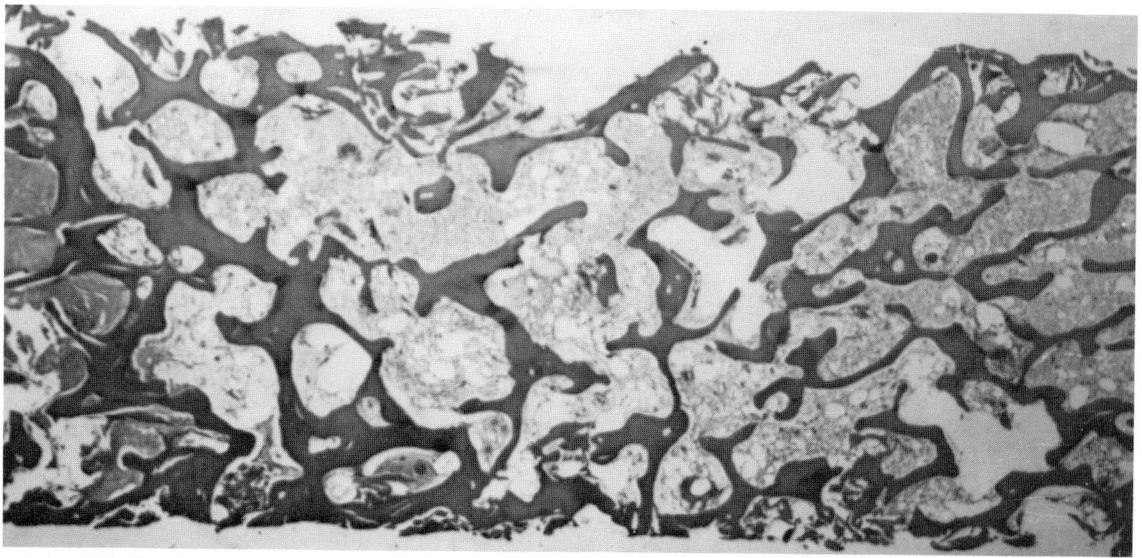

Fig.92.—Photomicrograph of a core specimen from a necrosis in Stage III, demonstrating to the left, the base of the sequestrum and underneath of the head and within the neck, a diffuse eosinophilic reticular necrosis with thin trabeculae.

nophilic reticular necrosis extending one to several centimeters in the specimens. In Type 3, the marrow necrosis is associated with clear trabecular necrosis with 50 to 100% of the lacunae empty. In Type 4, the preceding lesions also exist but foci of marrow fibrosis are encountered, and the dead trabeculae are increased in number and surrounded by living, newly formed bone.

This classification is morphological. It is tempting to give it significance in terms of evolution and to think that in ischemic necrosis of the femoral head, the lesions start by Type 1, go progressively to Type 2 and 3, and finally reach Type 4. It is probable that such an evolution exists, but we have not been able either to prove it or to confirm that this is always the case. It is possible that the eosinophilic reticular necrosis may be present from the beginning and in some cases that trabecular necrosis is simultaneous with medullary necrosis. It is even possible that osteogenesis occurs very early and constitutes an immediate reaction to a certain degree of ischemia. Since there may be a great variety both in the degree of initial ischemia and in the degree of progression, a wide variety of lesions may be seen. On all of these points, further experience is needed.

In spite of this uncertainty, there are certain facts that can be confirmed by this experience. Firstly, all types of lesions can be encountered in the same specimen. In the same biopsy, one can see areas of interstitial edema, hemorrhagic foci, areas of eosinophilic reticular necrosis, dead bone trabeculae, marrow fibrosis, and signs of reconstitution. Secondly, in the preradiologic stage of necrosis, although the predominant lesion is usually eosinophilic reticular necrosis of the marrow with or without trabecular necrosis (Type 2 or Type 3), it is not unusual to also observe, on the surface of some of the trabeculae, signs of bone reconstruction which are not radiologically evident. Finally, at all radiologic stages, necrotic lesions in the inferior part of the femoral head and neck are observed. This is particularly true at Stage III under the dense arcuate base of the sequestrum (Fig. 92). These three items are vitally important since they are not compatible with certain theories claiming that the necrosis is limited to a terminal arterial territory or to the femoral head itself. Furthermore, the findings are not compatible with the concept that the necrosis is the product of a sudden interruption of arterial flow in a given territory. These histopathological findings must be reconciled with any proposed pathogenesis. They can only be understood within the framework of a chronic and widespread ischemia. Moreover, this concept is not foreign since it is well known in two conditions with well-established etiologies caus-ing the necrosis, namely caisson disease, and the necrosis associated with sickle-cell disease.

It is true that in these conditions it is difficult to understand how a segment of the necrosis, that is the sequestrum itself, separates from the rest of the femoral head. However, sequestrum formation is a terminal event which unfortunately seems to be irreversible. The semiterminal type of distal circulation of the superior pole of the head may be a factor, as well as the effect of mechanical loading of the hip (maximal weight-bearing area). In this instance, one might compare the sequestrum formation with the dry and clearly delineated gangrene of the toes in arterial insufficiency of the lower extremities, where the femoral block is often present with reduction of the blood flow, not only to the toes, but to the whole leg.

METABOLIC SIGNS

OXYMETRY

Bone ischemia and its effect on the tissue impose changes in the composition of the blood within the bone. Besides the abnormal quantitative change (reduction of flow) that defines ischemia, one should look for qualitative changes of bone blood that are either causes or effects of the bone lesions. For instance, it can be argued that ischemia may directly be measured by the oxygen pressure in bone or that stasis, usually associated with ischemia, brings about changes in oxygen consumption or in the abnormal accummulation of CO_2. These are the reasons which prompted us to study blood gases in bone necrosis[23,166,352].

The technique has been reviewed in Chapter III. Femoral vein and femoral artery blood was always sampled simultaneously. Oxymetry has been carried out in 55 hips, 37 cases of INFH or ischemic coxopathy, and 18 cases of osteoarthrosis. Of the 37 cases of necrosis, 18 were confirmed histologically. Of the 19 non-operated cases, eight were radiographically typical (Stage III), and 11 were radiographically probable. The blood was taken from the intertrochanteric region in all cases. The intraosseous blood was slightly more acidic than the venous blood and considerably more than the arterial blood. Partial pressure of CO_2 was slightly higher in trochanteric than in arterial blood while the oxygen saturation was always higher in the trochanter than in the venous blood, sometimes reaching values near the oxygen saturation of the arterial blood (Fig. 93).

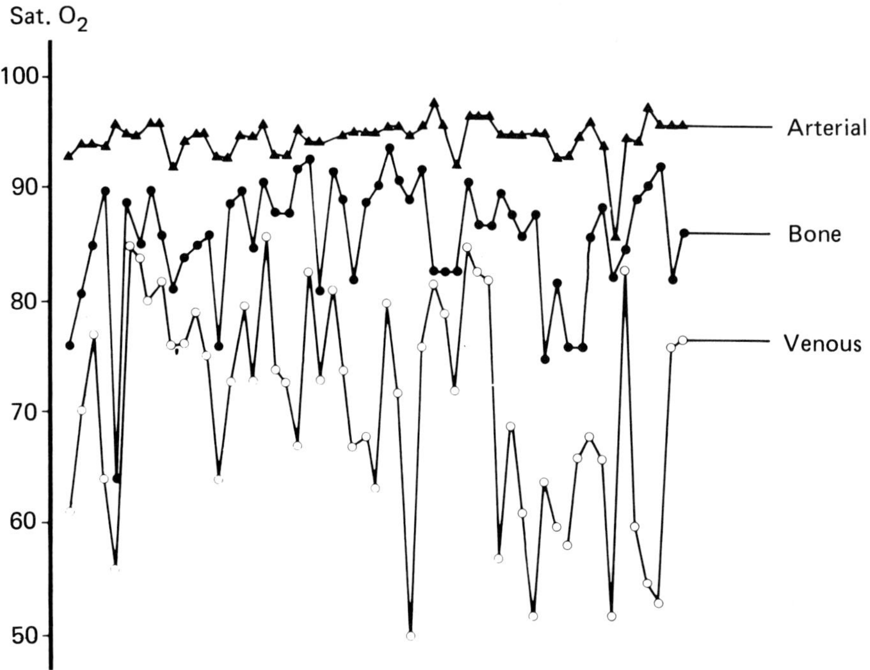

Fig.93.—Diagram of O_2 saturations measured simultaneously in the arterial, osseous, and venous blood in 55 patients. The O_2 saturation is always higher in the osseous blood than in the blood from the femoral vein.

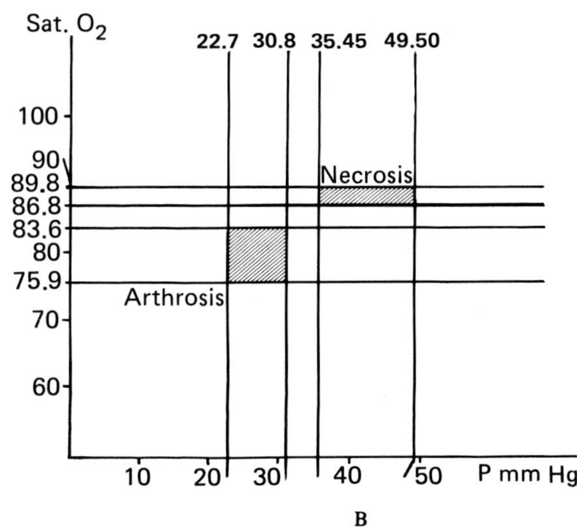

Fig.94.—This figure shows that the association of an elevated O_2 saturation with the high intramedullary pressure is much more common in necrosis than in arthrosis and vice versa.

TABLE XI
AVERAGE VALUES

	Pressure	O_2 *Saturation*
Typical necrosis	42.3 ± 6.8 mm Hg	88.3% ± 1.5
Arthrosis	26.7 ± 4 mm Hg	79.7% ± 3.9

In comparing those cases with necrosis and arthrosis (Fig. 94), the differences are statistically significant in relation to intramedullary pressure and oxygen saturation. There is a clear correlation between these two parameters. Table XI summarizes the values for both groups. By encompassing the means and ranges for both O_2 saturation and IMP, it can be seen that high IMP and O_2 saturation is characteristic of necrosis; lower IMP and O_2 saturation characterizes arthrosis (Fig. 94). From a practical point of view, this adds an additional means of diagnosis of ischemia in hip disorders. If the trochanteric blood has an O_2 saturation above 82%, this strongly suggests a necrosis or at least an ischemic coxopathy. The association of a high IMP with high oxygen saturation is even more significant. Therefore, this simple test can be added to the diagnostic measures and may be particularly applicable to sorting out early cases. Although there may be a practical application of these findings, they do require a pathophysiological explanation. The following hypothesis which is only theoretical explains the findings. At first, it seems paradoxical to find increased oxygen saturation in ischemic bone as compared to bone of patients with arthrosis. In fact, when we began this study, we expected to find the opposite. In any event, one has to also consider that our method of withdrawing intramedullary blood via the greater trochanter samples blood which is distal to both the arthrosic and the necrotic lesions. Is there a decrease in O_2 saturation in arthrosis? This was Madrigal's conclusion[294] from a study comparing 26 arthrosic hips with 40 normal controls. He withdrew blood from the femoral head at a time of surgical intervention under general anesthesia. The level of oxygen saturation was higher in the normals than in those with arthrosis. However, the absence of concomitant control of arterial oxygen saturation diminishes the significance of his findings. Is there an increased O_2 saturation in the necrosis? We prefer this interpretation since it is unlikely that there are bone blood changes so far distal to the main site of the arthrosic lesions while we know that ischemic lesions are evident throughout the bone and are at considerable distance from the area which later goes on to collapse. This increased saturation may be due to the stasis or to a defect in the utilization of oxygen.

These findings are considerably different from those of early ischemia of a traumatic origin, for example, fracture of the femoral neck where net reduction of arterial flow is an essential factor in the blood gas changes. Woodhouse[468] used an electrode which was capable of measuring oxygen tension directly. The method had been previously confirmed in a dog model showing that simple transection of the femoral neck did not change the O_2 partial pressure but that a rotation which twisted the ligamentum teres resulted in marked diminution of oxygen level. Using this method in 19 fractures of the femoral neck, he was able, in 17 cases, to measure a direct relationship between oxygen tension and the radiological and histological evolution of necrosis as observed six months later.

TABLE XII
TEMPERATURE COMPARISONS IN NECROSIS

Level	Mean Temperature (C°)
Trochanter	35.8
Head	35.2
Rectal	37

INTRAOSSEOUS THERMOMETRY

Table XII summarizes the findings according to the level of measurement in those cases with necrosis studied by intraosseous thermometry. In the majority of the cases, the temperature recorded has been between 34 and 35.5° with an upper limit of 36.1°. Intramedullary pressures varied between 30 and 70 mm Hg. Ischemic necrosis is strongly suggested when

TABLE XIII
TEMPERATURE COMPARISONS IN ALL CASES

Level	Mean Temperature (C°)
Trochanter	36.2
Head	36.3
Rectal	37.7

the temperature is below 36°C and the pressure above 30 mm Hg. A variety of other cases, including normal controls, arthrosis, and a variety of hip lesions, have been studied with the average temperatures recorded in Table XIII. The difference of .1° between the head and the trochanter compares to an average of .6° difference between head and trochanter in cases of confirmed necrosis. This difference in the case of necrosis would appear to be significant. In the non-necrosis cases, the temperature was higher in the head than in the trochanter while in cases of necrosis, the temperature was lower in the head than in the trochanter. Furthermore, in cases with sequestrum formation within the head, the temperature was always lower in the sequestrum than in the neighboring zones. The intramedullary pressure varies proportionally to the temperature in all cases except in necrosis where there is a disassociation with higher pressures being associated with lower temperatures. This temperature/pressure dissociation can form an additional basis for the diagnosis of ischemic necrosis of bone.

Evolution Of Ischemic Necrosis Of Bone

The evolution of Stage I necrosis will be considered in further detail in Chapter X, on treatment, since certainty of diagnosis in this stage of the disease requires histologic confirmation. However, the spontaneous evolution of femoral head necrosis diagnosed by radiography has been studied by several authors[101,276,337,357,392]. The conclusions of these authors are similar and can be emphasized by case illustrations. The first point to emphasize is that 50% or more of the cases of the patients with non-traumatic ischemic necrosis of the femoral head will eventually develop bilateral involvement. Since not all patients present initially with bilateral involvement, the initially non-involved hip can be viewed with a level of suspicion which aids early diagnosis.

Illustrative Case 11 (Fig. 95) - Mr. FRA..., a 42-year-old miner, presented initially in January, 1971, with a one-month history of pain in the right groin. He had suffered a significant injury in this region two months prior to the onset of pain. Even though the radiograph already showed advanced sclerosis with early collapse (Stage III), pain was rated as moderate and limitation of movement, minimal. A core biopsy was carried out on January 14, 1971, and histologically confirmed the diagnosis of bone necrosis (Type 4). This resulted in alleviation of pain for 11 months at which time reappearance of symptoms were associated with radiologic deterioration (Fig. 95). A pedicle bone graft was carried out in February, 1972, with a total hip replacement eventually being necessary in January, 1975.

In November, 1973, the patient presented with left hip pain for the first time. The x-ray was completely normal, although there was moderate, painful limitation of movement. Functional exploration in December, 1973, revealed a baseline pressure of 20 mm Hg with a sustained rise to 30 mm Hg on the stress test. The intramedullary venography revealed stasis, and the core biopsy showed a widespread eosinophilic reticular necrosis (Type 2). At latest follow-up in July, 1979, the hip remained asymptomatic and radiologically normal. Included among the probable etiologic factors was a diffuse arterial sclerosis demonstrated by arteriography. It is often the phenomenon of bilaterality which allows us to see cases of circulatory abnormality with no radiologic or even clinical signs similar to that reported by Marcus et al.[298].

The second feature suggested by many authors and confirmed in our series is that bilateral cases have a much worse prognosis with three-quarters of the cases undergoing spontaneous progression.

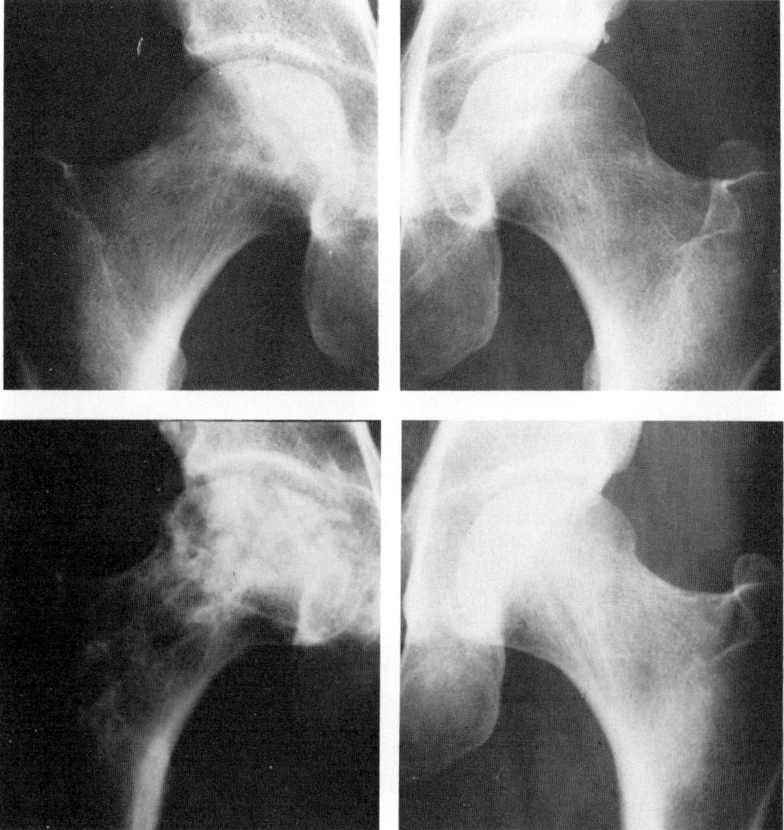

Fig.95.—Case 11
Upper x-rays (12-24-70): Clinical and radiological evidence of necrosis in Stage III on the right side. Lower x-rays (11-12-73): Radiologic deterioration of the right necrosis in spite of core decompression. Pain in the left hip in spite of normal x-rays: necrosis is suspected and was eventually proven by core biopsy.

Illustrative Case 12 (Fig. 96) - Mr. BLI..., a 51-year-old automotive mechanic, was seen for the first time in March, 1972, when he complained of the sudden onset of right hip pain beginning one month earlier. The pain began after lifting a heavy object and was severe and disabling. Although the range of movement of the hip was nearly normal, there was significant discomfort at the extremes of movement. The x-rays showed probable Stage II necrosis. The left hip was completely asymptomatic and with a normal exam, but areas of sclerosis could be identified in the head. A Strontium[87] bone scan demonstrated increased uptake on the right side.

Functional exploration of the right hip (4-18-72) showed a normal baseline intramedullary pressure but a positive stress test (increase from 20 mm Hg to 60 mm Hg). Phlebography showed considerable stasis and biopsy demonstrated diffuse medullary and trabecular necrosis. The core decompression did not prevent both symptomatic and radiologic deterioration which eventually resulted in total hip replacement on September 14, 1972.

Although the patient began to experience left hip pain in July, 1972, he only presented for examination in August. Radiographs then showed collapse of the left femoral head for which he also underwent total hip replacement at a later date. Among the possible etiologic factors in this case were hypertriglyceridemia, osteomalacia proven by iliac bone biopsy, and a history of high alcohol intake and smoking. This particular case is noteworthy for the rapidity of progression. Within five months, the disease successively affected the right hip and then the left hip. Within one month, the x-rays showed progression from near normal to collapse.

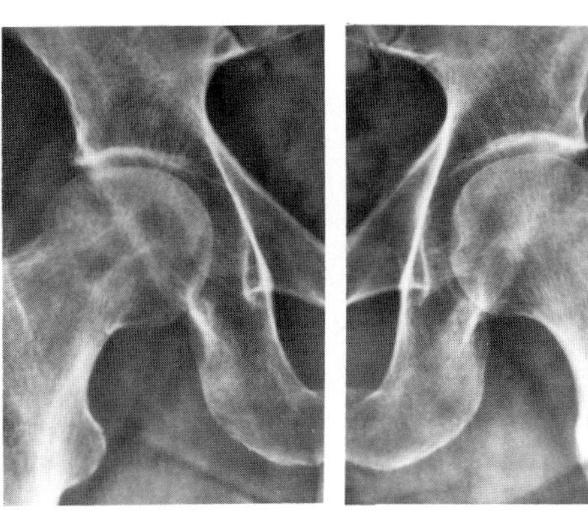

A: X-rays (5-8-72) Bilateral necrosis at Stage II with slight superior flattening of the right hip (beginning of the collapse)

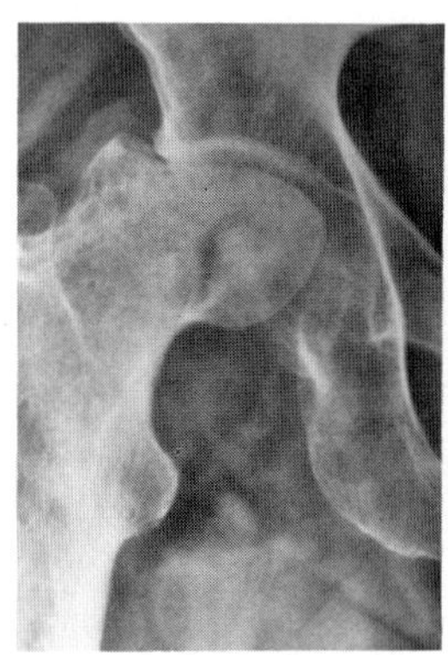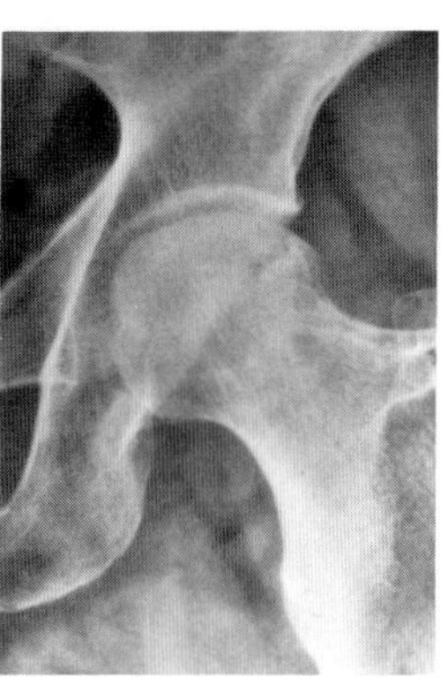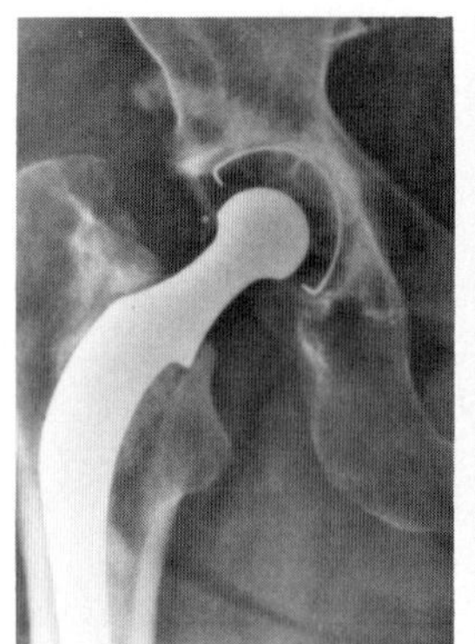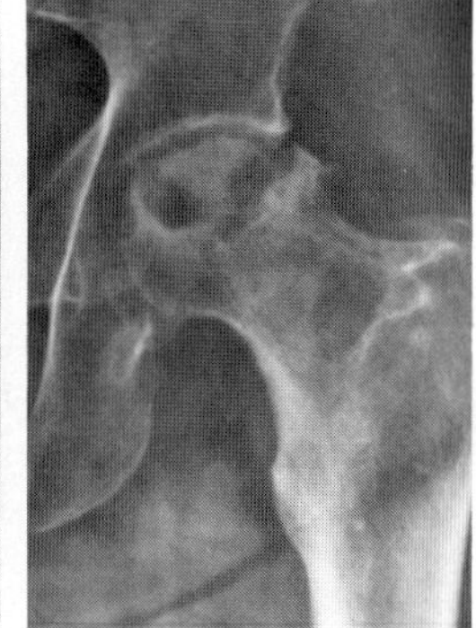

B: X-rays (8-28-72) Collapse of the right hip (Stage III) and superior flattening with slight collapse of the left hip.

C: X-rays (5-4-73) Right total hip replacement. Sequestrum with collapse of the left hip.

Fig.96.—Case 12

The final point mentioned by multiple authors concerning the progression of disease diagnosed by x-ray is that most cases go on to collapse. Merle D'Aubigné[310] observed such collapse in 20% of his cases in the first year while Coste et al.[101] noted that 72% progressed to collapse within two or three years of the onset of diagnosis. In rare cases, true head/neck fractures are observed as reported by Debeyre[117]. Benign, stable, or non-progressive cases are observed in about 20 to 30% of these series.

SUMMARY

Except for those cases with a well-defined anterolateral sequestrum, the radiologic diagnosis of necrosis remains uncertain. Some radiologic findings are, however, quite characteristic of bone necrosis, including the crescent sign (a subchondral radio-lucency); massive sclerosis or spotty sclerosis with an arcuate, superiorly concave, central, capital sclerosis; or cysts surrounded by a border of sclerosis. Nonetheless, for some stages and types of ischemic necrosis of bone, including all cases in Stage I, certain cases in Stage II, all cases characterized by osteoporosis, and certain cases in Stage IV, the functional exploration constitutes the only diagnostic method. We feel that this approach deserves more widespread understanding and use.

We believe that there are several reasons which explain the lack of a more widespread utilization of these techniques. Firstly, the traditional dependence of our specialty on x-ray for diagnosis of the bone lesions hinders the use of new techniques. Secondly, traditional orthopaedics has tended to view osteoarticular pathology in mechanical and not physiologic terms. Finally, the technique itself is a procedure which is too surgically oriented for the non-orthopaedist and too medically oriented for the surgeon. The area of application of this functional method of exploration includes not only non-traumatic ischemia as we have here described but also a variety of osteoarticular problems because of the frequency of secondary complicating ischemia.

From a practical, diagnostic point of view, it is not necessary to use all of the parameters described in this chapter. We suggest the following diagnostic steps when one encounters the problem of a painful hip without radiologic signs. These steps can be divided into three stages (Table XIV) correlated with the likelihood of positive diagnosis.

When one records an abnormally elevated baseline IMP or a significant hypertensive response to the stress test, phlebography is not necessary. Since these first two diagnostic tests are frequently positive, the diagnostic procedure is simplified. Also, phlebo-

TABLE XIV
STAGE I INFH
Three Levels of Diagnosis

First Level - suspicious *Clinical/X-ray*	*Triad of Suspicion* 1. Painful hip 2. Limitation of movement 3. Normal or near normal x-ray
Second Level - probable *Hemodynamic and/or isotopic*	*A. Vascular Exploration trochanter and head* 1. Elevated IMP 2. Positive stress test 3. Intramedullary venography- stasis reflux *B. Bone Scan* 1. Increased uptake
Third Level - certain *Histopathologic*	*Core Biopsy of Head and Neck* Signs of ischemia (stasis) and medullary trabecular necrosis (4 types)

graphy is quite painful. However, if the IMP is normal even after the stress test, it is preferable to carry out phlebography. It is possible to observe significant intraosseous stasis or derangement of the intraosseous drainage even in the face of normal IMP although this is quite unusual.

Radioisotope bone scan could be the initial investigation. Increased uptake of the isotope in the suspected hip is the equivalent of a positive hemodynamic exploration. The first two steps of the diagnostic procedure are then no longer necessary. Although the increased uptake is not specific, we have already explained the significance of this increased uptake and its correlation with our findings on the functional exploration, including biopsy.

Even though the bone scan is non-specific and does not depend upon a specific derangement in intraosseous circulation for its abnormality, it is our opinion that one is justified in the face of a positive bone scan to go directly to the third step of the investigation—namely, core biopsy. It should, however, be remembered that bone scan is considerably more expensive than the simple measurement of intramedullary pressure under local anesthesia. The biopsy specimen confirms the diagnosis but is also helpful in the prognosis of the specific case depending upon the extent and severity of the necrotic lesions.

ANALYSIS OF OUR PERSONAL SERIES

We began this chapter with an analysis of those elements and factors which characterize the ischemic syndrome in bone. This was taken from our experience and findings reported in the literature. A specific analysis of our clinical series of 136 patients with non-traumatic ischemic necrosis of the femoral head (INFH) serves to round out the picture. No cases of post-traumatic necrosis of the femoral head are included in this series, since they represent a group with known etiology[119]. On the other hand, most of the non-traumatic necroses which are seen have an uncertain etiologic association. This survey was undertaken in an effort to determine more precisely some of the etiologic associations. These 136 cases do not represent all of the non-traumatic cases of ischemic necrosis of bone which we have seen but only approximately one-half of them. However, those included in the series were analyzed under the most favorable conditions and met two criteria. Firstly, the diagnosis was established with certainty by histology of the femoral head on the core biopsy specimen. Only occasionally was histologic control not available in which case the diagnosis was made by radiologic evidence of a pathognomonic-appearing sequestrum (Stage III). Secondly, all cases were hospitalized patients for whom all of the data had been collected. Our computerized statistical survey used 80 separate parameters. The charts were transcribed onto perforated cards which could then be machine sorted. These statistics were analyzed by the Chi Square method. The most interesting results of this study are listed below[119].

AGE AND SEX DISTRIBUTION

There were 93 men and 43 women, constituting a more than 2:1 male/female ratio. There was a very great age spread, although a clear peak between 40 and 60 years encompassed 72 patients (52%). The 136 patients had a total of 181 hips involved with 45 bilateral cases (33%). There was no sex difference concerning bilaterality. Nearly as many right hips (89) were involved as left (92).

ETIOLOGY

The etiologically associated factors are listed in order of decreasing frequency.

Minor trauma - This includes injury which did not involve fracture of the neck, dislocation of the femoral head, nor fracture or dislocation of the acetabulum. There were 34 such cases (25.1%), of which nine were workmen's compensation. Only seven were bilateral (20.5%), which is clearly less than the general average of bilaterality. None of the cases involving workmen's compensation had bilateral necrosis.

Cortisone treatment - There were 22 such cases (16.1%), of which five were associated with rheumatoid arthritis. It is important to know that more than half of these cases were bilateral (59%), well above the general average.

Arteritis of the lower extremities - 22 cases (16%) -We have emphasized several times the association between arteritis and bone necrosis. This association has also been observed in connection with gangrene of the lower extremities. The importance of arteritis of the lower extremities and the etiology of necrosis of the femoral head seems unquestionable since, in our series, it has the same frequency as cortisone treatment.

Antecedent phlebitis - 22 cases (16.1%).

Hip dysplasia - 22 cases (16.1%).

Hyperuricemia (with or without clinical gout) - 22 cases (16%). This percentage is definitely above that of controlled subjects as we shall see subsequently.

Rheumatoid arthritis and other connective tissue disorders - 12 cases (9%) - This incidence is nearly the same as the percentage of patients with increased sedimentation rates, a point which will be a common denominator subsequently. Only two cases of definite SLE were encountered.

This etiologic composite is similar to that of other French series with the exception of arteritis, which is higher in our series. The incidence of bilaterality in cases involving cortisone treatment is not surprising, although, in those cases involving minor trauma, the 20% incidence of bilaterality was unexpected. Our survey does not mention caisson disease as we have never encountered it. There is one case of sickle-cell anemia in a West Indies negro and one case of Gaucher's Disease. Table XV summarizes the etiologic associations in our series.

CLINICAL SIGNS AND SYMPTOMS

The time interval between the first painful episode and the first consultation was less than six months in 59 cases and more than 12 months in 68 cases. Onset of symptoms was sudden in 82 of 159 cases where it could be established with precision, i.e., more than half of the cases. This point appears to us as being quite important and very characteristic of necrosis. A relationship exists between the rapidity of the onset and the time interval from the first pain to the first consultation. When the onset is rapid, the patient seeks consultation earlier.

In 113 cases (63%), the pain radiated to the groin which is typical for hip pathology and not simply characteristic of INFH. Radiation of pain to the knee was only encountered in 62 cases (35%). Night pain was present 39 times (21.5%), and the pain was exacerbated by cough in 15 cases. Hip stiffness on

TABLE XV

ETIOLOGY OF FEMORAL HEAD NECROSIS

Number of patients: 136
Sex: 93 men, 43 women (2M/1F)
Age: 72 patients between 40–60 yrs.
Bilateral: 33% (181 Pathological hips)

Etiological Factors	*Number of cases*	*Percentage*
Minor trauma (9 Workmen's Compensation)	34	25.1%
Corticosteroid therapy	22	16.1%
Arterial Disease of the lower extremity	22	16.1%
History of phlebitis	22	16.1%
Dysplasia	22	16.1%
Hyperuricemia (± gout)	21	16 %
Rheumatoid arthritis	12	9 %
Elevated sedimentation rate (above 20mm/hour)	50/122	40.9%
Hyperlipemia	15/96	15.5%
Hypertriglyceridemia	9/49	18.4%

first examination was quite variable; but, in 86 cases (out of a total of 181 hips), the limitation of movement was moderate with an average flexion of 90° ± 20°.

One last clinical item is the functional capacity of the patient. Sixty-six of 136 patients were forced to stop their activities whether housewife or professional duties, i.e., nearly 50%.

RADIOLOGICAL FINDINGS

The previous chapter defines our system of classification, which has value both from the point of view of type of treatment as well as determining prognosis. Table XVI summarizes this series according to stage. Six cases were difficult to classify. It is interesting to detail the type of the bone texture changes. Intracapital or intracervical sclerosis was observed in 84 cases (46.4%). Cysts were present in 45 cases (24.8%). We wish to underscore the frequency of the cystic type. Of course, joint space narrowing was present in all cases with Stage IV and in all ischemic coxopathies.

LABORATORY FINDINGS

The abnormalities most frequently encountered were as follows. Acceleration of the sedimentation rate (above 20 mm in the first hour) in 50 cases of 122 or in 40.9% of the cases was observed. This surprised

us; and, in fact, in a great proportion of these cases, we have not been able to find a cause for this abnormality. However, one has to remember the relative frequency in these cases of gout, of phlebitis, and of inflammatory arthritis, as well as the presence of inflammatory foci in the synovial membrane[14,16]. This "touch of inflammation" seems to have been neglected in most reports. Hyperuricemia was found 21 times in 122 cases or in 17.2% of the cases. Hyperlipemia (greater than 9 gm/liter) was found 15 times out of 96 cases or in 15.5% of the cases. Hypertriglyceridemia (greater than 1.50 gm/liter) was found nine times in 94 of the cases (10.9%). Since this survey, we have conducted a comparative study between the patients afflicted with osteoarthrosis and those with INFH. That study proved that hypertriglyceridemia is found more frequently in INFH cases than in osteoarthrosis at a statistically significant level[37].

FUNCTIONAL INVESTIGATION

Hemodynamic Data

Measurement of the IMP taken 133 times has shown that the IMP was equal to or above 30 mm Hg in 96 cases (72%). Let us recall that the pressure was taken in most cases in the trochanteric region at a distance from the more severe lesions. Phlebography was performed 111 times in the trochanteric region and was abnormal 106 times (95%). This statistic

TABLE XVI

HISTOGRAM OF THE RADIOLOGIC STAGES

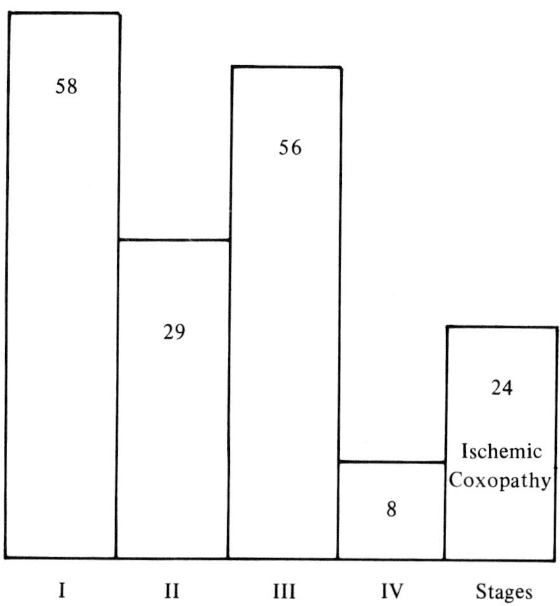

emphasizes once more the practical and theorical importance of the phlebographic stasis which is almost constant in the necrosis, being present from the beginning of the necrosis.

Histological Data

Histological examination has been performed on specimens from 158 cases and has allowed us to classify our cases according to the histological type which we have already described—Type 1 - 19 cases, Type 2 - 41 cases, Type 3 - 66 cases, Type 4 - 31 cases.

It is interesting to compare the radiologic stages with the histologic types as shown in Table XVII. An analysis of this comparison leads to several conclusions. In the preradiologic stage, there are significant numbers of cases (7 of 54) where either trabecular histologic changes or evidence of reconstruction exist even though this reconstruction is not seen with the standard roentgenographic films. However, it is at this radiologic stage that Type 1 histologic lesions are most frequently seen. Necrotic lesions are widely disseminated, of small volume, and probably reversible.

At radiological Stage III, trabecular necrosis is more often encountered than in the preceding stages. This applies, as well, to the signs of reconstruction. On the other hand, reconstruction signs are rarely observed in the ischemic coxopathies.

If the histological factors are grouped by etiology,

TABLE XVII

Relationship Between
Radiologic Stages and Histological Types

Histologic Types	*Number of Cases*				
4	7	6	13	4	1
3	15	8	29	3	11
2	18	10	4	0	10
1	14	2	2	0	1
Radiologic Stages	I	II	III	IV	Ischemic coxopathies

it can be seen that in the arteritic, hyperuricemic, and cortisone group, the histological lesions are often of the Type 3 and 4, i.e., advanced. On the other hand, in the minor trauma and post-phlebitic groups, the lesions are often of Type 1 and 2 and, therefore, much less severe. These facts suggest that the mechanism of ischemia may be different for these two groups of patients. In the first group, it could be direct, secondary to a decrease of blood flow as a consequence of an arteriopathy. In the second group, it could be due to an indirect cause, by embarrassment of the venous drainage, or intraosseous hemorrhage.

CHAPTER VI

DIFFERENTIAL DIAGNOSIS OF BONE ISCHEMIA AND NECROSIS

It is not possible in this chapter to draft all the potential differential diagnoses at Stage I of the disease, since this would entail a review of all periarticular and osteoarticular pathology. At the pre-radiologic stage, the beginning of any pathologic condition is possible. The whole diagnosis rests then on the results of complementary paraclinical examinations, including contrast arthrography (synovial chondromatosis, adhesive capsulitis, and arthrosis), synovial biopsy (inflammatory arthropathy and pigmented villonodular synovitis), and the functional exploration of the bone. In this chapter, we will discuss, however, two conditions which, in spite of their own identities, have a common background with an ill-defined relationship to osteonecrosis. These conditions are reflex sympathetic dystrophy and arthrosis.

REFLEX SYMPATHETIC DYSTROPHY

The firm diagnosis of reflex sympathetic dystrophy must be based upon clinical, radiographic, and pathologic criteria. There can be a remarkable overlap in many or all of these areas with the osteoporotic type of Stage II bone necrosis which we have previously discussed. However, careful analysis can usually differentiate between the two conditions.

CLINICAL EVALUATION

A great range of presentations is possible with reflex sympathetic dystrophy. There is frequently some precipitating event, including trauma, which may seem quite trivial, or neurological or cardiopulmonary diseases, which usually have some sudden onset or exacerbation. The post-traumatic variety is known under a variety of terms, including post-traumatic osteoporosis, acute bone atrophy, Sudeck's dystrophy, etc. In general, the pain and joint stiffness are out of proportion to the other physical findings. The joint involved may be edematous, and there may be either increased or decreased local skin temperature.

Radiographic findings are very similar to the Stage II osteoporotic type of necrosis which we have previously described. The osteoporosis, however, is generally more intense, diffuse, and occasionally has a microcystic appearance. The standard laboratory examination contributes nothing to the diagnosis except the documentation of a complete absence of systemic signs of inflammation. The bone scan invariably shows increased isotopic uptake which is inevitably intense. We have carried out the functional evaluation of the bone involved, since it appeared to us that this condition was, above all, a vascular phenomenon. These findings will be presented in a separate section. Concerning the bone scan, Riffat et al[362] reported interesting findings in scanning patients with a focus of reflex sympathetic dystrophy and comparing these with the hemodynamic findings in the contralateral joint. He reported increased uptake in some joints which were not clinically involved, other areas of hemodynamic abnormalities which were neither clinically or radioisotopically involved, and some areas of significant osteoporosis but without symptoms. His report suggested that the existence of clinically silent lesions may be quite extensive and that the syndrome of sympathetic dystrophy may be more generalized than was previously believed. Obviously, any attempt to explain the pathophysiology of this condition requires a deeper understanding of the regulation of bone and joint blood flow.

PATHOPHYSIOLOGY

Everyone agrees on the vascular nature of this condition because the osteoporosis conforms to the territorial vascular unity of the joint. However, regarding the mechanism of the circulatory problem, several hypotheses exist. Leriche[280] proposed an initial phase of vasoconstriction followed by vasodilatation. The latter was the reason for the apparent increased vascularization of the joint, producing a pseudoinflammatory picture in the affected part.

Huet and Huguier[209] put forth the hypothesis that the syndrome could be understood in terms of reflex capillary stasis. Rohner[366] suggested that the bone was ischemic on the basis of diminution in size of the intraosseous arteries. There was, however, no data available, prior to the studies which we are reporting below, concerning the status of the intraosseous circulation. Since it is obvious from the clinical course that one is dealing, in most instances, with a reversible problem, it appears that there are sufficient arguments to incriminate a dysfunction of vasomotor regulation of the joint with opening of arteriovenous shunts under the control of the autonomic nervous system. In this sense, reflex sympathetic dystrophy represents a neurovascular adaptation syndrome. It is also probable that the circulatory changes are not the same in the different clinical phases as described by Sudeck: hypertrophic, dystrophic, and atrophic.

We have carried out the functional hemodynamic exploration of bone in 29 cases of reflex sympathetic dystrophy[140,145], including 10 hips, 13 knees, 3 wrists, 2 feet, and 1 shoulder. Intramedullary pressure was nearly always abnormally elevated. In 25% of the cases, the baseline pressure was normal, but the stress test was *always* positive. In the hip, the baseline pressure was elevated in the femoral head, in several instances, while normal in the trochanter. The stress test in the head increased the intertrochanteric pressure and vice versa, but this interaction was not constant. Intramedullary venography was equally abnormal and almost constantly exhibited diaphyseal reflux with intramedullary stasis, which documented the stagnation of the circulation and the difficulty in venous drainage. This intraosseous stasis seems to be a key element in the vicious cycle in which edema, fibrosis, and anoxia have a noxious inter-relationship. It should also be pointed out that, in several cases of the hip, a functional hemodynamic investigation of the contralateral side demonstrated significant intramedullary pressure abnormalities and abnormal venograms on hip that were clinically, and even radiologically, normal.

A core biopsy is considerably more difficult to carry out in osteonecrosis of the porotic type or reflex sympathetic dystrophy since the bone is very soft and friable. The bone marrow often appears liquified. During extraction of the biopsy specimen, one often observes a thin, grayish-yellow or salmon-colored fluid leaking out from the biopsy opening. Because the bone is friable, it is difficult to remove from the trephine and obtain a good specimen. Therefore, in these cases, it is best to use the double trephine with the slotted inner tube which gives the best possibility of obtaining a good specimen.

The histology of the specimen shows, in the majority of cases, marrow lesions of vascular origin characterized by intrasinusoidal plasmostasis, interstitial edema, hemorrhage, and fibrosis. In a recent analysis of ten core biopsies of cases of RSD of the proximal femur biopsied 1-3 months after the onset of symptoms, seven cases showed evidence of bony reconstruction (new bone formation, trabeculae lined with osteoblasts) in marked contrast to the marked osteoporosis[14a]. However, in four cases considered as reflex sympathetic dystrophy, the biopsy showed extensive necrotic lesions either of the marrow or of both the marrow and the trabeculae which place them quite similar to the Type 2 and Type 3 lesions of those cases considered to be bone necrosis. The osteopenia is also marked. Although the mechanism of this change is not well understood, one case operated on one month after the onset of clinical symptoms showed marked osteoclastic resorption of trabeculae.

In 80% of the cases, we have been able to document a spectacular decrease in pain following the core biopsy. This has permitted the introduction of physical therapy with improvement in joint range of movement and a more rapid recalcification of the epiphysis.

Illustrative Case 13 - Mr. JON..., a 41-year-old male, experienced the onset of left hip pain in April, 1971, following a minor accident. The patient also suffered from asthma and had been taking Prednisone in varied doses for the previous three years. In June, 1971, he underwent partial gastrectomy for ulcer disease. The post-operative period was benign, but he experienced increasing hip pain. The movement of the hip was limited and painful. X-rays showed considerable diffuse osteoporosis involving the entire left femoral head and acetabulum. The outlines of the femoral head itself were hardly visible (Fig. 97). The trochanteric intramedullary pressure was normal at 25 mm Hg but increased to 48 mm Hg after a saline injection. Core biopsy (8-13-71) revealed severe extensive medullary stasis but with no necrotic foci. The pain disappeared completely immediately following the core biopsy. Two months later, the hip was both clinically and radiologically normal.

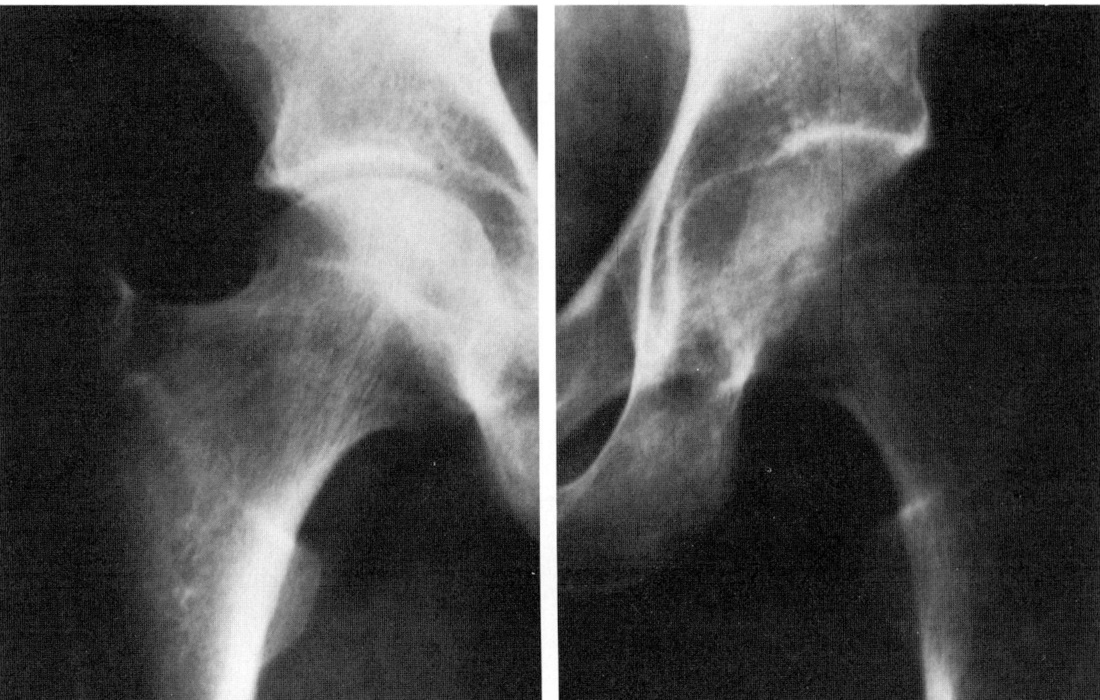

A: X-rays (July 71). Diffuse demineralization of the left hip affecting the acetabulum and the whole upper end of the femur: the outline of the head is obscured with an indistinct joint line.

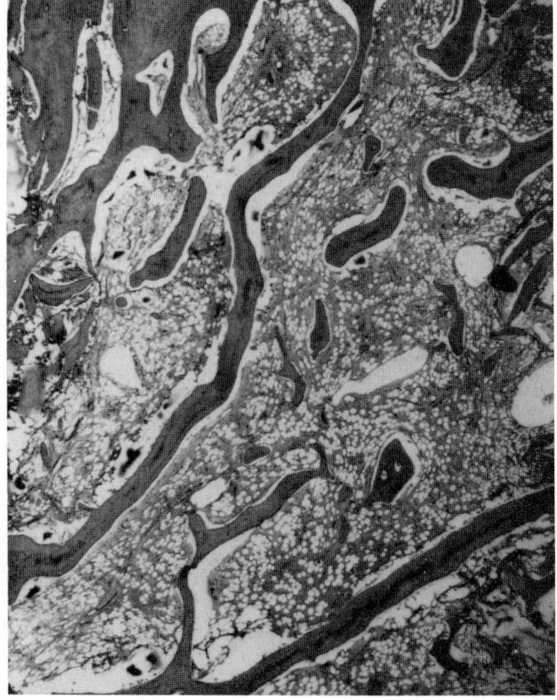

B: Osteopenia of the bone trabeculae and intercellular stasis.

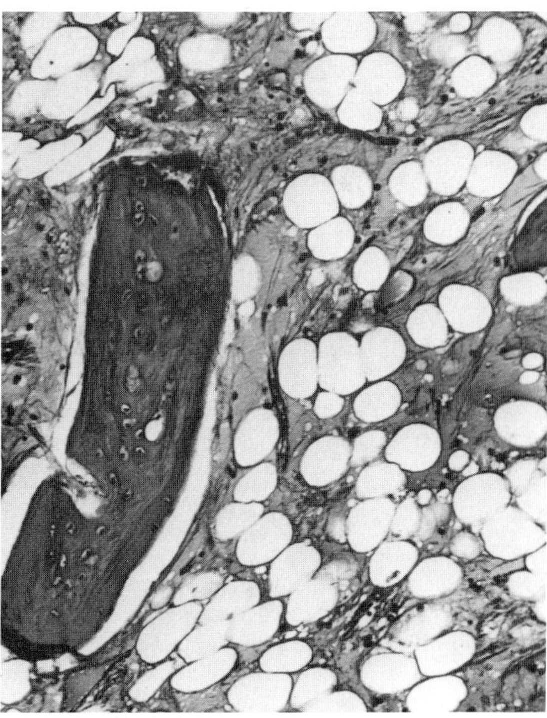

C: Bone marrow at a high magnification: the lipocytes are separated by amorphous material. The live trabecula is surrounded by reticular fibers.

Fig.97.—Case 13

Illustrative Case 14 - Mr. MAU..., a 36-year-old white male, had the sudden onset (in February, 1975) of left hip pain made worse by exercise. All laboratory tests, including sedimentation rate, were normal. One month later, the pain had increased and became constant, with pain radiating down the anterior aspect of the leg. Night pain was also present. There was moderate, painful limitation of movement in all directions. X-rays showed diffuse osteoporosis with blurring of the outlines but with no other abnormalities on either the lateral film or on tomography. There was considerable tenderness over the greater trochanter. On March 20, 1975, functional investigation showed a baseline pressure of 38 mm Hg in the trochanteric region and 65 mm Hg in the head. The saline test elevated pressure to 80 mm Hg. Phlebography showed intraosseous stasis. The biopsy specimen showed loose fibrosis, interstitial edema, and the presence of histiocytes, osteoblasts, and osteoclasts. By May, 1975, the patient had recovered full range of movement of the hip and by July, 1975, had both clinical and radiologic healing of the lesion. In October, 1976, the patient had a similar episode in the right hip which was treated non-operatively. At last follow-up, in 1979, the patient remained completely cured.

DISCUSSION

Initially, we would like to dispel the confusion of RSD with a condition reported as transient osteoporosis of the hip. Curtis et al[108] reported six cases during pregnancy under this rubric. DeMarchi et al[297] described six cases of which two presented with an ipsilateral reflex sympathetic dystrophy of the foot. In their cases, they reported a rapidly evolving course with signs of necrosis, resorption, and reconstruction at bone biopsy and speculated on the possibility of an intraosseous circulatory problem. Hunder et al[216] reported nine cases with eight synovial biopsies and four bone biopsies also showing signs of necrosis, hemorrhage, and reconstruction. Of his nine cases, four had other joint involvement (one in both feet, one in the shoulder, one in the opposite hip, and one in both knees). We cannot accept that these reports represent an independent clinical syndrome, and we do not believe that they have made a good case for rejecting the diagnosis of reflex sympathetic dystrophy. All of the particulars of the cases so described can fit very well within the nosologic framework of reflex sympathetic dystrophy as demonstrated by many workers. This is also the opinion of Lequesne[273].

To our knowledge, Rutishauser et al[277] have been the only investigators to have thoroughly described the histopathological substratum of this condition. He describes vascular and marrow changes arranged in dystrophic foci consisting of dilatation of the venous sinus, intrasinusoidal plasmostasis, interstitial edema, the disappearance of the hematopoietic cells, and the replacement of the lipocytes by a reticular, fibrous marrow. In addition, thickening of the arterial walls can be observed. Obviously, this picture recalls, very well, the changes discovered in cases of early INFH. Histopathology alone cannot untangle the difficult nuances in this diagnosis in which there may be some mixed cases. Moreover, the natural tendency of sympathetic dystrophy to resolve and osteonecrosis to progress may not always be followed in any individual case.

The real problem concerns the relationship between reflex sympathetic dystrophy and osteonecrosis. The unitarian point of view would hold that reflex sympathetic dystrophy should be considered as an acute and abortive osteoporotic type of necrosis. The dualist point of view must explain why a typical reflex sympathetic dystrophy with definite clinical and radiologic criteria may be accompanied by authentic Type 2 medullary necrosis or even Type 3 histologic changes with trabecular necrosis. We reject the nosologic concepts which limit themselves to clinical and radiological data. This is a criticism which could be leveled at the contemporary French School (Rénier, DeSèze, Ravault, Serre, Louyot, and Lequesne). One must return to the healthy anatomical/clinical comparisons in order to understand the basis upon which all clinical and radiological signs rest. This is exactly what the Geneva School under Rohner[366] has done in a notable report which underlines three important points. Firstly, there is a basic similarity in the histopathologic findings to what one has already described in Type 1 necrosis. Secondly, in both cases, the vicious cycle centers on the stasis-ischemic axis which may lead to marrow trabecular necrosis as it is sometimes observed in severe, longstanding cases of reflex sympathetic dystrophy. However, ischemia and stasis are not synonymous with necrosis, as proven by the fact that, in the majority of cases of reflex sympathetic dystrophy, there is no necrotic lesion. It appears that bone marrow is more easily regenerated at the level of large, well-vascularized metaphyses, such as the knee, than in poorly vascularized epiphyses, such as the femoral head. This perhaps explains the crossover between necrosis and reflex sympathetic dystrophy of the hip.

There are two histologic aspects which are fairly characteristic of reflex sympathetic dystrophy and are evident early in the process. As Rutishauser[277] pointed out, there are foci of dystrophic changes both in the intramedullary vessels and the marrow itself associated with an important local disturbance in bone turnover, leading to very thin trabeculae. The intraosseous vessel walls increase enormously in thickness with the parietal cells assuming an epithelioid appearance. It is not possible to determine whether these vessels are permanently blocked or only intermittently or temporarily non-functional.

This histologic description has lead Rohner[366] to conceptualize that decrease in bone blood flow distal to these narrow arterioles leads either to severe ischemia with necrosis and liquefaction of the marrow or to a more moderate ischemia with a fibrillar transformation of the marrow with hemorrhagic foci.

We believe that reflex sympathetic dystrophy and ischemic necrosis of bone are two different conditions with different primary causes for the vasomotor alterations and that they differ, also, in the mechanism by which the deteriorating pathophysiologic cycle occurs. However, the two conditions are similar in the histological consequences that result from the pathophysiologic changes. We also believe that certain forms of RSD may be severe enough and persist long enough to result in actual necrosis of both bone and bone marrow. In that case, it could then be an etiologic factor in the necrosis. This could happen in certain types of diffuse osteoporosis (Stage II). It could also be one of the reasons for severe prolongation of the dystrophic syndrome and their sequelae in certain recalcitrant cases reported by Leriche[280].

ARTHROSIS[154,155,158]

We have seen that arthrosis can be an end-stage complication of femoral head necrosis even though the cartilage degeneration appears at the last stage of the disease process (Stage IV). In addition, arthrosis itself can simulate necrosis because of the erosion of the superior portion of the femoral head in the end stages of arthrosis. We have also seen that some types of necrosis, which we have designated as ischemic coxopathies, simulate arthrosis, suggesting the possibility that some of the so-called "iodio-pathic" or primary arthroses may be of vascular origin. Furthermore, the complexity and diversity of both the presentation and evolution of these two conditions hinders the degree of precision with which the diagnosis can be made. The clinical presentation is of some help in directing the examiner to the correct diagnosis associated with peripheral ischemic factors, e.g., night pain and sudden onset of symptoms favoring ischemia. The x-ray may be very helpful in suggesting either an arthrosic process (dysplasia or joint space narrowing) or a necrosis, but it must be underlined here that there is only one truly pathognomonic picture, that is the sequestrum formation with an intact joint space (early Stage III). Even late stage arthrosis can give the appearance of a false sequestrum when there has been disappearance of the joint line and deformity of the joint outlines. If the diagnosis of longstanding disorders of the hip is based only on the x-ray, it will remain poorly defined. The functional investigation permits a deeper penetration into the responsible factors in any particular hip disorder whereby syndromes can be identified permitting more refined etiologic considerations rather than simply lumping all conditions under a single end-stage rubric.

TABLE XVIII

	IMP	*Probability*
Arthrosis	28.8 ± 4	p 0.01
Necrosis	42.3 ± 6.8	

INTRAMEDULLARY PRESSURE IN ARTHROSIS

Hemodynamic abnormalities are virtually absent at the onset of the dysplastic coxopathies. They exist mainly in advanced cases with marked joint space narrowing and obvious reactive new bone formation or in the non-dysplastic coxarthroses which are often labeled "primary." We have carried out a statistical comparative analysis on the results of intertrochanteric IMP in 46 necroses and 57 arthroses with a certain diagnosis being supported either by a pathognomonic x-ray picture or by histology. Fifty percent of the necroses have demonstrated abnormal baseline pressures compared to 29% in the arthroses with 77% incidence of positive stress test in the necroses and 47% in the arthroses[21]. The results are summarized in Table XVIII. In the arthroses, the hemodynamic changes are more pronounced in the so-called primary cases and in the more advanced cases.

Arnoldi et al.[29] also studied the IMP in arthroses. They found the average IMP at the level of the femoral neck was 29.7 mm Hg greater in the arthroses than the average pressure at the same level in the normal hip. Likewise, normal IMP was 6.8 mm Hg above the average femoral vein pressure while in the coxarthrosis the average difference was 36.5 mm Hg. However, all of the studies were carried out in advanced arthrosis so that it was impossible to conclude whether these vascular abnormalities were present early or only at the late stages.

The same authors, however, carried out a similar study in the knee, comparing four groups of patients who had had meniscal lesions. Group I had normal x-rays and was without pain suggesting arthrosis. Group II had the radiographic changes of arthrosis but was without arthrosic pain. Group III also had pain at rest but was without radiographic evidence of arthrosis. Group IV had both arthrosis and pain at rest[28]. IMP was measured directly, both in the femur and tibia, and showed significant increase, progressing from Group I to Group IV with no significant difference between the pressures of the femur and tibia. In Group IV, the averages recorded were 47 mm Hg in the tibia and 41.8 mm Hg in the femur compared to 18.4 mm Hg and 18 mm Hg, respectively, in Group I. Arnoldi singles out Group III (pain at rest without arthrosis) and asks two questions. Are vascular problems early signs of a developing arthrosis? Is it possible to stop the process before lesions of the articular cartilage occur? He proposed cortical fenestration based on the same principle as our core decompression. Our work suggests "yes" as an answer to the first question and "perhaps" to the second, although our experience is not yet of sufficient length to make that definitive. These observations also suggest the possibility of an ischemic gonopathy corresponding to our group of ischemic coxopathy.

RADIOISOTOPIC BONE SCANNING

Muheim and Bohne[324] demonstrated by bone scans of the knee that the rate of strontium fixation is significantly higher in necrosis than in arthrosis. By comparing the bone scans of 72 normal hips, 75 hips with arthrosis and without necrosis, and 48 hips with osteonecrosis, Crutchlow[104] demonstrated that the rate of isotope uptake is higher with the more advanced necrosis and that necrosis with a "secondary" arthrosis could be separated from other arthroses either primary or secondary from any other cause since there was a statistically significant difference between the groups. In the necroses, the absolute scan values are higher; the ratio of uptake of

superolateral to inferomedial is higher; the ratio of acetabulum to femoral head is lower. Danielson[113] has confirmed these findings in the hip, while Anderson[6] reported similar findings in the knee. Both from the radioisotopic and functional investigational points of view, arthrosis and necrosis of both the hip and the knee can be differentiated, keeping in mind that a secondary, end-stage arthrosis may follow from an osteonecrosis.

HISTOLOGY

The unequivocal separation of the two syndromes is on the basis of tissue examination, and one wonders why it is not used more often. The most important reason is probably the lack of awareness of the ischemic coxopathy syndrome. Everyone is content with the generic diagnosis of arthrosis, and curiosity does not lead any further. The second reason is that diagnosis based on x-rays reveals only advanced cases requiring surgical treatment; and, in these conditions, the etiologic repartition is of little practical value. Although, from the surgeons point of view, this may explain the lack of interest in the microscopic examination of femoral heads after total hip replacement, it does not excuse it. The possibility of an earlier diagnosis leading to a non-replacement, therapeutic intervention should change this attitude.

The histopathological examination lends certainty to the diagnosis in most cases. Our experiences are based not only on femoral heads taken at arthroplasty but also on core biopsy, either taken alone or in a systemic fashion in the course of osteotomies for arthrosis. Even from a macroscopic point of view, by examining the excised pieces, the individuality of the two diseases can be distinguished, even down to their end-stages. Slabs of the femoral head, cut in the coronal section, can be superimposed on a phantom outline of the femoral head which approximately reconstitutes their original contour. The degree of wear and deformity is quite different in appearance. In the arthroses, the sphere flattens .3 cm on the average while widening .5 cm by marginal osteophyte proliferation. In the necroses, on the other hand, the superior deformity is three to five times greater (1.6 cm on the average) with insignificant marginal proliferation. This fact alone emphasizes the destructive nature of the necroses. Arthrosic wear is, therefore, limited, more regular, progressive, and mainly arising from a superficial necrosis of the contact area proportional to the functional demands. This is wear and tear produced by friction of the bony surface which is devoid of a protective cartilage covering (Table XIX). The wear of the necrotic head is more abrupt and extensive, pro-

TABLE XIX

DIFFERENTIAL DIAGNOSIS BETWEEN ARTHROSIS INFLAMMATORY ARTHRITIS,
AND NECROSIS BY MEASUREMENT OF THE REMOVED FEMORAL HEAD (Meric [307])

	osteoarthrosis	*osteonecrosis*	*inflammatory joint disease*
	Segment A =0.3 cm	Segment A =1.6 cm	Segment A =0.4 cm
	Diameter B + 0.5 cm	Diameter B essentially normal	Diameter B essentially normal
Typical form			

Segment A—height difference between the pathological specimen and an estimation of the original height as measured in a prolongation of the axis of the neck

Diameter B—diameter of the pathological specimen measured on a line across the geometrical center of the original femoral head and perpendicular to the long axis of the neck

duced by destruction in the depth of the tissue with collapse of the section of the femoral head at the level of the pressure cone. The destruction of cartilage is secondary and related both to the subchondral ischemia and the incongruency of the surfaces (Fig. 98).

From a microscopic point of view, the differential diagnosis between arthrosis and necrosis is also quite easy with examination of the biopsy specimens. Arthrosis shows evidence of stasis, edema, medullary fibrosis, chondroid islands, and thickening of trabeculae, but it never shows either extensive medullary necrosis except for small islands on the surface. Sequestrum formation never occurs. The appearance of stasis and medullary fibrosis accounts for the circulatory abnormalities demonstrated on the hemodynamic tests (Fig. 99). Very rarely, one encounters borderline cases which are difficult to interpret. Arthrosis and necrosis can, therefore, usually be easily differentiated on a histologic slide, and this is a view not clearly expressed in publications on this question.

histological point of view even if hemodynamic and isotopic investigations seem to underline certain points in common. Nevertheless, even for these diagnostic modalities, there are statistical differences between the two conditions. Thermography and oxymetry findings presented earlier also confirm their individual identity. Differential diagnosis, however, based on a single x-ray is unreliable and deceptive. The same picture may be called destructive coxar-

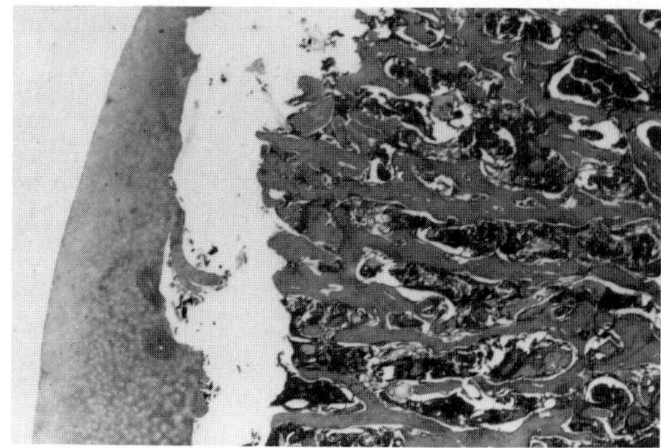

Fig.98.—Necrosis of the femoral head. Cartilaginous sequestrum of irregular height with cellular changes. Beneath the cleavage plane, the dense sequestrum reveals complete bone marrow necrosis.

CONCLUSIONS

Arthrosis and necrosis are two separate conditions. They are fundamentally different from a throsis by some and necrosis by others. Streda[431] reported 161 radiologic pictures of "sequestra" on 235 cases of severe coxarthrosis for an incidence of 68.5%; however, in these cases, there was no histological confirmation of necrosis. Therefore, these were not truly sequestra but only gave such a radiologic appearance.

How should we classify the cartilage lesion in the particular type of necrosis represented in ischemic coxopathy? Is it an arthrosis secondary to vascular origin or simply ischemic chondrosis? We prefer the second concept. There is, however, a place for true mechanical arthrosis with an ischemic necrosis as we have described in relation to trauma and dysplasia.

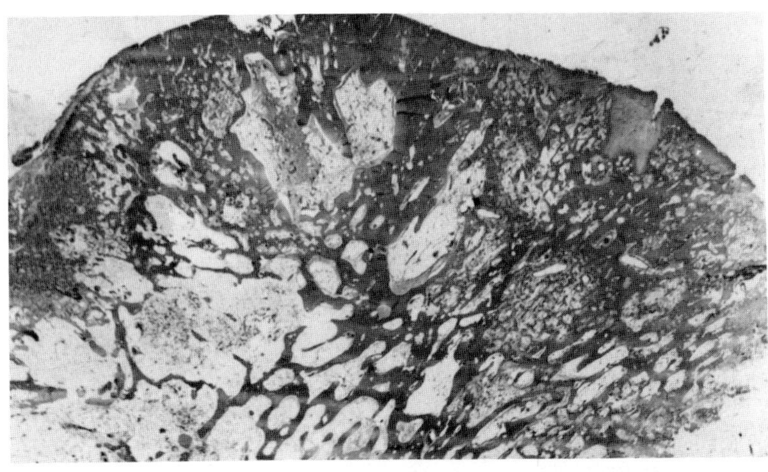

Fig.99.—Macrophotography of histological slide of an arthrosic femoral head.

A: Deformity of the outline with almost complete disappearance of the cartilage; multiple fibrous cysts and sclerosis in the weight-bearing cone.

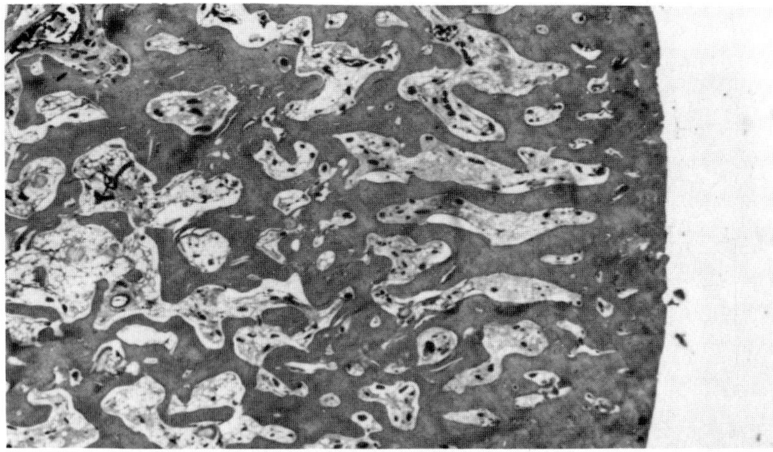

B: Complete eburnation with sclerosis of the weight-bearing cone and vascular stasis in the narrowed bone marrow spaces.

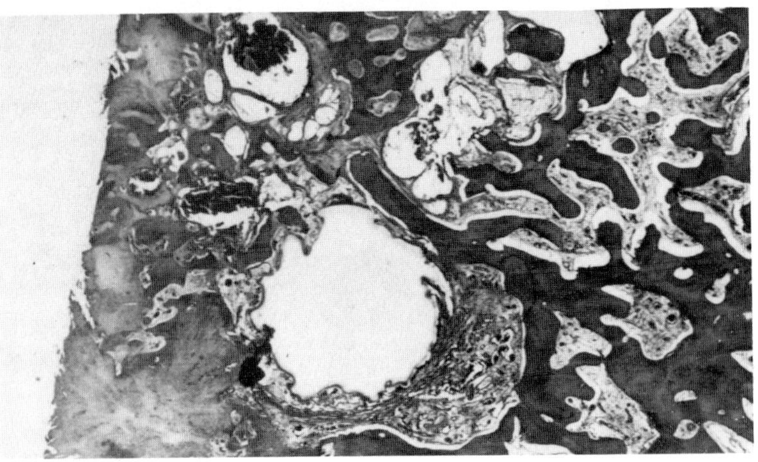

C: Magnification of a cyst lined by a layer of fibrous tissue. The vascular channels are engorged. The cyst is separated from the abraded surface by a fibrous plug.

CHAPTER VII

BONE NECROSIS OF KNOWN ETIOLOGY

The next two chapters detail that which is known about specific kinds of bone necroses. In Chapter VII, the causal relationships are clear and generally widely accepted. In Chapter VIII, a causal relationship can be implied, but the relationship is unclear or perhaps, in some instances, even disputed. These two chapters are based upon our personal experience and do not include the problem of necrosis in children (post-fracture following CDH reduction or Perthes' Disease). For the same reason, certain classes will be discussed in more detail than others, e.g., arteriopathy is much more frequent in our series than caisson disease and sickle-cell anemia. Although both of these later conditions comprise clear-cut examples of bone necrosis, they are simply not frequent in our area, and our experiences are limited.

MAJOR TRAUMA

Included in this section are fractures of the femoral neck, dislocations of the hip, and fractures of the acetabulum. Although we are not including a great number of details from our statistics involving secondary post-traumatic necroses, we are discussing them in this chapter because they constitute an important source of information concerning bone necrosis. For instance, we know the exact time of injury and often the type of vascular lesion as well, e.g., the ligamentum teres is ruptured in dislocations. The transosseous metaphyseal pathways are disrupted in undisplaced fracture of the femoral neck, and the superior epiphyseal vessels are interrupted in displaced femoral neck fractures or with impacted valgus fractures. To some extent, the topographical systematisation of the vascular lesion has, for the study of necrosis in general, almost the same value as in the experimental situation. This gives us information on the frequency, the radiologic and clinical evolution, and prognosis, as well as opportunities for hemodynamic, metabolic, radioisotopic, and histopathologic evaluation. In some cases, also, whole femoral heads are retrieved at the time of arthroplastic procedures. Any femoral neck fracture or hip dislocation is equivalent to an experimental ischemia. There is really no better model in a pathological study of the effects of ischemia on all the parameters that we have so far discussed.

FRACTURES OF THE FEMORAL NECK

A survey of the world literature concerning the statistical frequency of necrosis following femoral neck fracture averages at about 30%[62,86,285,308,358]. However, it must be understood in this review that the diagnosis of necrosis has been made by x-ray alone. Therefore, the percentage is based solely on radiographic criteria. We have already seen how deficient these criteria are in the diagnosis of necrosis. Therefore, the percentage represents only a gross evaluation of advanced disease. Authors who have reported their criteria on histopathological or biological criteria report a much higher incidence. Sevitt[393] found 21 necroses in 24 cases assessed at autopsy. Woodhouse[469] documented decrease in vascularization, as judged by tetracycline uptake, in two-thirds of his cases. Similarly, Boyd and Calandruccio[62] observed a decrease in radioactive phosphorus fixation by autoradiography in two-thirds of their cases. Others have reported similar findings in the 65-66% range[88,185,344]. This again confirms the deficiency in radiographic evaluation for frequency of ischemic complications of fracture. Contrary to what might be expected in the young patient, the "benignity" of the fracture and choice of treatment are no guarantee against necrosis. The percentage is the same. Functional investigation of the bone may offer some usefulness. Arnoldi and Linderholm[27] systematically studied IMP in the head and in the femoral neck in 92 cases of fresh fractures of the femoral neck after reduction. In fresh cases, the tip of the trocar must be placed at a distance of at least 2 cm from the fracture line. In 25 extracapsular pertrochanteric fractures, the tracing from the head and neck both exhibited similar pulsatile tracings, indicating an intact arterial and venous circulation. In 16 valgus fractures of the femoral neck, all the tracings had pulsatile pressure recordings, but in four cases, the head pressure was much higher (> 20 mm Hg) than pressure at the level of the neck. This suggested venous blockage within the head. On 61 varus fractures of the femoral neck, 36 showed intact arterial vascularization in terms of pulsatile pressures, while 15 (29%) exhibited a tracing in the head without pulsation. In seven cases only, there was complete blockage of the arterial pathway, i.e., tracings with no pulsations and very low pressures. In the other eight cases, there was only a suggestion of decrease in the arterial pulsation associated with venous obstruction. In summary, 29.8% of the femoral neck fractures showed signs of circulatory disturbances with venous abnormalities appearing to these authors more frequently than arterial interruptions.

These studies were done on fresh fractures. It would be interesting to repeat the same study with longer follow-ups, as we have had the occasion to do in some cases two or three years after fracture. In one such case, although there were no radiographic signs (Stage I), there was both pain and increased IMP in the femoral head. Reticular necrosis of the marrow extended from the fracture line to the end of the core specimen. It appears, however, that in much longer follow-ups, even with a well-delineated sequestrum, the pressure within the head, and outside the sequestrum, may become normal, as we have seen in one case of post-traumatic necrosis four years after fracture.

Venography—The posterior vein of the femoral neck is usually absent and stasis is present in the head for a variable duration. These results do not have absolute value since 20% of the cases demonstrating necrosis had normal intraosseous venograms. Venography is, however, significant and is a definite way of demonstrating both the blocked venous drainage and the prolonged stasis of the contrast medium. Hulth[210,211,212,213] has given an account of his technique using this method to determine viability of the femoral head after fracture of the femoral neck. Two milliliters of contrast material is introduced in the center of the head three days following fracture.

The venogram is said to be positive if the normal drainage veins are injected of which there are two possible routes of drainage—one going through the ligamentum teres or obturator vein and the other, through the circumflex and femoral veins. Negative venograms consisted of non-visualization of the extraosseous veins. In 43 cases, 12 negative venograms were all associated with subsequent necrosis. Ten necroses occurred, however, with 31 positive venograms. Harrison[198] arrived at similar conclusions, recommending that venography be carried out 10 days after the initial surgical procedure. Eberle[131,132,133], with an experience of 280 venograms following femoral neck fracture, arrived at similar conclusions finding a 90% incidence of necrosis with negative visualization of the extraosseous veins.

Radioisotope uptake—Several different radioactive tracers have been used, including the following: P^{32} measured in bone by a sensor following intravenous injection[61,62,448], I^{131} measured at the level of the heart following intraosseous injection[218], Na^{24} measuring decay-curve at the groin following injection into the head[260], and Sr^{85} given as an intravenous injection prior to surgery and comparing isotopic fixation counts at both the trochanteric level and the head per unit weight with the specimens being taken at the time of surgery[86]. The latter method gives a ratio between femoral head and trochanteric counts. On 30 cases of fresh fracture using this technique in 23 successful applications, 14 cases had a head/trochanter ratio greater than one. With a follow-up of one to three years, all 14 have healed without necrosis. Nine cases had a head/trochanter ratio of less than one-half. Eight cases developed necrosis and one a non-union, although, on the latter, the head specimen had not been examined.

DISLOCATION OF THE HIP

According to all authors, fracture-dislocations result in a much higher incidence of necrosis than simple dislocation[118,442]. Early reduction is the best preventive treatment. If reduction is done more than 24 hours after the dislocation, there is nearly a 100% incidence of necrosis, while, if it is done in the first few hours, the percentage reported ranges from 20 to 30%[428]. Stewart and Milford reported 14 cases of necrosis on 90 non-operated hips (15.5%) and 11 necroses on 28 operated cases (40%). However, these authors classify sclerosis of the femoral head and narrowing of the joint space as arthrosis and not necrosis. We can not justify this conclusion of diagnosis without a biopsy, and it is quite probable that, in fact, their percentage of necrosis is much higher. In our own series of 96 cases (32 simple dislocations and 64 fracture dislocations), we have observed 30% necrosis in the simple dislocations and 54.6% in the fracture dislocations. Among these cases are included six cases of osteonecrosis at Stage I which have only been diagnosed by means of the functional investigation of bone. Seventeen cases of post-dislocation necrosis (5 simple dislocations and 12 fracture dislocations) were evaluated by IMP measurement from two months to 9 years after the injury. The baseline IMP was normal in seven cases at the level of the trochanter. In five of these, the saline test was positive. In the other two, the IMP in the head was very high. It was in one of these cases that our all time highest IMP, following stress test, was recorded at 120 mm Hg!

Venography - Venography before and after reduction has demonstrated objectively functional obstruction of the venous drainage either by torsion or compression. If the reduction is too late, irreversible thrombosis is likely to occur. This explains the better prognosis in those cases reduced in the first few hours and immediately aspirated. Occasionally, we have seen subchondral pooling of dye in the superolateral corner which suggests impaction fractures of the trabeculae in this region which are not evident radiologically. The elasticity of the articular cartilage in the subchondral bone would mask the impact at the time of dislocation by recovering its overall form. The usual venogram showed drainage via the circumflex vessels, although there may be abnormalities in both the course and caliber of the vessels; the ligamentum teres vessels did not visualize. Eberle[133] found a 50% incidence of necrosis (in cases which failed to show normal venous drainage).

ACETABULAR FRACTURES

In a recent report on 302 operated fractures of the acetabulum, Judet and Letournel[238] observed only 21 cases of necrosis (6.95%) with a follow-up of three to 18 months and 16 cases of arthrosis on 244 follow-ups (6%). It is possible that these percentages will become higher with time. In our personal series of 60 cases of acetabular fracture, we have seen a 35% incidence of radiologically evident necrosis. This rises to 50% if one includes those cases which could be considered questionable (six cases corresponding to Stage I). The frequency of osteonecrosis was higher in patients over 50 and in patients with more serious fractures.

Intramedullary pressure - This has been carried out in 12 cases with seven normal baseline pressures in the trochanteric region. However, in these seven cases, elevated pressure could be recorded after the stress test or by measuring the pressure in the femoral head (five cases). In four cases of normal baseline head pressure, two exhibited positive stress tests. The two with normal stress tests were in Stage III. However, separation of the subchondral bone of the head can lower intramedullary pressure by placing the cancellous epiphyseal tissue in communication with the articular cavity.

Venography carried out in nine cases showed stasis of the contrast material in the head with absence of filling of the posterior veins of the neck but only rarely with diaphyseal reflux.

SUMMARY

The study of necrosis after major trauma leads us to the following conclusions. The functional investigation of the hip will take on an increasingly important role in detecting the preradiologic types of necrosis and those with non-pathognomonic radiographic changes. Radioisotopic and uptake studies with the Sr[87] at the stage of probable necrosis, seen several months after trauma, showed parallel and overlapping results with those of the functional investigation of the hip. There was increased uptake in all cases of necrosis in whatever radiologic stage or histologic type. As with functional exploration of the hip, this examination allows diagnosis in the preradiologic stage (Stage I). Type of trauma and time interval do not appear to have any particular relationship to the validity of the radioisotopic scanning investigation.

Certain clinical signs should also alert the clinician to the possibility of complication of the injury by necrosis. Increased pain and limp, instead of the usual steady improvement following trauma within the first year, is the most important sign. There also may be a considerable time interval between the trauma and the subsequent necrosis. We have observed 22 cases with necrosis more than five years following injury. We do not feel this time interval should be used for an argument to deny the responsibility of the injury for the necrosis. There is often a clear dissociation between both degree of pain, which can be considerable, and the minimal limitation of movement. Relative increased density of the femoral head, which is observed a few months following fracture of the neck, is probably secondary to vascular exclusion of the head as well as regional post-traumatic osteoporosis of those parts which remain well vascularized. Any difficulty associated with the metallic implants should also be interpreted in light of possible ischemic complication. This can be documented if the functional investigation of the hip is done, in these cases, before removal of the internal fixation devices. Intraosseous hypothermia with a temperature of less than 36°C in the head is also compatible with necrosis[355].

The problem of post-traumatic arthrosis, as well as that of arthrosis in general, needs to be completely reviewed in light of the functional investigation in the post-traumatic situation. There are several possible combinations and permutations, since either the cartilage or the blood supply may be injured singly or in combination. With a pure cartilage lesion, the functional investigation is normal. When the functional investigation is positive in post-traumatic arthrosis, it is difficult to say whether the cartilage lesion is secondary to the bone necrosis (ischemic post-traumatic coxopathy) or whether the two lesions, circulatory and cartilagenous, are coincidently associated and both secondary to the injury. We believe that all three of these combinations are possible. We have seen examples of post-traumatic necrosis in the femoral head which occur late and are associated with progressive joint space narrowing, a condition which seems to be quite similar to the ischemic coxopathy described earlier. Histological data from Jacqueline[220,222] confirms this cartilage pathology following fractures of the femoral neck.

CAISSON DISEASE

Bone necrosis is the most common pathological manifestation when the human body is subjected to compressed air for varying intervals of time. Divers who are compelled to breath compressed air while working under water are the individuals most often affected. Uncontrolled resurfacing, i.e., rapid decompression, results in nitrogen gas coming out of solution in both blood and interstitial tissue. This produces gas emboli or extrinsic compression of the vessels within the bone marrow, both resulting in vascular obstruction. Faulty decompression may be experienced acutely either as painful episodes, the "bends," or as a late sequellae, as in osteonecrosis. Prolonged dives seem to be particularly involved, and the joints involved usually include the hips and shoulders. A third of the cases are bilateral. The interval between episode and clinical manifestation may vary from a few months to several years. The present regulations of the Workmen's Compensation Board accepts ten years without contest. In France, the most recent works are those of Jaffres et al[225], and Fournier and Jullien[169]. The latter workers did an exhaustive study on the radiologic manifestations based on 200 cases, describing essentially the same features that we have observed in the non-traumatic INFH.

There are, however, some radiologic features which seem to be more common in decompression-related necroses. Periosteal appositional new bone formation seems to be more common than in the primary necroses. This has also been noted with necrosis associated with sickle-cell disease. Perhaps

this is related to the more massive ischemia in which anoxia and increased intramedullary pressure play an important role. Fournier and Jullien[169] noted that joint line changes occur very late. We have been impressed, however, by their frequency. To be convinced, one has merely to measure the joint line in all films presented by these authors and note in over 50% of the cases, even in an early stage, that joint space narrowing is present either globally or segmentally in the superomedial or superolateral areas. This suggests a local and early change in the cartilage, the evolution of which is probably very slow and may be misleading with regard to the true nature of cartilage involvement. In contrast to other forms of bone necrosis, the radiologic signs frequently appear to be present in a preclinical phase of the disease in a great number of cases. Although even in the other forms of necrosis of bone, asymptomatic radiologic lesions exist, particularly in cases of bilateral disease, although they are not especially common except in decompression necrosis. Amako[4] in systemically examining 450 divers from Ohura, found 70.6% incidence of asymptomatic radiologic lesions, he also pointed out that symptoms exist in 19.3% of the cases without radiologic lesions. This corresponds to our Stage I cases. His four-stage classification is similar to ours, and he advocates bone grafting in the beginning of Stage II before collapse of the epiphysis. His histologic observations are similar, as well, with marrow necrosis and relative preservation of the cartilage which, nevertheless, may also show some evidence of necrosis.

SICKLE-CELL ANEMIA

In this condition, a hereditary hemoglobinopathy characterized by the presence of hemoglobin-S in the blood, is associated with bone necrosis. This pathologic hemoglobin is the result of a genetic defect which is transmitted as a Mendelian dominant. It mainly affects the Negro race of the tropical region of Central Africa between the 15th parallel of the North latitude and 20th parallel of the South latitude. In the Congo forest, 40% of the population is affected. Because of population migrations, it is also encountered in Southeast Asia, India, the Mediterranean Basin, the West Indies, and the North American continent. With the homozygotic type, a very serious and progressive anemia results in few patients living after the age of 40. With the heterozygous type, with at least 50% of the normal hemoglobin-A in the blood (sickle-cell trait), there are usually long latency periods which may be interrupted by painful paroxysmal hemolytic crises. These painful crises are usually related to phases of sickling in which the red cells become deformed, usually in the presence of low oxygen, producing blockage of small vessels, thrombosis, and infarctions. The sickling is reversible if oxygen content is increased, and the episodes may vary considerably in both intensity and duration. Either homozygotic or heterozygotic types may be affected with sickle-cell osteonecrosis.

At the University of Kinshasa, bone crises accounted for 20% of the consultations associated with sickle-cell disease, which was more than for anemia (13%) or gastroenteritis (17%). Kabakele[241] devoted his thesis to the early diagnosis of sickle-cell related bone necrosis. He was able to distinguish two separate types of osteoarticular manifestations of sickle-cell disease. The acute manifestations either presented with articular localization masquerading as a pseudorheumatic type or with a bone location with pain in the long bones. Seventy percent of cases initially manifest their disease with the latter type of osteo-articular complaint, usually presenting with negative x-rays in spite of the intensity of the clinical signs. This manifestation sometimes was accompanied by very marked pain and fusiform swelling of the extremity. When visiting Dakar, we were astonished by the paucity of radiographic signs in spite of the dramatic symptoms whereas several months later the same patients demonstrated structural changes, including microcysts, periosteal new bone formation, and, later on, sequestra. This seemed to have a striking similarity to the findings in Stage I of osteonecrosis, and we suggested that they carry out functional investigations of bone as both a diagnostic and a therapeutic tool. This has been done by Kabakele, at the National University of Zaire[241], who has been able to confirm, step by step, all which we have published concerning these Stage I cases encountered in France[153].

The chronic presentation usually represents epiphyseal osteonecrosis, affecting mainly the hip and, less frequently, the shoulder or other joints. Chung and Ralston[91] presented 13 cases and a review of the literature concerning necrosis of the femoral head. In SS disease, Cockshott[93] found no cases in his 120 patients. Siegling[414] found 4% incidence in 170 cases with SS disease while Tanaka[435] reported 12% on 51 cases. Lejeune et al.[269] collected 71 cases from the world literature, adding a single additional case. In SC disease, reported statistics varied from 20 to 68% incidence of bone necrosis.

In addition to the typical metaphyseal/epiphyseal localization for other forms of bone necrosis, there are several other skeletal abnormalities which are characteristic of bone changes associated with sickle-cell anemia. In common with other congenital hemolytic anemias, cortical-thinning, enlargement of the medullary cavity, osteoporosis, and thickening of the cranial vault with a brush border are seen. Vertebral changes include diffuse osteoporosis and flattening of the vertebral bodies, sometimes giving the typical codfish appearance (80% of the cases). The long bones may also show osteosclerosis with thickening of the cortex and narrowing of the bone marrow (particularly in the adult). Such changes are usually seen in the tibia, fibula, and femur. Bone infarctions may also be seen characterized by radiolucent lacunae surrounding an opaque bone island. Periosteal new bone formation may also be observed in the metaphyses. For many authors, the typical, even diagnostic, criteria of sickle-cell anemia combines vertebral osteoporosis with localized bone infarction.

There is, in addition, a peculiar affectation of bone which seems to find expression mainly in sickle-cell patients. The sites of bone ischemia and infarction seem particularly susceptible to a Salmonella-type osteomyelitis. This adds to the severity of the necrosis. It is possible that early preventive treatment of either the bone crisis or the necrosis in the early stages could prevent some of the osteomyelitic sequelae, thereby improving the prognosis.

Illustrative Case 15. - Serge L..., a 21-year-old black male from Guadalupe, had the diagnosis of sickle-cell anemia made at the age of one with the onset of painful nodular swelling in the hands and feet. Since then, he has had recurrent episodes of joint pain affecting mainly the hips, knees, and spine. He had never had any respiratory, genital, urinary, neuropsychiatric, or hemolytic problems. He presented on February 23, 1974 with a history of pain in his right hip, occurring in a mild crisis-like pattern mainly at night. Physical examination showed only a slight limitation of movement, and the patient was only moderately functionally limited. The x-ray showed Stage III necrosis of the right hip with seqestrum formation and collapse of the superior pole. Laboratory exam showed a very strong sickle-cell test with 95% hemoglobin-S in 5% hemoglobin-F. A functional investigation was carried out, recording 100 mm Hg IMP in the trochanter and 72 mm Hg in the head, whereas in the sequestrum, the pressure was 50 mm Hg and non-pulsating. Venograms showed severe stasis. The core biopsy demonstrated necrosis of Type 3 and 4, whereas the cartilage over the sequestrum showed degenerated and necrotic chondrocytes in decreased numbers mainly in the superficial layers (Fig. 100). On the left side, the intramedullary pressure measured 60 mm Hg in the trochanter and 72 mm Hg in the head, with venography showing stasis in the head. A core biopsy carried out showed Type 3 necrosis that was much less extensive than on the right hand side. Surgery to the right hip included a pedicle bone graft plus a Voss-type tenotomy. Follow-up at three years showed full, painless range of movement and a patient without symptoms.

This case is an excellent demonstration of the concept of latent pathology. The paradoxical opposition of a clinically and radiologically normal hip, in spite of major hemodynamic changes, with unques-

tionable osteonecrosis clearly establishes not only the authenticity of Stage I but also the existence of a completely asymptomatic Stage I. It is also interesting, from a more general point of view, that the electron-microscopic examination of the cartilage from the right hip showed evidence of degeneration of the cartilage covering the sequestrum, suggesting the ischemic origin of the cartilage necrosis and, therefore, the role of bone circulation in the nutrition of the cartilage.

Kabakele[241] was able to carry out 65 functional investigations in sickle-cell osteonecrosis, particularly in the femur and tibia. He also demonstrated this complication of sickle-cell disease in Stage I (bone pain) with no radiologic signs. Two examples from his series demonstrate the use for this new diagnostic approach.

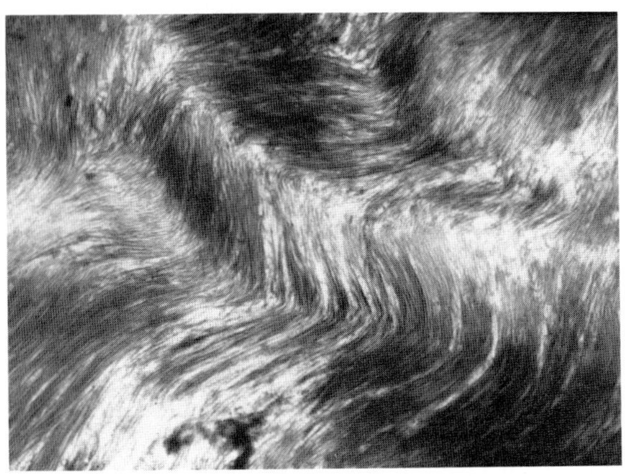

A: Superficial layer (C1) with very marked fibrillar density.

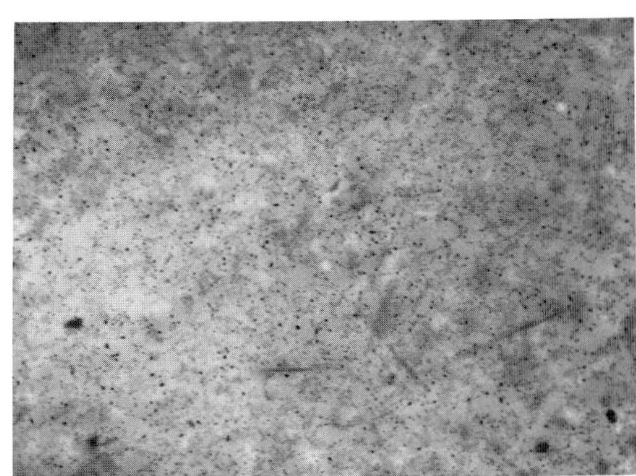

B: Middle layer with complete disappearance of the fibrillar material.

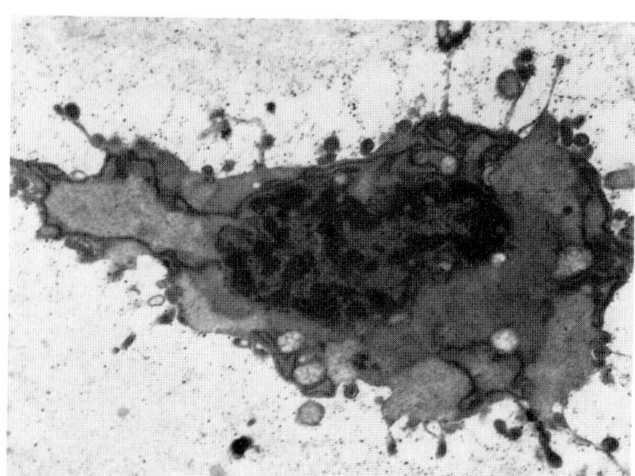

C: Degenerated chondrocyte of the middle layer (C2): amorphous aspect of the cytoplasm with disapperance of the organelles.

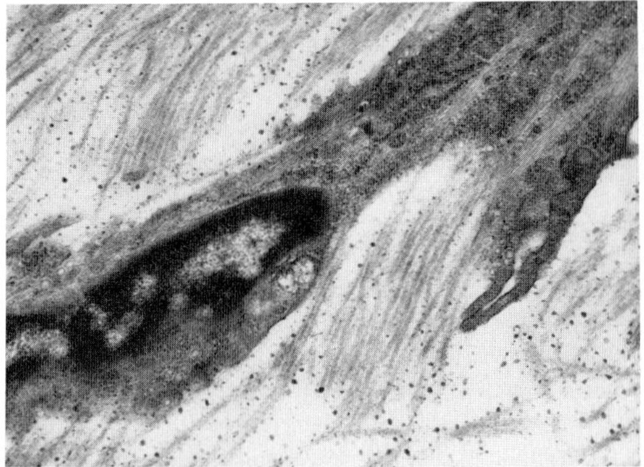

D: Degenerated chondrocyte of the superficial areas; partial disappearance of the nuclear membrane. Notice the continuity of the cytoplasmic fibrils with the extracellular fibers.

Fig. 100.—Electron microscopic aspect of the cartilage overlying the sequestrum.

Illustrative Case 16. - A three and one-half-year-old black girl with SS disease was presented initially at the age of one and one-half with swelling of the hands and feet. In 1970, she had three crises with hyperthermia, cough, dyspnea, hepatomegaly, and abdominal pain. At the last crisis, pain in both knees and severe pain in the left femur appeared. The x-ray was normal with the exception of slight periostitis. Hemodynamic exploration of the left femur showed baseline intramedullary pressure of the distal metaphysis at 40 mm Hg with a stress test to 72 mm Hg. Venography showed spectacular stasis with pooling of the dye along the whole length of the diaphysis (Fig. 101). Bone biopsy showed extensive marrow necrosis with areas of fibrosis and trabecular necrosis. In follow-up, the pain disappeared the evening of surgery, and, since then, the patient has been crisis-free on the operated femur.

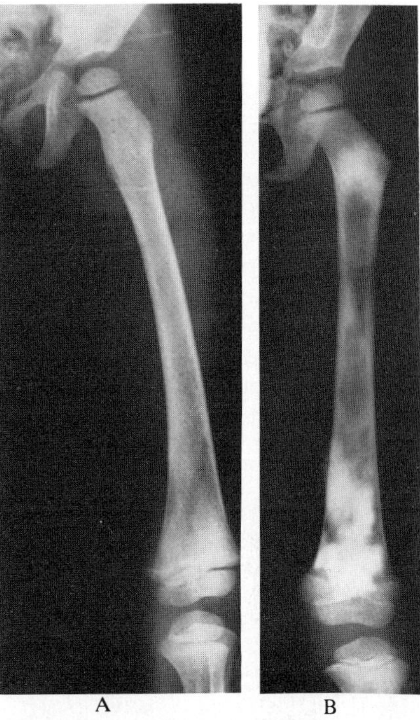

Fig. 101.—Case 16. A: X-rays of the normal appearing left femur. B: Massive intraosseous stasis.

Illustrative Case 17. - This is a 15-year-old black female with SS disease. At the age of nine, the patient had a fracture of the left femoral neck after a fall. At age 13, an episode of bone pain with hyperpyrexia was experienced in both hips. In 1970, three crises affected the hips, both legs, and the chest. Hemodynamic exploration of the tibia revealed a baseline diaphyseal medullary pressure of 20 mm Hg with a negative stress test. Phlebography demonstrated considerable diaphyseal stasis with absence of efferent veins (Fig. 102). Bone biopsy revealed trabecular necrosis and almost total marrow necrosis with small hemorrhagic foci. Immediately after the operation, the patient had complete disappearance of pain from the operated site. In spite of occasional episodes of arthralgia around the knee, the operated tibia has not been affected in subsequent episodes.

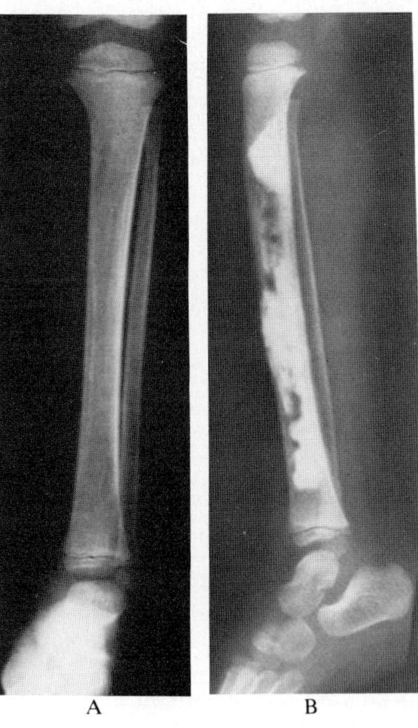

Fig. 102.—Case 17. A: Normal appearing tibia. B: Massive intramedullary stasis of the whole tibial diaphysis.

POST-IRRADIATION
BONE NECROSIS

This etiology and the cortisone-induced bone necrosis constitute the two most important and interesting groups of iatrogenic osteonecrosis. This is far from a "historical" section. Although there has been considerable improvement in radiation techniques since this remarkable therapeutic tool was introduced by Walsh in 1897[459], this complication of anti-tumor therapy has not yet been eradicated. Ewing[138] described "radiation osteitis" in detail in 1926. This is a good term since the necrosis which is probably the most important complication of radiation is accompanied and followed by dynamic and progressive changes of the bone, producing a complex composite of local changes. One has only to recall that sometimes reconstitution of bone follows a well-conducted irradiation for a bone metastasis to realize that the effect of radiation is not only necrosis but that it also allows, and even stimulates, osteogenesis.

Bone necrosis most often follows treatment of genital cancer in women, including the cervix, body of the uterus, ovaries, fallopian tubes, and vagina. For this reason, clinical patient cases mainly involve the pelvis. The irradiation usually includes the pelvic lymph nodes and the bony structures surrounding the pelvis, which are often commonly a part of the target area. Bone tissue appears to be particularly vulnerable because of its high coefficient of x-ray absorption, which is two times higher than soft tissues. This is due to the high concentration of particles with a high atomic number, namely calcium and phosphorus. The greater the total dose received, the greater the danger of radionecrosis. Baclesse[33] studied fractures of the femoral neck following irradiation for lesions of the cervix, encountering eight fractures in 100 patients treated by intensive radiotherapy with total doses from 3,900 to 4,300 rads. On the other hand, Kottmeier[257] reported no fractures of the neck with lower doses in the range of 2,000 rads. The percentage of obvious radiologic bone lesions rarely reaches 6%. Baclasse[33] reported an incidence of 0.58% on 2,163 patients, while Peck[340] reported an incidence of 2.7% on 1,027 patients.

Since 1960, the use of cobalt therapy raised the hopes of seeing this complication disappear completely. With Cobalt[60], the absorption of radiation by the bone tissue is less than with radiation emitted by lower energy machines. However, radiation through multiple ports produced a central nucleus of an extremely high dose which may coincide with the bony pelvis[128]. In fact, there are bone necroses with cobalt therapy, and their incidence is not very different from radionecrosis following conventional radio-therapy. Lalanne and Fajbisowicz[261] compared two series of patients finding 2.5% osteonecrosis following conventional radiotherapy and 2.1% following cobalt therapy. Delouche et al.[120] had similar findings with an incidence of 2.37% of 821 patients treated by cobalt therapy. Although the percentages are similar, it is clear that the higher depth doses are being delivered by cobalt therapy.

It must also be recognized that the percentages reported are obviously less than the true incidence since the above authors are only reporting on radiologically obvious lesions, and it is certain that all histologic lesions of bone necrosis are not visible on radiographs. Radiologic evaluation and clinical examination, obviously, will miss a great number of histologic lesions, the incidence of which remains to be studied.

Radiographic Findings

Post-irradiation fracture of the femoral neck was the first radiographic abnormality to be reported. It is usually a fracture of a very special type, localized subcapitally, progressive, incomplete, or, at least, often impacted. The fracture line is visible as a notch at the superior border of the femoral neck near the head and extending for a few millimeters into the bone. The head angulates inferiorly, resulting in a coxa vara with impaction of the femoral neck into the lower part of the head. The bone changes consist of both the development of the alteration of radiolucent and radiodense zones within the femoral head and neck and some disorganization of the trabecular pattern. The favorable prognosis of these impacted fractures will be reviewed in a later section.

It is only more recently that we have recognized aspects of radiation necrosis which are similar to the idiopathic necroses of the femoral head. A central area of sclerosis with superior concavity may or may not be associated with collapse of the superior outline of the head. These are typical of the features of Stage II and III of the idiopathic necroses. When there is only slight calcification of the head, it is difficult to be certain that one is dealing with bone necrosis. In such circumstances, it is only the functional exploration of bone that permits this confirmation (Case 20).

Acetabular lesions are less often reported and, perhaps, indeed, are less common. However, Delouche et al.[120] reported 11 cases. The diagnosis can be assumed when the acetabulum appears abnormally radiodense or spontaneously fractured. Frequently, these two features co-exist. The site of fracture can be either in the floor or in the roof of the acetabulum. Acetabular lesions are often associated with other pelvic lesions. The prognosis is not always favorable, particularly if the patient continues with weight-bearing, producing a protrusion of the femoral head into the ilium.

Advanced lesions of the ischiopubic rami[373], featuring sclerosis and fracture lines with or without displacement and with or without healing by hypertrophic callus, are also seen. However, they usually run a favorable course. Lesions of the sacrum and the sacroiliac joint are more easily missed. They are often simple incidental radiologic findings of sclerosis on one side or the other of the sacroiliac joints. Of course, this represents a late and indirect sign of necrosis.

Other than a fracture of the neck, the hip may show a lesion which gives the appearance of an ischemic coxopathy. In some of our cases, the articular cartilage of the hip was affected as well. A feature which has not previously been sufficiently emphasized. The joint line narrowing may be the only sign, or it may be associated with osteoporosis or sclerosis of the central part of the femoral head. In such instances, one can speak of an ischemic coxopathy. In other instances, one sees collapse of the femoral head and formation of a sequestrum, the typical appearance of the classic Stage IV. In either case, the condition may be even confused with an inflammatory hip disease or arthrosis. The term "postradiotherapy coxarthrosis" used by Meary et al.[306] and Mourgues et al.[323] corresponds to this description.

Clinical Features

Post-irradiation necrosis may either be discovered because the patient experiences pain and disability or the lesions may be incidently encountered on follow-up x-rays. Occasionally, the patient presents with symptoms very suggestive of hip involvement, but the x-rays are normal (Case 20). To us, such presentation suggests at least the possibility of a preradiologic stage of necrosis, but it could also be the earliest stage of a bone metastasis in a patient who has been previously treated for cancer. This is the most common and the most difficult diagnostic problem. The physical finding may be altered from other bony lesions about the pelvic girdle, particularly fractures of the ischiopubic rami. In these cases as well, metastasis should be ruled out. It is obvious that, in such cases, positive diagnosis is essential, since it would be ridiculous to treat a lesion which actually had been produced by previous irradiation with more irradiation simply because metastasis is suspected. In general, with necrosis, the pain diminishes or disappears when weight-bearing is relieved. The radiologic lesions have a tendency to evolve towards healing if there was a fracture and to sclerosis if there was no fracture.

Physical examination can often detect a tender spot in the pelvis at the site of a lesion. In the case of necrosis, there is no surrounding soft tissue swelling. It is helpful that most genital metastases are not of the sclerosing type. On the one hand, radiolucent areas can be produced either by metastasis or by necrosis. Metastasis can be more likely suspected if the outlines are poorly defined, and the bone structure has disappeared. Other physical findings in cases that we have encountered include evidence of lymphatic edema, peau d'orange, and sclerosis of the skin over the abdominal/inguinal region which documents a type of radiodermatitis, indicating the intensity of the irradiation to the skin and suggesting the possibility of underlying bone lesions. When the radiographic and clinical considerations are inconclusive, a needle or core biopsy should be carried out as the most simple and efficient means of arriving at the diagnosis. Post-irradiation bone lesions are like those seen with other idiopathic ischemic necroses, They are not visible radiologically at their onset. In the future, we must attempt to establish the diagnosis in the preradiologic stage. In those cases that we have treated, a method of functional and hemodynamic exploration has proven to be of the same value as in other types of necrosis.

Illustrative Case 18. - Mrs. SOL..., a 72-year-old white female, was treated surgically for carcinoma of the body of the uterus in November, 1968, followed by conventional radiotherapy in two stages, first in March, 1969, and then in September, 1969. She received a total skin dose each time of 3,500 rads per field through a total of four fields, two anterior and two posterior. The second dose was for recurrence of the tumor. In July, 1970, the patient presented with right groin pain and a limp. X-rays at that time showed only increased density of the left S-I joint. Two months later, the patient was hospitalized because of increasing disability. At that time, the right lower extremity was in external rotation, and the range of motion of the hip was very limited. X-rays showed a subcapital fracture of the neck with interomedial displacement of the head and impaction. A needle biopsy of the iliac crest confirmed osteoporosis and bone marrow necrosis, but with no evidence of metastasis. Intramedullary pressure at the level of the trochanter showed a baseline reading of 33 mm Hg with an increase to 60 mm Hg following the injection of 3 ml of saline.

Following one month of bedrest, the pain decreased, and the patient underwent physical therapy and resumed weight-bearing. Nonetheless, the hip remained stiff and slightly painful on weight-bearing. The x-ray in October, 1972, demonstrated significant joint line narrowing, signifying involvement of the articular cartilage.

Illustrative Case 19. - Mrs. PIL..., a 36-year-old white female, had a hysterectomy in July, 1966, followed by intrapelvic radium implantation and cobalt therapy to the left ilio-inguinal region because of carcinoma of the cervix with involvement of the lymphatic nodes. In January, 1967, she had the rapid onset of left groin pain with radiation to the knee. Symptoms were increased by coughing. At the time of initiation of symptoms, the x-ray was normal. She was seen by us for the first time in May, 1972, at which time there was definite limitation of movement of the left hip (flexion to 100°). X-rays revealed a flattening of the superior surface of the femoral head, which was best seen on a lateral view. There were also marginal osteophytes and increased density of the femoral head. The joint space was preserved (Fig. 103). A core biopsy was undertaken on 6-15-72, at which time, IMP was elevated in the head (32 mm Hg) and increased to 40 mm Hg following the stress test. Diffuse medullary necrosis was seen on the histologic section of the removed specimen. The patient has had less pain since the procedure and has had clinical and radiologic stabilization of her condition seven years from the core biopsy (May, 1979).

Fig. 103.—Case 19. A: (1967) Normal x-rays (onset of symptoms). B: (1972) Superior flattening, marginal osteophytes, thickening of the femoral neck, sclerosis of the femoral head, and good joint space. Core depression. C: (1975) Three years later, stabilized by core decompression.

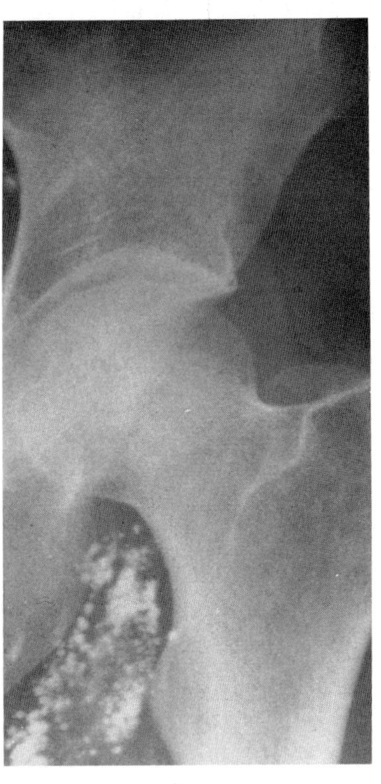 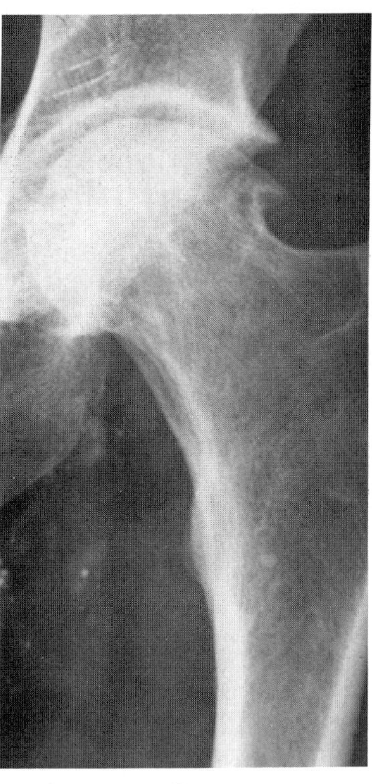 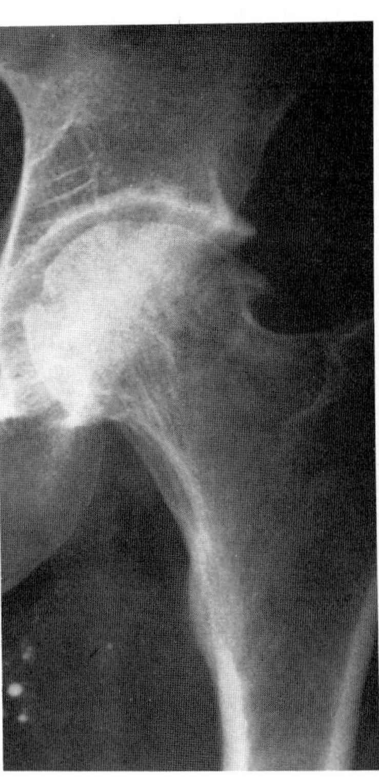

A   B   C

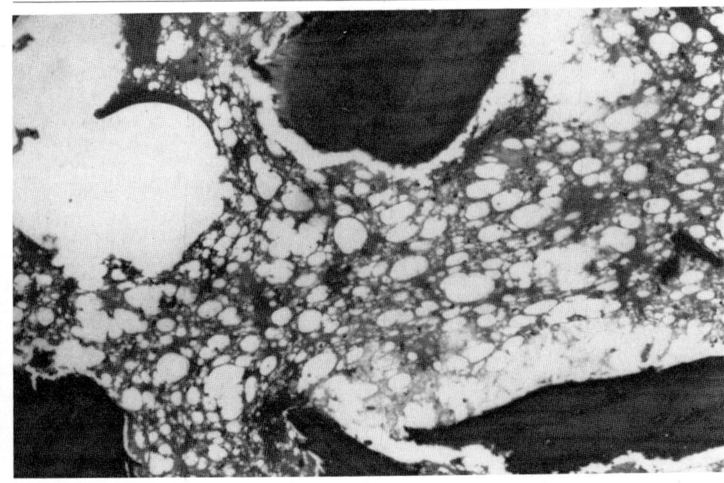

Fig. 103.—D: Histology of the lesions: diffuse eosinophilic reticular necrosis.

D

Illustrative Case 20. (Fig. 104) - Miss FON..., a 35-year-old female, developed carcinoma of the vulva which was treated by surgical excision in 1968. In August, 1969, a local recurrence was treated by cobalt therapy using three fields, right inguinal, left inguinal, and vulvoperineal regions, with a total dose of 6,000 rads. In February, 1970, the patient had the sudden onset of bilateral inguinal pain and difficulty in walking. She was first hospitalized for this in May, 1970. Examination did not reveal any local recurrence. There was skin sclerosis in the pubic, superpubic, and inguinal regions. Examination of the hips showed marked limitation of movement with flexion to only 80° and virtual elimination of abduction and rotation. Radiographs, on the other hand, were completely within normal limits. Hemodynamic exploration was carried out with the right trochanteric IMP recorded at 57 mm Hg with an increase to 70 mm Hg after the stress test. Although this represented a strong suspicion of necrosis, the patient improved

Fig. 104.—Case 20. A: (May 1970) Painful stiffness of both hips with normal x-rays. B: (December 1972) Two months after bilateral forage. Notice the marked lysis of both pubic bones.

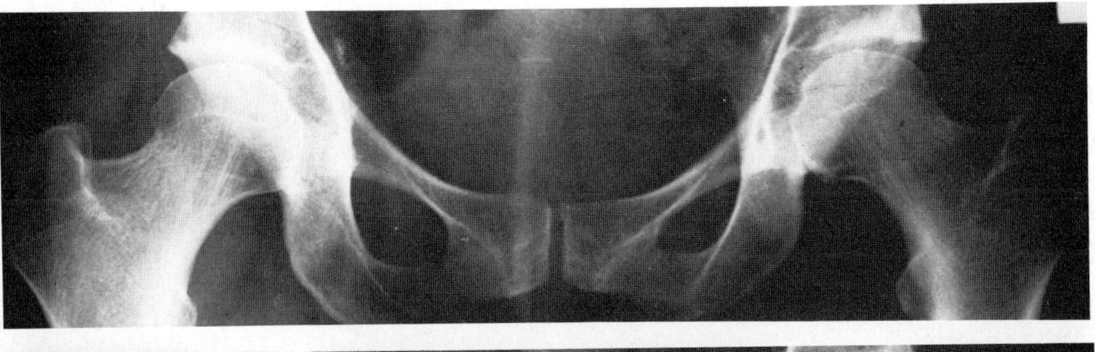

A

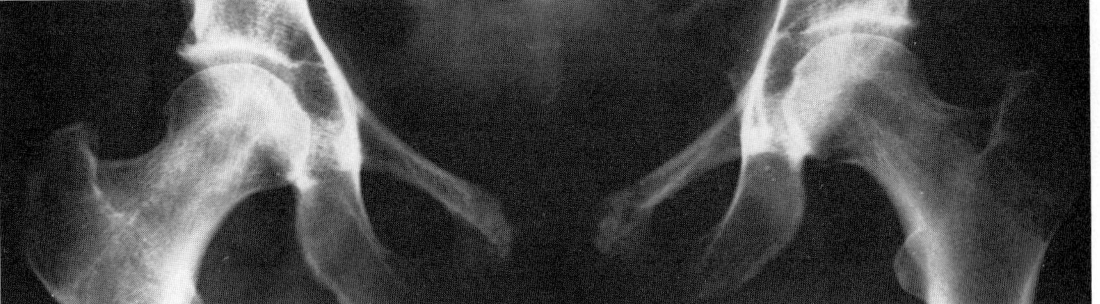

B

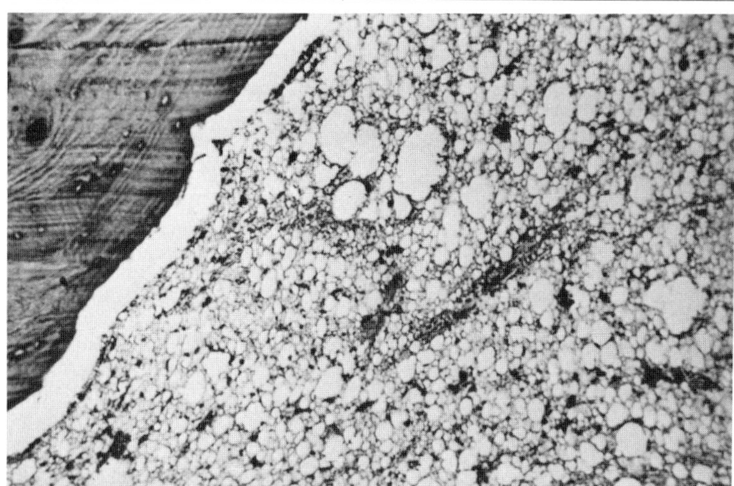

Fig. 104 C: Massive eosinophilic reticular necrosis.

C

considerably after a period of rest and resumed her normal activities for the next two years. In April, 1971, new x-rays of the pelvis showed an important lytic structural lesion of the pubis with separation of the pubic symphysis but with a normal femoral head. In June, 1972, the patient experienced recurrence of bilateral hip pain, and bilateral core decompression was carried out. The histological lesion was typical for bone marrow necrosis Type III (Fig. 104c). After a seven-year follow-up, the patient is asymptomatic without radiologic progression.

Pathophysiology

It is possible to observe at least three different types of lesions in the femoral head: subcapital fracture, necrosis similar to the idiopathic type, and ischemic coxopathy. Each of these could result from separate mechanisms. The exact mechanisms are not well understood. The initial target point of the irradiation may be either cellular or vascular. Any of the cells present may be implicated, including the hematopoietic cells, the fatty marrow as we have observed it, the osteoblasts[111]and, finally, the vessels of bone marrow themselves. Several authors[112,254,284] have demonstrated that irradiation may produce both parietal vascular lesions (sclerosis and calcification) as well as intra-arteriolar thrombosis. Post-irradiation bone necrosis may, therefore, be either primary, i.e., resulting from the direct action of the irradiation on bone marrow and osteoblasts, or secondary to a reduction in arteriolar flow by obliteration of the intramedullary vessels. We should emphasize that the material which we have studied following core biopsy in our patients shows the same typical lesions of those obtained in cases of idiopathic necrosis, particularly the eosinophilic reticular necrosis of the fatty marrow. In most cases, however, necrosis is not complete, which explains the radiologic signs of osteosclerosis and the histologic signs of regeneration. If the radiologic picture of necrosis or ischemic coxopathy is mainly produced by a vascular mechanism, the subcapital fracture is probably secondary to osteopenia due to slowing of bone turnover by direct inhibition of the osteoblasts by the irradiation. In this sense, it is a "stress fracture."

As for the cartilage changes, there may also be two mechanisms for its subsequent demise. Although cartilage tissue is generally held to be radioresistant, there may be subtle changes in the chondrocytes from a direct reaction to the ionizing radiation which then promotes earlier break-down, or the changes in the chondrocytes may be secondary to necrosis of subchondral bone and subsequent alteration in joint mechanics.

BONE NECROSIS OF ARTERIAL ORIGIN

In this section, we will discuss bone necrosis secondary to non-traumatic arterial disease, of which there are three main types. Atherosclerotic lesions with secondary thrombosis and/or emboli are considered as a sequella of hypertension and are best known for sites of localization at the aortic bifurcation, the external iliac, femoral, and popliteal arteries. Inflammatory arteritis is present in such conditions as periarteritis nodosa, systemic lupus erythematous, and allergic arteritis. The third type of stenosing arteritis, so-called Buerger's disease, is characterized by uniform, wide-spread reduction in the luminal size of arteries. The spasmodic characteristic of these arteriopathies is not always apparent. Also, it appears that, in certain cases of this type, there may be an underlying congenital narrowing of the arterial tree[464]. In all of these cases, the diseases result in reduction in blood flow to the organs served by the arteries involved. The lesions produced depend upon the severity of the ischemia and the characteristics of the ischemic tissue. The changes range from reversible cellular hypoxia to sudden and definitive cell death. Furthermore, when the ischemia is chronic and partial, the affected tissue "reacts," i.e., undergoes adaptation and histologic change. Finally, the obliteration of a terminal artery may produce an infarction of the area of irrigation.

Experimental Background

Bone tissue also suffers complications of ischemia as proven by numerous animal experiments studying the effect of arterial ligation on bone tissue. This experimental work has been the origin of our understanding of the arterial side of bone blood supply. They will be discussed in some detail in the chapter devoted to experimental bone necrosis. In this introduction, we shall only describe experimental facts concerning epiphyseal ischemia and its repercussion on the articular cartilage.

The destruction of the epiphyseal artery by stripping may produce massive epiphyseal necrosis, but the revascularization and repair of the bone is rapid and effective. This explains why, in certain experiments, the articular cartilage itself is seldom altered. However, Holdsworth[207] noted changes consisting of cartilage thinning and poor staining with toluidine-blue, thought to be secondary to reduction in metabolic activity of the chondrocytes. According to Brookes[70], this ischemic joint cartilage is reversible because of the rapidity of epiphyseal repair.

The study of epiphyseal cartilage lesions showing epiphyseal ischemia has been studied by Rutishauser and Taillard on the rabbit[379]. They noted both thinning and softening of the articular cartilage with replacement of cartilaginous structures in the superficial layers by fibrous tissue which they refer to as "vascular pannus." In these cases, we can then speak of true ischemic coxopathy as meaning that the effects of ischemia, involving both bone and cartilage at the same time, produces a truly articular disease. Concerning bone and articular lesions produced by non-traumatic ischemia in man, the most significant publications have been done on the phalanges of patients undergoing amputation for arteritic gangrene of the foot. Jaffe and Pomeranz[224], as well as Brookes[69], have been mainly interested in the cortex which becomes less radiodense as it is weakened by three types of change: a.) The vascular channels become enlarged, b.) Notches appear in the outer cortex associated with the presence of new vessels, and c.) Many lacunae in the cortex are empty. This direct sign of osteocytic necrosis is of value only if the empty lacunae are numerous, since we know that it is normal to see a certain percentage of empty osteocytic lacunae. Two quite contradictory phenomenon are then seen. On the one hand, cellular disappearance with widening of the lacunae suggest osteocytic osteolysis and, secondly, vascular proliferation with perivascular resorption. It is possible that these two phenomenon are sequential, and the observations are merely being made together at the time of amputation, since reduction of arterial flow is seldom complete, allowing for compensatory responses as the blood flow gradually decreases.

Brookes interprets these findings in the following way. Initially, medullary ischemia decreases cortical metabolism, bringing about a decrease in pH and an increase in pCO_2. The changes stimulate vascular-neogenesis from the periosteal vessels. In the second phase, there is a reversal of blood flow with blood flowing from the periosteum towards the bone marrow. This is a vascular response to supplement the marrow ischemia. Microangiography has confirmed increased density of periosteal circulation in these ischemic bones. Medullary and epiphyseal lesions have not been as well studied in these experiments. According to Brookes[69], neither medullary infarction nor articular lesions could be identified.

Sherman and Selakowich[402] studied ten tibiae amputated because of distal gangrene. In one case, the bone was almost entirely dead. In another case, the authors observed lesions involving both cancellous and cortical bone. In the cancellous bone, there were foci of medullary necrosis in contact with bone trabeculae which were also dead. Elsewhere, there were foci of fibrosis and edema, a macrophagic histiocyte response, and medullary revascularization of the angiomatous type. In the cortex of those cases where periosteal vessels were preserved, many lacunae were filled with capillaries causing the cortex to resemble cancellous bone, an observation also made by Brookes. Of course, these anatomical, pathological descriptions only show the status at a particular moment in the disease where the battle at the tissue level may have been going on for months or years with local successes and failures in reacting to the increasing ischemia.

NECROSIS OF THE FEMORAL HEAD BY PROVEN ARTERIAL PATHOLOGY[18,19]

Before our first published work on this form of osteonecrosis in 1971, similar cases in the literature were unusual. However, Hughes, Schumacher, and

Sparbaro[215] reported a patient with advanced osteonecrosis of both femoral heads associated with complete block at the aortic bifurcation. Since our original five cases, we have encountered additional cases of proven bone necrosis with unquestionable arterial involvement, expanding our experience to a total of 18 cases. In this series, there were 12 men and 6 women with an age range from 27 to 78 years of age (mean - 51). Fifteen of 18 patients were over 40 years of age. Arteriography was carried out on 17 of these patients showing typical arteriosclerotic disease in 13 patients and a stenosing arteritis in four. Seven cases were bilateral, giving a total of 25 femoral heads with proven bone necrosis. Seven patients were in Stage I (biopsy proven), four in Stage II, nine in Stage III or IV, and five with ischemic coxopathy. IMP was measured in 19 cases and was abnormally elevated in 14. Venography was carried out in nine cases and demonstrated intramedullary stasis. Core biopsy was carried out 15 times, showing marrow necrotic lesions in six cases and both marrow and trabecular necrotic lesions in nine cases.

Illustrative Case 21 (Fig. 105). - Mr. ABA..., a 56-year-old male, was managed medically for obstructive arterial disease of the lower extremities (absent right femoral pulse). In May, 1964, the patient complained of left groin pain following a fall, with the pain exacerbated by walking or hip movement. Examination at that time revealed stiffness of the left hip with flexion limited to 90° and absence of internal rotation. The initial x-rays showed left hip osteonecrosis (Stage III) and slight flattening of the superior pole of the femoral head on the right. Several months later, a femoral arteriogram confirmed bilateral femoral arterial obstruction from atheromata. A left distal femoral metaphyseal infarction was also visualized. Bilateral sympathectomy was performed. In January, 1966, because of increased symptoms in the left hip, a core biopsy of the left femoral head was followed by a pedicle bone graft. Histology confirmed the existence of abnormal bone marrow throughout the specimen with many areas of granular and fibrinoid necrosis. In other areas, the bone marrow space was filled with fibrous tissue. The trabeculae were irregular and often thickened. Some of them were totally necrotic, while others were alive showing evidence of reconstruction with both osteoblasts and osteoclasts. Although the arterial disease stabilized, the bone lesions worsened. By 1970, there was almost total ankylosis of the left hip with little pain. The right hip progressed to a clear Stage III, necessitating total hip replacement in May, 1973.

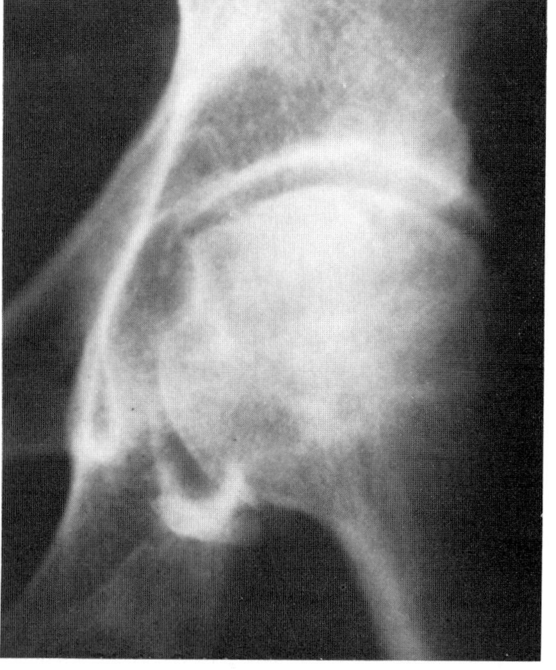

A

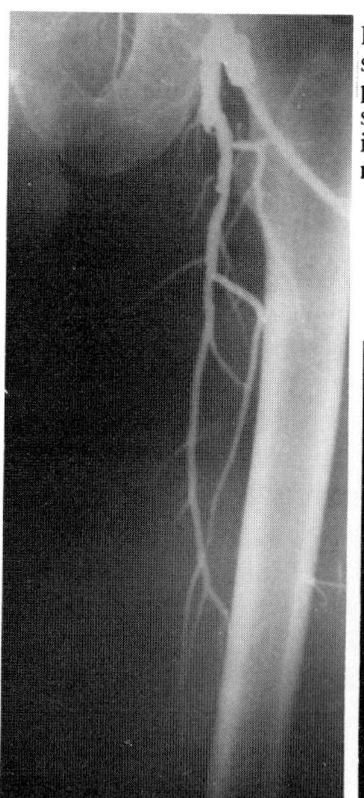

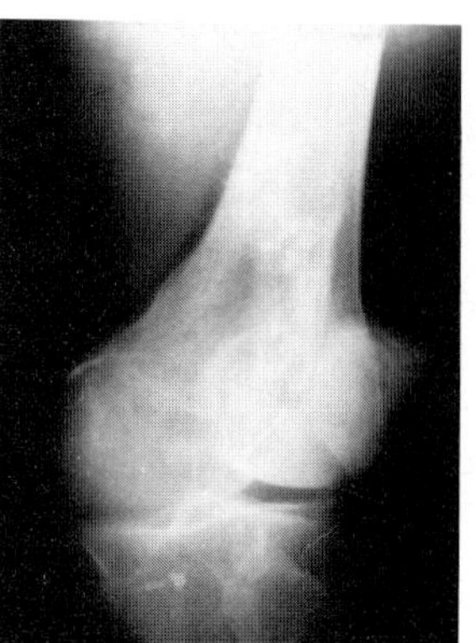

Fig. 105.—Case 21. A: Necrosis with sequestrum. B: Complete block at the origin of the superficial femoral artery with infarction of the inferior femoral metaphysis.

B

Illustrative Case 22. - Miss EAR..., a 65-year-old woman, began with the onset of pain in the right thigh with ambulation in 1965. She was seen for the first time in March, 1968, with pain and disability in both lower extremities. Physical exam showed significant restriction of movement of both hips. The x-rays showed bilateral INFH, Stage II on the left, and Stage III on the right (Fig. 106). Bilateral core biopsies were carried out with measurement of IMP in April, 1968. IMP was 30 mm Hg in the right and 22 mm Hg in the left with positive stress tests bilaterally. The biopsy on the right showed some trabecular death in the femoral head, but the necrosis was incomplete. In the neck, there was the same picture with hemorrhagic areas. On the left, there was necrosis with microfractures of trabeculae in the head and in the neck. Three months later, the patient was clinically improved. The radiologic signs were unchanged. In March of 1969, the patient was asymptomatic relative to the hips but was having vasomotor problems in both feet. The patient was seen again in November, 1970, presenting with typical intermittent claudication after 150 meters. Arteriography confirmed femoral blockage on the right and stenosis of the common iliac artery. In December, 1970, an iliofemoral, popliteal thrombo-endarterectomy was performed together with a right lumbar sympathectomy. At follow-up in October, 1971, the left hip was clinically normal three years after the core biopsy. The right hip remained painful.

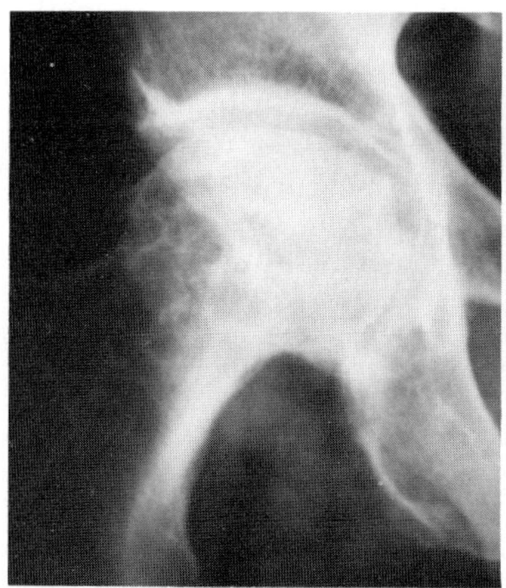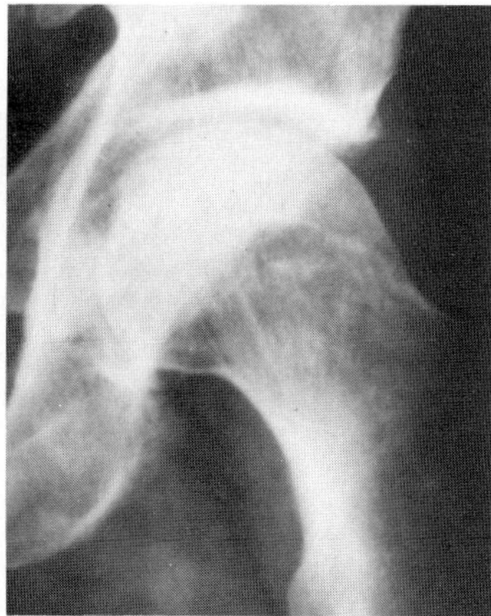

Fig. 106.—Case 22. X-rays showing a necrosis at Stage III on the right and Stage II (sclerosis) on the left.

Illustrative Case 23. - Miss JAM... (Fig. 107), is a 27-year-old female with Buerger's disease involving all four extremities. She had the onset of left groin pain in April, 1967 which, nonetheless, did not interfere with her duties as a teacher. The symptoms continued until she was hospitalized in January and again in March, 1969, in Paris; because abnormality in her left hip was suspected. She was first seen by us in April, 1969, when left hip involvement was of concern. Range of motion was decreased; flexion was only to 90°. The right hip was normal. X-rays showed a slight but definite superior joint line narrowing with three subchondral microcysts near the fovea on the left (Fig. 107). IMP in the left trochanter was 32 mm Hg with prolonged elevation to 50 mm Hg and severe pain following injection of saline. On the right, the IMP was normal, but the stress test was painful. In January, 1970, a biopsy of both bone and synovium on the left was carried out showing nonspecific synovitis, diffuse marrow, and trabecular necrosis (Fig. 107). The diagnosis of inflammatory hip disease was ruled out in favor of necrosis of the ischemic coxopathy type. In follow-up, the left hip became painless at one month post-op, but the vasomotor symptoms of the Raynaud type, particularly in the hands, became more clear. Oscillometric examination revealed diminished pulses at the groin and absent pulses distally. Arteriography confirmed the diagnosis of Buerger's disease with marked narrowing of the entire arterial tree in the lower extremities. In May and June, 1970, a left adrenalectomy and bilateral lumbar sympathectomies were carried out with a disappearance of the vasomotor problems to the lower extremities.

In April, 1971, the patient still had some discomfort of both hips, although the movement in the left hip had improved to 130° flexion. The joint space narrowing and microcysts persisted on the left.

Because of continuing Raynaud's phenomenon in the upper extremity, bilateral cervical sympathectomies were performed. Four years following the core biopsy, because of continuing hip pain and increased joint line narrowing, a total hip replacement was carried out on the left.

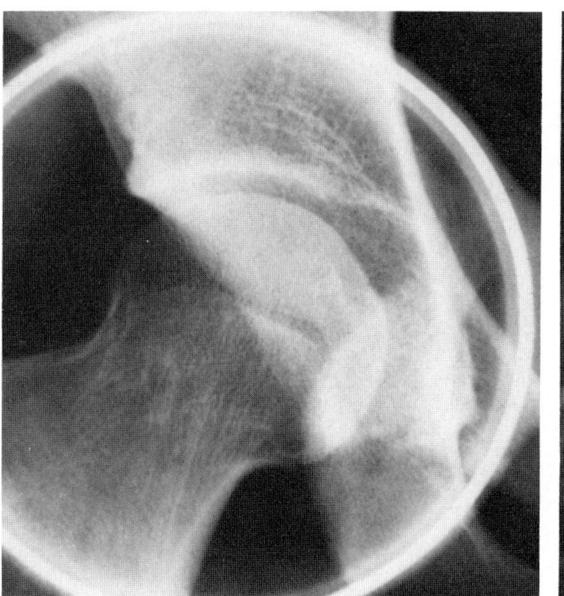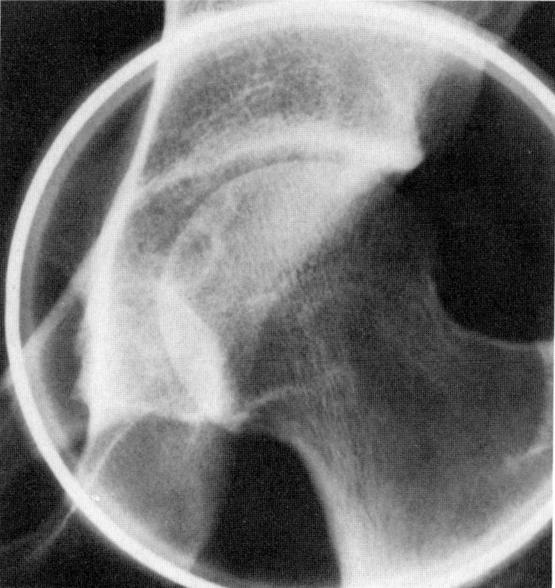

A: Left hip narrowing of the joint space with a subfoveal microcyst.

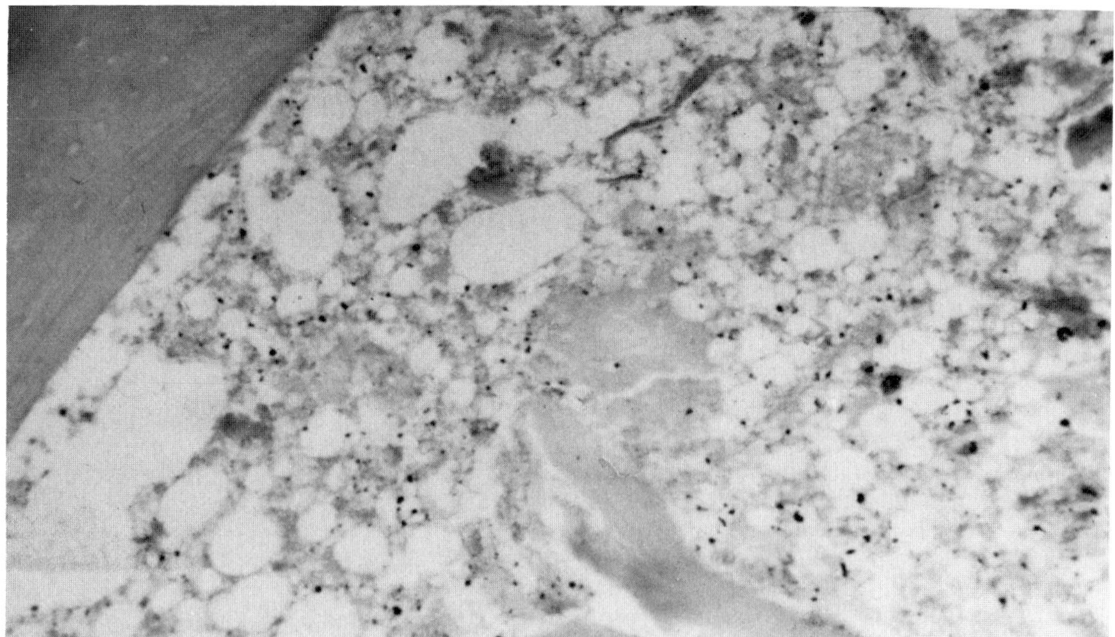

B: Total necrosis of bone marow with partial trabecular necrosis.

Fig. 107.—Case 23.

Illustrative Case 24 (Fig. 108). - Miss LAU..., a 31-year-old nurse, experienced two separate episodes in 1967 and 1968 of left-sided radicular pain associated with a cold sensation and severe dysesthesia. Myelography was normal at each episode. Each event was followed by thrombophlebitis and treated by heparin. Beginning in 1969, she experienced night-time muscle cramps and, from 1970, periodic urinary incontinence.

She presented to us in 1970 with painful limitation of left hip motion with no appreciable x-ray changes except for questionable dysplasia (Fig. 108A). Intramedullary venography revealed gross stasis of the contrast media of several hours duration (Fig. 108B). A general medical work-up, including arteriogram,

confirmed the diagnosis of Buerger's disease with a very narrowed arterial tree (Fig. 108C). Bilateral lumbar sympathectomy and left adrenalectomy relieved both the lower extremity symptoms and improved the left hip discomfort. Histology of a biopsied arteriole confirmed the first stage of Beurger's, disease with subintimal fibrosis. In 1972, at the time of presentation with left hip pain, the x-ray showed evidence of sclerosis in both proximal femora (Fig. 108D). Core biopsy revealed Type 4 necrosis. There had been no further radiologic progression, and she continued without symptoms. The patient was followed up in 1979, and the clinical and radiologic findings are unchanged.

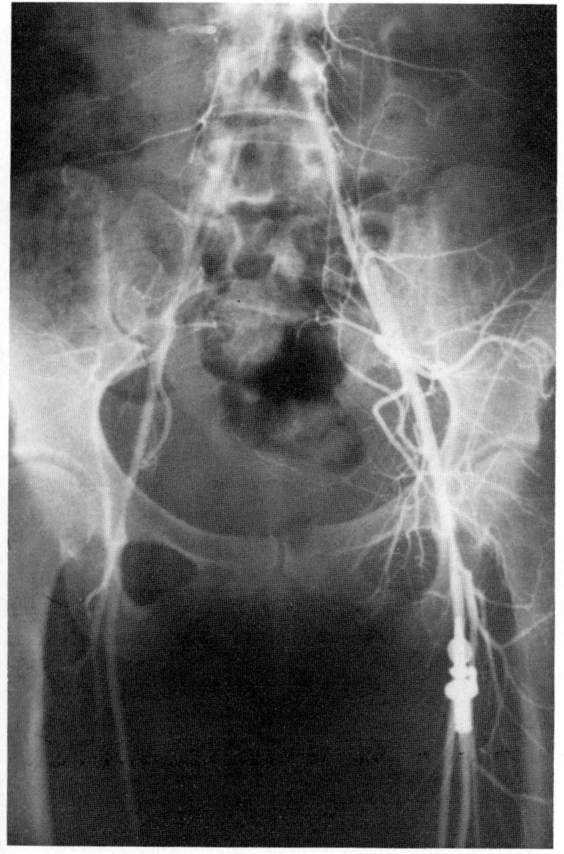

C

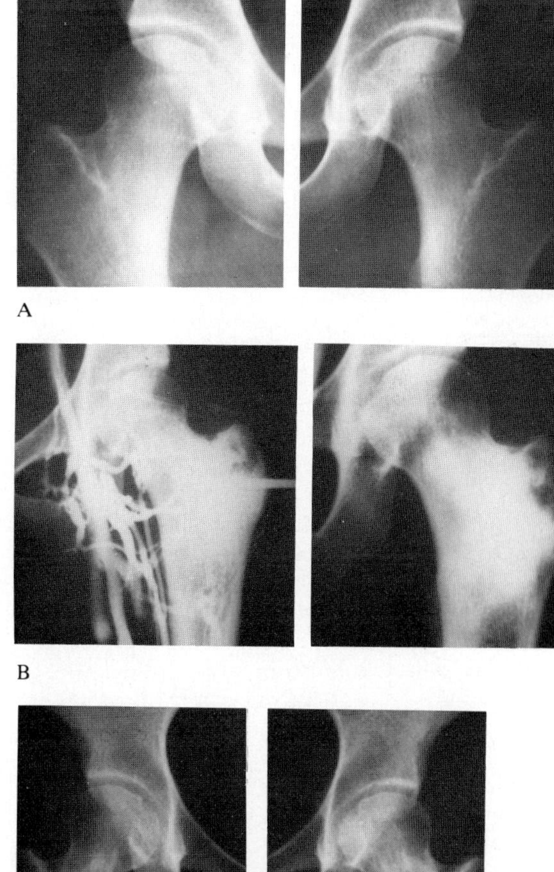

A

B

D

Fig. 108.—Case 24. A: November 1970: normal hips with bilateral coxa valga. B: Phlebography. Massive stasis of the whole metaphyseal region (at the end of the injection and after 15 minutes). C: Arteriography. Thin, poorly filling arterial network. D: Present status: sclerosis around the core tract canal and in the upper part of the diaphysis.

Through individual case experiences as reported above and confirmed by the publications of Hipp[204,205] and Jung, Kehr, and Hamid[239,240], we know, with certainty, that some high arterial lesions from the aortic bifurcation to the division of the common femoral artery can be associated with INFH. However, it remains to be proven that the association occurs with significant frequency. The question is put in doubt because of the work of Ravault et al.[353], who studied 1,000 aortograms without finding a single case of radiologically evident INFH. We have done a similar study on 159 aortographies and have found two cases of femoral head necrosis at Stage III with marked collapse and a sequestrum formation of the superior pole, i.e., a 1.2% incidence. Furthermore, on these aortographies, we have noted interesting changes in the femoral head, specifically, 5 cases with sclerotic borders, 7 cases of flattening of the femoral head, 14 cases of superomedial joint line narrowing, and 25 cases with localized sclerosis. It should be emphasized that the radiological examination of the hips is sub-optimal with the aortograms because the x-ray techniques are not ideal for bone.

For these reasons, we were prompted to undertake a comprehensive clinical and radiologic review on all cases with arterial disease admitted to the vascular surgery service for a period of 18 months. This investigation has been done by one of our rheumatologists (Millet[239]), who personally took the clinical history, performed the physical examination, and requested and examined the x-rays, after which, he discussed them with one of us. This work on 138 patients with arterial disease, all of whom had an arteriogram, confirmed the arterial disease with precision as to its nature and location. There were 113 men and 25 women from 40 to 79 years of age, of which 80 patients ranged from 50 to 69 years of age. The clinical examination revealed a very interesting feature. Sixty-six patients (47.6%) exhibited in one or both hips one or several of the three clinical signs that we were looking for, i.e., spontaneous pain, induced pain, objective limitation of movement. These clinical features were more common in the group of 48 patients with proximally located arterial lesions (between the aortic bifurcation and the division of the common femoral) being present in 66% of this subgroup. The x-rays of the 138 patients revealed radiological changes of one or both hips in 59 patients (42.8%). Again, these radiologic changes were much more common in subjects with proximal arterial lesions (29 of 48 cases). These x-ray changes can be summarized in the following way: 5 cases of INFH in Stage II and III (3.6%), 14 cases of probable necrosis at Stage II (10%) (In these cases, there

were either sclerotic areas, sclerotic islands, or cysts with sclerotic borders), 14 cases (10%) with a stiff, painful hip but radiologically normal (possibly Stage I necrosis), and 26 patients (18.8%) with superomedial joint line narrowing. Sixteen of these 26 patients had clinical signs of hip disease.

Eleven patients had pertrochanteric phlebography carried out. In eight of them, there was obvious stasis of the contrast media five minutes after injection, and the stasis persisted for at least six hours in three patients. On the three patients with no stasis, there was an abnormal diaphyseal reflux. The phlebography was, therefore, abnormal in all 11 cases. Similar findings have already been reported by Schobinger[385]. It can be concluded from this study that the hips are involved in patients with arterial disease. Furthermore, the lesions observed suggest either the classic type of bone necrosis or the special type that we have described under the name ischemic coxopathy, as evidenced by the superomedial joint narrowing. It is possible that the small percentage of Stage III necrosis may be due to the fact that patients with peripheral vascular disease and intermittent claudication walk less than patients without arterial disease.

Conclusion

We believe that, from now on, it is time to take a prospective attitude in the face of these necroses that we should know about and recognize. The experimental data and the clinical observations are of sufficient value to warrant a systematic investigation of these necroses and ischemic coxopathies in these patients with peripheral vascular disease. Phemister was already of this opinion[343]. Pain and disability in such a patient should not be assumed to be produced only by muscular ischemia. The joints should be carefully examined in these patients. One often finds a painful stiffness suggesting involvement of the joint as a whole—epiphysis, articular cartilage, synovial membrane, capsule, and tendons. Leriche[280] had already reported clinical observations of knee stiffness in cases with lower extremity peripheral vascular disease. Superomedial joint-line narrowing may also be a sign of vascular damage of the hip.

Only the functional exploration can document the existence of bone ischemia at its onset while the x-rays are normal. The transosseous phlebography also permits the diagnosis of reduction of the arterial flow, although the measurement of the IMP is a simpler method and devoid of complications. Our histopathological data, although as yet insufficient, indicates that the lesions of arterial origin are similar to those from other etiologies.

It is important to systematically search for signs of bone necrosis in all patients with peripheral vascular disease. Likewise, all patients with suspected or proven INFH should be carefully examined for peripheral vascular disease, including pulses, evidence of temperature differences, trophic changes, or Raynaud's phenomenon. Any absence of pulse in the lower extremity, under these circumstances, would warrant arteriography. The latter, ideally, should include a general aortography to visualize large trunk lesions and selective arteriography of the hip, focusing attention on the posterior circumflex and retinacular arteries.

GAUCHER'S DISEASE

Most cases of Gaucher's Disease are the chronic non-neuropathic type (Type 1) with symptoms appearing for the first time in either childhood or adult life. This hereditary defect in the metabolism of glycocerebrosides results from a deficiency in Beta glucosidase resulting in an accumulation of the glycocerebrosides. The surplus then accumulates in the reticuloendothelial cells forming typical "Gaucher's cells" which are found in abundance in the liver, spleen, lymphatic nodes, and bone marrow. The clinical course is usually chronic with splenomegaly, with or without hypersplenism (leucopenia, thrombocytopenia) and bone lesions. The bone manifestations were first described by Brill in 1904[173]. The Gaucher's cells fill the bone marrow impinging on the lumen of the capillaries within the bone and reducing intramedullary circulation. Strictly speaking, there is no real encroachment on the bone trabeculae or the cortex, but the cortex becomes deformed with growth by the mass of the abnormal cells. The trabeculae react to the ischemia by proliferation and necrosis. Radiographic evidence of bone pathology is present in 50-75% of Type 1 cases. The most widely recognized sign is the characteristic enlargement of the distal femoral metaphysis (Erlenmeyer flask deformity). However, radiologic signs compatible with bone necrosis at Stage II and Stage III are not uncommon. In children, the radiologic appearance is similar to that of Perthes' Disease[262]. Clinical symptoms may or may not be present. Pathological fractures have been reported. In childhood and adolescence, bone involvement can produce acute episodes of intense pain with fever, leucocytosis, and local inflammatory changes suggesting osteomyelitis. Each crisis may last a few days or a few weeks and spontaneously regress, but they may quickly subside after decompression[173].

The pelvis, the long bones, the phalanges, and the ribs are most commonly affected. Destructive vertebral lesions have also been reported. Under light microscopy, the Gaucher's cells are very characteristic with cell diameter from 20-100 microns, an eccentric nucleus, and cytoplasm containing irregular fibrillar material, which under polarized light gives the appearance of crumpled paper. The intracellular material is stained by PAS and Mallory trichrome. The cells are rich in acid phosphotase.

Illustrative Case 25 (Fig. 109). - Mrs. PUJ..., a 23-year-old woman, underwent splenectomy for "tumor" in 1944; no histology is available. When seen by us for the first time in 1966, she complained of pain in the left groin of one year's duration with recent increase in severity forcing her to stop working. Passive movement of the left hip was restricted to 60° flexion. X-rays showed diffuse sclerosis of both femoral heads with an intact subchondral outline on the right. The left femoral head was deformed, and the joint line was narrowed. Blood chemistry findings were normal, including lipid levels. Bilateral core biopsy (1-21-67) showed typical Gaucher's cells and evidence of marrow and trabecular necrosis. On the basis of the histology, the diagnosis of Gaucher's disease, Type 1, could be established. In February, 1969, her right knee became painful, and x-rays showed sclerosis and collapse of the medial femoral condyle. February, 1970, three years after the core decompression, the right hip remained asymptomatic with unchanged x-rays (Stage II). The left hip also was less painful than before the decompression, and its radiologic appearance was little changed from that seen in 1967 (Fig. 109). This patient was last seen in 1978, at which time both the radiologic and clinical aspects of her condition remained unchanged.

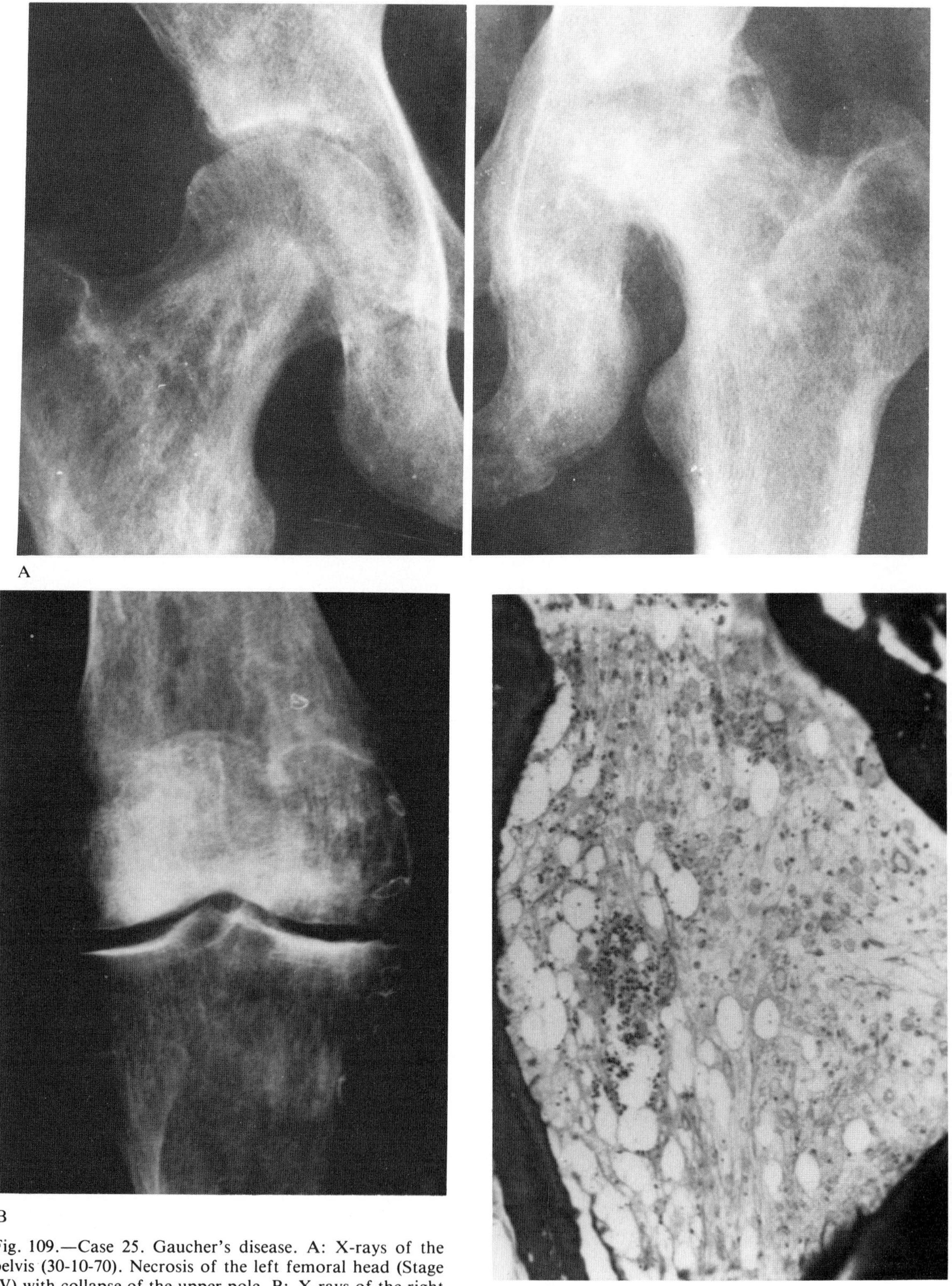

Fig. 109.—Case 25. Gaucher's disease. A: X-rays of the pelvis (30-10-70). Necrosis of the left femoral head (Stage IV) with collapse of the upper pole. B: X-rays of the right knee (3-7-70). Necrosis of the medial condyle. C: Histological section showing Gaucher's cells encroaching on the marrow space.

CHAPTER VIII

BONE NECROSES WITH PROBABLE ETIOLOGIC RELATIONSHIPS

In the preceding chapter, the etiologic agents were clearly associated with the subsequent necrosis. In this chapter, the etiologic associations are less certain. By virtue of temporal association or increased incidence in groups of patients exhibiting the particular characteristics, a common, but not proven, association has been generally accepted. In many of these instances, the pathophysiologic relationship between the causal agent and the subsequent necrosis is either poorly understood or under dispute.

BONE NECROSIS FOLLOWING MINOR INJURY

Bone necrosis associated with major injury, including fractures and dislocations, represents a clear-cut and little-disputed causal relationship to the subsequent necrosis. In this section, we are concerned with injury which is not manifest initially by any detectable radiologic abnormalities. There are basically two separate types of injury: direct contusion, either in the groin, indirectly through the greater trochanter, or through trauma to the flexed knee (dashboard injury) or the feet (vertical fall); and torsional injuries, usually forced abduction or internal rotation. Most series have reported minor trauma as a possible etiologic factor, although without great conviction. The percentage of cases to which minor trauma has been attributed to play a

role varies from 6-36% depending on the series[300,391,394,458,473]. The attitude of most authors, alleging that the trauma has only precipitated symptoms in an underlying necrosis, is not helpful to an understanding of its potential, true relationship. Some authors have had second thoughts concerning the role of minor injury in precipitating subsequent bone necrosis[159,279]. Lequesne et al.[275] reported eight cases of post-contusion necrosis of the femoral head diagnosed on radiologic criteria alone. In our own experience, minor injury is part of the presenting history in 25.1% of patients. It is important to establish a cause-and-effect relationship of trauma to subsequent bone ischemia and to elucidate the mechanism of the circulatory disturbance. From a medical-legal point of view, it is important to establish the relationship of minor injury to the necrosis in order to protect both the patient and responsible third parties.

A review of the detailed information on 20 cases, for which we have attributed minor injury to be a cause, sheds some light on the problem. Thirteen cases had trochanteric contusion; three, a vertical fall landing on the feet; and four, a torsional injury. Two of our cases also had fracture of the ischiopubic ramus. It is important to use all possible parameters in assessing the magnitude of the injury. Such things as deep hematomas or superficial ecchymosis, pain and immediate functional disability, fracture at a distance, etc., should be considered. Males predominate because of the exposure to trauma. Manual workers are also in the majority (13 of 20). Three patients in the series had asymptomatic hyperuricemia above 7.0 mg/100 ml. Apart from one patient who had cortisone eight years previously for psoriasis, there were no potentially predisposing factors other than the history of injuries.

In 16 out of 20 cases, pain was experienced coincident with the injury and persisted until the first examination. In three other cases, the pain appeared less than one week after the injury. There was, however, always some interval between the functional exploration of bone and the injury: four to six months in five cases, six to twelve months in four cases, one to two years in six cases, and two to three years in five cases. Pain was felt in the groin with a tendency to radiate toward the knee in two-thirds of the cases. Some patients had a sciatic-type pain. The discomfort tended to be moderate with intermittent, acute exacerbations. Night pain was sometimes present. In half of the cases, there was significant limitation of movement in the range of 60° flexion and 20° abduction. Even with normal movement, however, pain could be elicited at the extremes and on internal rotation.

At the time of presentation with symptoms, ten patients had normal radiographs, three showed diffuse demineralization suggesting reflex sympathetic dystrophy, five cases were in Stage III, and two cases were in Stage IV. In the ten patients presenting with normal x-rays, biopsy provided histologic evidence of necrosis.

The specific findings on the functional exploration of bone for the 13 cases with normal x-rays or simple osteoporosis are reviewed in Table XX. In all cases, the histologic examination confirmed the diagnosis of ischemia or necrosis. In every case but No. 5, at least one of the other parameters of the functional evaluation was also abnormal.

Histology was available for review in 17 of the 20 cases. The most frequent lesion seen was eosinophilic reticular necrosis in 14 out of 17 cases (Type 2 and 3). In nine cases, there was also necrosis of the trabeculae (Type 3). One case showed features of bone reconstruction (Type 4). Specimens from this group of patients, however, showed evidence of intramedullary hemorrhage more frequently than other groups independent of the interval from the injury (even after three years). We have tried to exclude the possibility that the hemorrhage was an artifact of taking the core by only counting hemorrhage seen in the center of the specimen with features of organization. These histologic lesions do appear to

be more characteristic of the post-traumatic osteonecrosis and were seen in all cases of Type 1, half of the Type 2 cases, and only once in Type 3.

Discussion

From our experience, we conclude that osteonecrosis is a possible sequelae of relatively minor injury and that such lesions may initially present with a completely normal x-ray. When the injury is slight, it is usually held that it is not responsible for the subsequent necrosis but only precipitates symptoms of necrosis. The necrosis then bears only a coincidental relationship to the injury. When the trauma was severe, it was certainly possible that trabecular microfractures, which would not appear on x-ray, have occurred. When the condition is bilateral in spite of unilateral injury, predisposing causes are usually suspected. The injury is not usually held responsible for the entire clinical picture. This concept is suspect, however, because post-traumatic reflex sympathetic dystrophy on both the functional exploration level and on the basis of bone scanning has been shown to sometimes involve both sides even though only one side sustained the injury. We feel that bilateral involvement cannot arbitrarily exclude the possibility of the injury being responsible for the necrosis. The exact mechanism of the injury, previously documented clinical and radiologic evidence of the integrity of the femoral head, evidence of the intensity of the injury, and the absence of other etiologic factors must also be taken into consideration. The immediate and rapid onset of articular symptoms following injury would favor implicating the injury as an etiologic factor.

We have already seen in other forms of necrosis that there may be a long latency period of several months, or even several years, between the predisposing episode and the diagnosis of the necrosis. Therefore, a significant time delay between the injury and the subsequent necrosis should not, in and of itself, exclude the possibility of a cause-and-effect relationship. In this regard, it is interesting to note that the Workmen's Compensation Board, which previously accepted only a five-year interval between diving and osteonecrosis to label the diving as responsible, extended that latency to 10 years in 1957 and to 20 years in 1967.

A particular medical-legal dilemma exists with Stage I bone necrosis. We have seen too many experts exclude the possibility of injury-related necrosis on the basis of examining a single x-ray. Sometimes the patient is accused of malingering or of hysterics. Functional exploration of bone or a bone scan could provide objective verification of their complaints.

TABLE XX NECROSIS OF THE FEMORAL HEAD AFTER MINOR INJURY
HEMODYNAMIC AND HISTOLOGIC EVALUATION (13 cases)

Observation No.		1	2	3	4	5	6	7	8	9	10	11	12	13
Increased IMP	Trochanter	+	+	+	+	±	+	0	+	0			0	0
	Neck or Head		+	+			+	+		+	+			
Abnormal Intramedullary Venography			+		+	±	+		+	+	+	+	+	+
Histologic Type		1	1	1	3	3	3	2	2	3	2	1	3	3

Illustrative Case 26. - MR. B..., a 50-year-old farmer with no prior hip symptoms, sustained a direct blow to the right greater trochanter in a traffic accident. X-rays were taken on the day of the accident, showing a completely normal femoral head. One month later, the pain persisted, but the x-rays remained normal. Four months later, with continuation of pain and disability, the x-rays showed a typical sequestrum in the femoral head with joint line narrowing (Stage IV, Fig. 110). This case shows several important features. There was no history of clinical symptoms prior to the injury. Pain began immediately at the time of the accident and persisted continuously through the appearance of the radiologic lesion. The pre-radiologic status of this almost experimental situation was documented at the time of injury and one month later. The rapid and nearly total joint space narrowing suggested post-traumatic cartilage necrosis directly related to the injury and not secondary to the underlying bone ischemia.

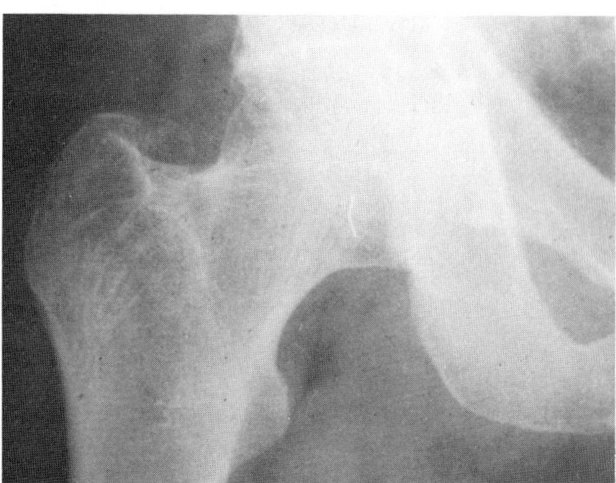

A

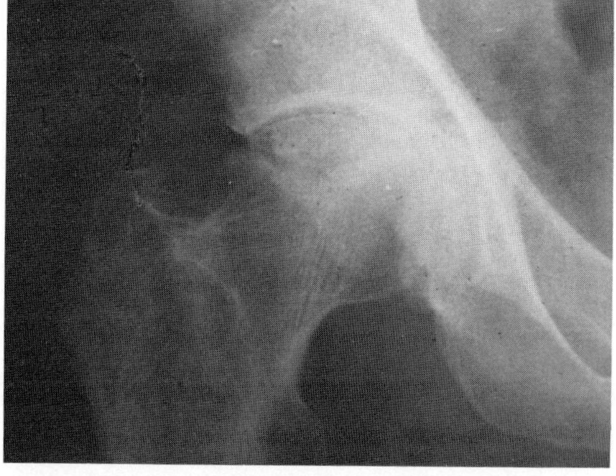

B

Fig. 110.—Case 26. A: X-rays of the right hip on the day of the accident: normal. B: X-rays of the same hip four months after the accident. Necrosis already in Stage IV with a well-defined sequestrum and joint-line narrowing.

Illustrative Case 27. - Mr. BR..., a 41-year-old male laborer, sustained a fall at work in February, 1963, following which he complained of pain in the left groin. The right hip became painful in June, 1963. Thirteen months later, at the time of examination in our clinic, there was 75% painful reduction of hip movement on the left hip and 50% reduction on the right. The x-rays at the time of presentation showed Stage III necrosis on the left with a massive sequestrum in a superior pole (Fig. 111). On the right, there was early collapse in the weight-bearing zone with early sequestrum formation. The functional exploration showed stasis and moderate reflux with all venous drainage passing through the circumflex vein. Biopsy showed bone and medullary necrosis with dense fibrosis. In spite of the advanced stages of lesions, core decompression resulted in remarkable clinical improvement, and the patient has not required other surgical intervention.

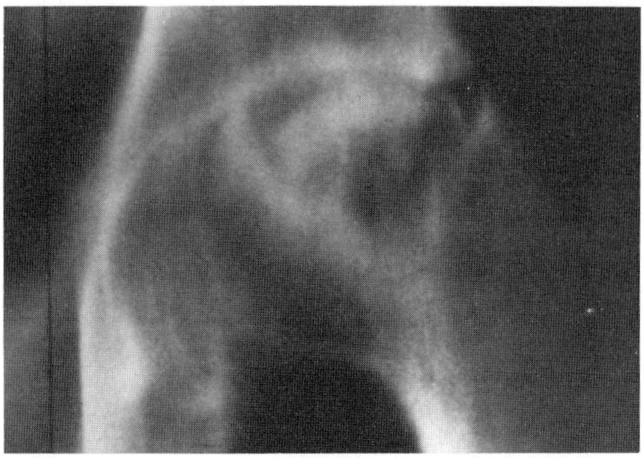

A

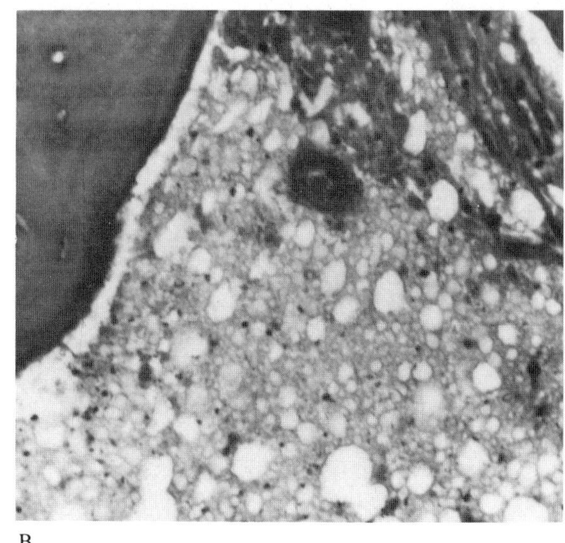

B

Fig. 111.—Case 27. A: X-rays of the left hip 13 months after an accident demonstrating a necrosis at Stage III-IV with collapse of the sequestrum. B: Forage biopsy revealed eosinophilic reticulated necrotic lesions of the bone marrow just under the sequestrum.

Illustrative Case 28. - Mr. CAZ..., a 54-year-old mechanic, sustained a significant contusion in the region of the left trochanter on July 2, 1970, following which increasing pain appeared in the left hip. He was treated for sciatica with a plaster jacket and epidural injection because of the radicular nature of his symptoms. Nonetheless, permanent pain persisted in the region of the left knee. In September, 1973, painful limitation of movement of the left hip was still present. X-rays were completely normal. Functional exploration was carried out on April 4, 1974, with IMP measuring 30 mm Hg in the greater trochanter and rising to 52 mm Hg with the stress test. Femoral head pressures measured 70 mm Hg without pulsation. A venogram did not visualize the circumflex veins. All the drainage flowed through the posterior vein of the neck. There was considerable medullary stasis. Specimen from the core biopsy showed massive medullary necrosis, Type 2, with many necrotic cysts in the areas of medullary necrosis. The clinical result was spectacular with disappearance of night pain immediately after surgery. The hip regained nearly normal range of movement within a few weeks. Two months after the core decompression, he was able to return to work as a mechanic. At last follow-up in 1979, the patient was asymptomatic.

Illustrative Case 29. - Mr. BE..., a 17-year-old student, sustained a bad fall while ice skating, twisting the leg into wide abduction. The pain in the right groin was so severe that he fainted. Although he only limped for a few days after the injury, he had continuous discomfort. Five months after the injury, the pain was severe. Examination of the right hip showed considerable stiffness (flexion to 105°). X-ray showed diffuse demineralization of both the right femoral head and acetabulum (Fig. 112). The IMP at that time showed a baseline pressure of 17 mm Hg rising to 85 mm Hg with the stress test. Venography showed obvious stasis. A diagnosis of reflex sympathetic dystrophy was suspected, but the biopsy specimen on January 15, 1970, showed diffuse medullary necrosis as well as necrosis of the few bone trabeculae (Fig. 88B). Since the decompression, the pain has disappeared completely. At follow-up in December, 1975, the hip showed slightly decreased ROM but was asymptomatic. He has resumed activities, including sports. X-rays of the right hip showed normal bone density but slight joint space narrowing (Fig. 112). When last seen in 1978, there had been no change in the clinical or radiologic picture.

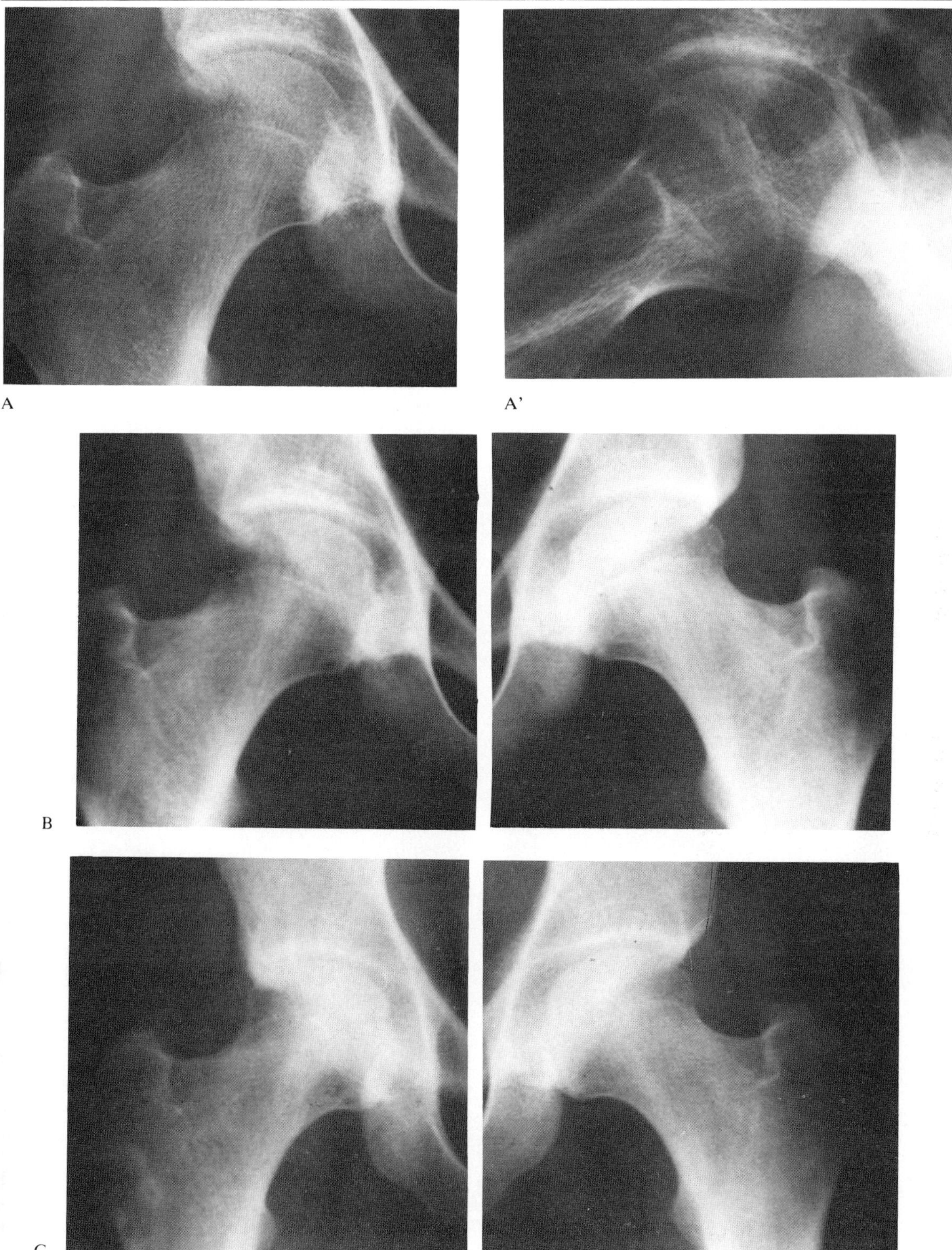

Fig. 112.—Case 29. A: AP and lateral views of the right hip six months after the accident (notice the integrity of the outline of the femoral head). B: X-rays of the pelvis done in the same period reveal the osteoporosis of the symtomatic hip (R) compared to the opposite side. C: X-rays of the pelvis done six years after the core decompression do not show abnormalities except for a very slight joint-line narrowing.

CORTISONE-ASSOCIATED NECROSIS OF BONE

Of all the undesirable sequelae of exogenous corticosteroid therapy, bone necrosis was the last to be recognized. Hench predicted all of the complications of cortisone treatment with the exception of bone necrosis, which was first reported in 1957 by Pietrogrande and Mastromarino[347]. Bloch-Michel reported the first cases in France[53]. Since cortisone is widely used and bone necrosis is not particularly rare, it may be questioned that there is a causal relationship between the steroid administration and bone necrosis. The low incidence of bone necrosis in patients with rheumatoid arthritis, many of whom have taken prednisone in the 5-15 mg range for years, is also striking and brings the causal relationship into question. However, in the renal allograft group of patients who receive high daily doses of cortisone, the incidence of bone necrosis is high and, as suggested by Harrington et al.[196], seems to be dose related. With high dosage, necrosis occurred in over half of the cases. Many hypotheses have been put forward regarding the pathogenesis of steroid related bone necrosis; although, as we shall see, none are truly satisfactory. The mechanism remains in doubt, and the missing link between the condition, the steroid treatment, and the necrosis remains to be determined[365].

The list of diseases and disorders treated by exogenous steroid administration is long and varied. It includes the connective tissue diseases from rheumatoid arthritis to systemic lupus erythematosus, encompassing dermatomyositis, periarteritis nodosa, and scleroderma. Hemoglobinopathies and gout are two general conditions occasionally treated by steroids. Many cutaneous conditions such as pemphigus, eczema, urticaria, and many bronchiopulmonary conditions, particularly asthma, chronic bronchitis, and pulmonary fibrosis, are treated by either intermittent or long-term treatments. Occasionally, head injury and acute, overwhelming viral infections are also treated with large doses of cortisone. Acute and chronic hepatitis and some ocular conditions are treated as well and are reflected in our series. The role of steroids in immunosuppression in the renal allograft patient has already been referred to.

In general, the oral route has been used for administration, but, on occasion, intramuscular and periarticular injections with slow release of cortisone are involved. One wonders if cutaneous application of steroids over a long time in widespread areas for dermatologic conditions could cause a bone necrosis.

Most frequently, the daily dose is high, usually above 20 mg/day, prednisone equivalent, and often as high as 60 mg/day. This dose is not always continuous, and it is impossible at this point to determine if the intermittent cortisone therapy is less dangerous for a necrosis than continuous treatment. In the early reported cases, treatment was of at least six-months duration and usually for one to two years. It appears now, however, that shorter courses of treatment are also capable of producing necrosis. We have seen a case of acute hepatitis with only six weeks of cortisone· followed by INFH. Recently, Good[185] attributed bilateral INFH to a 16-day course of ACTH.

There is a great variation between cases, regarding the interval between the onset of treatment and the appearance of signs and symptoms of bone necrosis. In general, the necrosis is not manifest before the end of the first year after the onset of treatment and frequently not before the end of the second year, independent of whether the treatment is continuous or intermittent. Nonetheless, some earlier cases of necrosis have been observed within six months of the onset of cortisone therapy. Cruess et al.[103] reported a case with early clinical signs two and one-half months after the onset of treatment in a patient with renal transplantation.

The incidence of bone necrosis in the patient population with renal allografts is remarkable, over 30% in some series. Cruess et al.[103] found ten cases of femoral head necrosis in 36 patients surviving six months or more after transplantation. Murray[330], reviewing 339 allografts carried out between 1964 and 1971, found that 14% of these patients exhibited x-ray changes compatible with the diagnosis of necrosis. On the other hand, in a group of 68 patients with a daily dose of prednisone equivalent of more than 100 mg/day for less than three weeks, the percentage of bone necrosis was 34%. Arfi et al.[8] found an 18% incidence of bone necrosis in patients with renal transplant surviving more than one year. The severity of the problem is compounded by the fact that numerous sites are often involved in the same patient. Murray[330] reported 94 affected joints in 46 patients and Arfi[8], 4 locations in 29 patients. Collapse of the femoral head with sequestrum formation also seems to take place early in the disease. Furthermore, the fact that these patients cannot have their steroids terminated means that the presumed etiologic cause remains.

Clinical signs frequently precede radiologic signs —by six months, according to Murray[330], by two months, according to Cruess[103], and by one month, according to Arfi et al.[8]. Nonetheless, it is possible to see patients with radiologic signs of necrosis in Stage III who are not symptomatic. When one encounters a renal transplant patient with hip pain and a negative x-ray, the existence of a necrosis is very likely, and functional exploration can document the pathophysiologic changes. Since core decompression can favorably influence the outcome in Stage I, as has been demonstrated[146], we believe that this surgical intervention is mandatory in such cases.

PERSONAL EXPERIENCE

Our experience with 15 cases of histologically proven femoral head necrosis and associated with steroid therapy documents some of the findings and problems in this group of patients. (Table XXI).

Functional Exploration

Ten of these 15 cases had IMP measured in the trochanter. In two cases, measurement was bilateral. Of these 12 measurements, eight were over 30 mm Hg. In three of the remaining four, the stress test was positive. Five cases had trochanteric intramedullary venography which showed stasis in all cases. Histologic examination was possible in all cases, either after core biopsy or total hip replacement. Medullary necrosis of the reticular eosinophilic type was present in all cases, although there was a particular feature in some cases. Instead of a fine homogeneous reticular pattern, large degenerated lipocytes showed thick, irregular eosinophilic walls with the cytoplasm divided by eosinophilic bands.

There was, occcasionally, the appearance of newly formed blood vessels. We have only seen this feature in cortisone-related necrosis (Fig. 113). Trabecular necrosis was evident in most cases. Evidence of trabecular reconstruction was seen in five cases, while a definite osteopenia was present in ten cases. In the single case of renal transplantation, histologic evidence of hyperparathyroidism was also clearly present.

TABLE XXI

STEROID–ASSOCIATED NECROSIS
OF THE FEMORAL HEAD

1. Age, Sexes, Localization	
Sex:	12 men, 3 women
Ages:	*average* 54; *range* 27–75
Bilaterality:	8 cases
Other sites:	2 cases

2. Radiology, Biology		
Radiologic Stages		*Associated Blood Findings*
I:	2 cases	Dyslipoproteinemia: 4 cases
II:	1 case	Positive Rose–Waaler: 2 cases
III & IV:	12 cases	Hyperuricemia: 1 case
		Cryoglobulinemia: 1 case

3. Medical causes for Cortisone Treatment	
Pulmonary:	6 cases
Rheumatologic:	4 cases
Neurologic, Dermatologic, Immunosuppression, Pathologic, Ophthalmologic:	1 case each

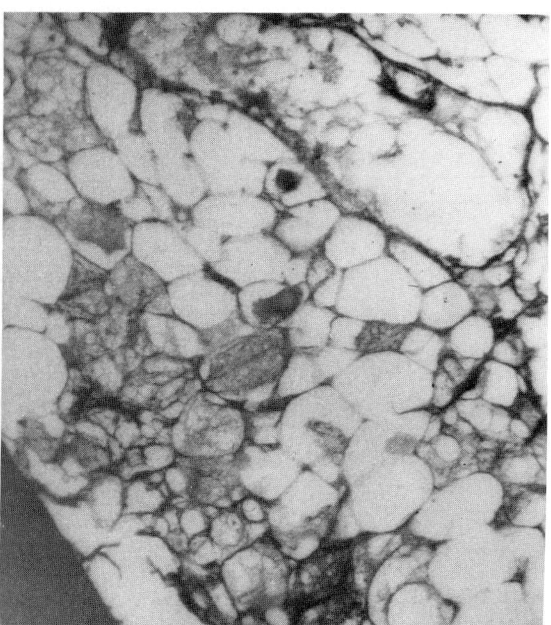

A
Fig. 113.—Cortisone-related bone marrow necrosis. A: A reticular pattern is seen within the lypocyte membranes.

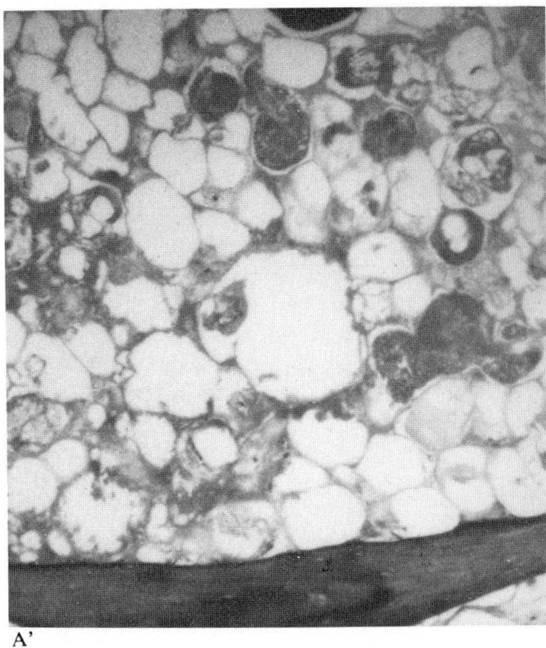

A'

B: Dense fibrinoid depositing inside the lypocyte membranes.

All of the commercially available corticosteroid preparations had been used, including prednisone, methylcortisone, dexamethasone, triamcinolone, and betamethasone. It is sometimes difficult, retrospectively, to determine the daily dosage, but in 13 of the 15 cases, it was greater than 10 mg of prednisone equivalent daily. In two cases, it had never been more than 5 mg/day (1 gouty arthritis, 1 rheumatoid arthritis). The minimum duration of the treatment was 45 days (1 hepatitis, 1 dermatitis). In all other cases, it was of several months and, sometimes, several years duration.

It is not always possible to precisely ascertain the interval between the onset of cortisone treatment and the first appearance of signs of bone necrosis, since some patients have taken several short courses of cortisone prior to beginning a more regular or continuous treatment. In two cases, corticosteroid therapy had been started several years prior to evidence of bone necrosis. In one case, there was only a six-month interval. In more than half of the cases, the earliest signs began during the steroid treatment, but, in one case, symptoms appeared two years after termination of the steroid therapy.

Illustrative Case 30. - Mrs. ZAR..., an 18-year-old patient, had post-puerperal septicemia with Clostridia perfringens, during which time six peritoneal dialyses were performed. In March, 1972, at the age of 27, she had polyradicular neuritis affecting the cranial nerves for which she was treated with cortisone in a dose ranging from 20-30 mg (prednisone equivalent) daily for three months. By June, 1972, her neurologic symptoms had subsided. By September, 1972, the initial symptoms appeared in the left hip with pain radiating to the knee; symptoms were worsened by walking. Her physician first thought that this represented recurrence of her neurologic condition since she had previously experienced radicular pain in her extremities. Cortisone was restarted but was discontinued after three months because of gastrointestinal bleeding. We first saw her in January, 1973, at which time she had severe left hip pain as well as night pain. Physical exam showed moderate restriction of movement with flexion to 100° and abduction of 15°.

The radiograph showed that the left hip had already advanced to Stage III with sclerocystic changes in the femoral head and superior collapse but without joint line narrowing. All laboratory tests were normal. At the time of core biopsy, on February 1, 1973, the IMP was recorded at 90 mm Hg. Histologic examination of the specimen showed both marrow and trabecular necrosis (Type 3). The decompression resulted in temporary clinical improvement. The return of symptoms lead to total hip replacement on February 27, 1974.

Illustrative Case 31. - Mr. RO..., a 73-year-old white male, was seen initially in April, 1972, with a one-month history of pain in both hips which began suddenly. For the previous year, he had been treated with daily cortisone for asthma. Physical exam showed only very slight reduction in range of movement of the hips. X-rays showed diffuse, mild osteoporosis with a normal femoral head contour and joint line spaces. Trochanteric intramedullary pressure recorded 25 mm Hg for a baseline but a rise to 80 mm Hg with the stress test, even though only 3 ml were injected. A subsequent injection of saline elevated IMP to 100 mm Hg. All laboratory findings were within normal limits. The patient decided not to undergo the recommended core decompression. He continued with cortisone therapy until June, 1972, and was seen again in our clinic one month later because of increasing hip pain. At that time, restriction of movement was much greater and left hip pain more severe, requiring the use of canes. He had no night pain. X-rays showed sclerosis on the right side without collapse (Stage II) and collapse with sequestrum formation but preservation of a good joint space on the left (Stage III). The patient had progressed from Stage I to Stage III on the left in three months. Bilateral core decompression was carried out in November, 1972. At two-year follow-up, the clinical status was unchanged, but x-rays showed progressive joint space narrowing on the left and the appearance of a mixed sclerotic cystic lesion. We anticipate that this patient will require total hip replacement when the clinical symtoms justify such an intervention.

Illustrative Case 32. - Mr. TO..., a 36-year-old university professor, afflicted with familial glomerulonephritis (Alport's syndrome), received a renal allograft on March 12, 1972. He was treated postoperatively with azathioprine (100-150 mg/day) and prednisone (30-40 mg/day) for several weeks, then with a tapering dosage. Ten months following the kidney transplant, he complained of pain in his left hip. Movement was restricted in both hips. The x-ray showed typical Stage III lesion on the left and Stage II on the right. Core decompression was carried out on February 15, 1973, on the left and was followed by marked reduction in symptoms. In April, 1973, the patient experienced the onset of right hip pain and in July, 1973, right shoulder pain. IMP measurements of 32 mm Hg in the trochanter and 46 mm Hg in the femoral head on the right on July 3, 1973, were followed by a core biopsy. The patient also had a needle biopsy of the liver because of hepatitis with elevated transaminase. The liver biopsy was normal. The bone biopsy revealed areas of marrow and trabecular necrosis with areas of markedly increased bone turnover, compatible with an associated hyperparathyroidism (Fig. 114). Clinically, the patient's discomfort was markedly reduced, and the improvement has been maintained through the most recent follow-up in 1979.

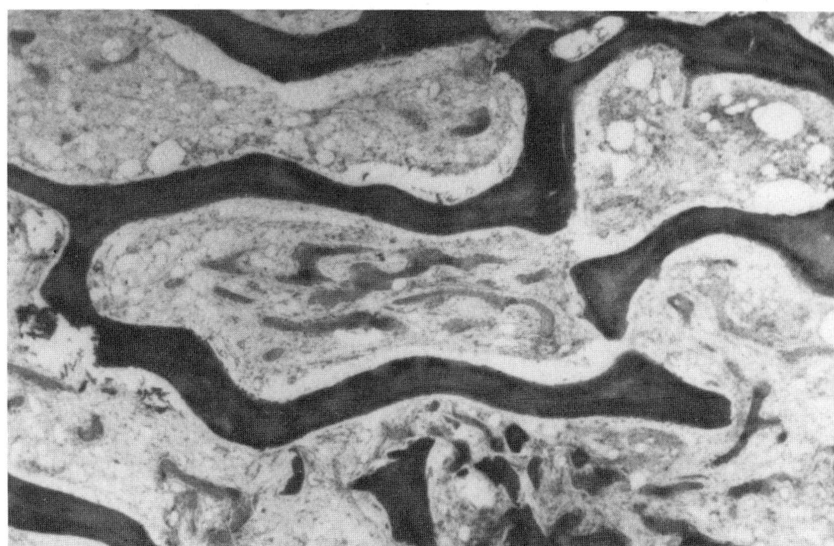

Fig. 114.—Case 32. New bone formation within bone marrow space.

PATHOGENESIS OF CORTISONE-RELATED BONE NECROSIS

The actual mechanism by which cortisone may produce bone necrosis remains ill defined, although some hypotheses have been put forth. Arfi et al.[7] have published a good review. It has been suggested that the necrosis might be secondary to multiple and accumulated microfractures, which themselves are secondary to a cortisone-induced osteoporosis. Osteoporosis and osteomalacia are often produced by cortisone treatment even in young, adult males. However, the necrosis occurs earlier than the osteoporosis and after a smaller total dose. Furthermore, it is difficult to explain why these multiple microfractures might occur in the shoulder. To our knowledge, these microfractures have not been objectively demonstrated histologically. Nonetheless, osteoporosis is often associated with cortisone-related necrosis, as we have seen in our personal experience.

Another possible mechanism has been suggested by Jones et al.[230,231,234] who hypothesize that repeated microembolization of fat accumulate in the small vessels of the femoral head resulting in ischemia and eventual bone death. The source of the microemboli is supposedly from fatty liver changes induced by cortisone. Cortisone treatment also causes lipid metabolism abnormalities which are reflected in serum lipid changes. Histologic demonstration of intravascular fat in subchondral vessels has been claimed by Fischer, Bickel, and Holley[161,162] and by Cruess et al.[103]. However, there is no proof that such microembolism has come from the fatty liver. Such emboli would have to first cross the pulmonary capillary bed before reaching the bone. In addition, the demonstration of microemboli in the subchondral circulation in the human material has been in advanced stage disease where some collapse was present. The possibility that such fat comes from intramarrow fat forced into the vessels at the time of collapse of the bone cannot be ruled out. Furthermore, the histologic evidence of bone and bone marrow necrosis is abundant throughout the femoral head and neck region corresponding to the extensive hemodynamic changes involving the entire proximal femur. In such circumstances, we do not believe that the necrosis is secondary to obstruction of the terminal arterioles in the subchondral region of the femoral head.

Direct arteriolar and venous causes cannot be disregarded. Cortisone treatment leads to hypercoagulability with the possibility of venous thrombosis. The fragile equilibrium of the intraosseous circulation, which results from the semi-closed compartment nature of bone, may explain that microthrombosis could bring about an irreversible stasis leading to necrosis. In our cases, the stasis was widespread, early, constant, and associated with increased IMP.

In the case of bone necrosis associated with renal allografts, multiple factors are probably involved. Necrosis has been recorded in patients who have renal insufficiency and have been treated by dialysis but have never received cortisone[34]. Patients with transplants are usually taking immunosuppressive drugs other than cortisone. These patients often continue with renal insufficiency and usually have some element of secondary hyperparathyroidism. These findings suggest to us that cortisone-related necrosis may depend upon several associated mechanisms, since its incidence is greater when these factors are multiple. Bone necrosis in patients with systemic lupus erythematosus is another good example of multifactorial involvement.

NECROSIS OF THE FEMORAL HEAD ASSOCIATED WITH GOUT AND HYPERURICEMIA

Recent evidence linking gout, hyperuricemia, and bone necrosis is somewhat surprising. It also lends support to those who feel that those diseases which have been recognized for a long time and seem to be well understood should be periodically reassessed in the light of new ideas. The first report of this association was by Mauvoisin, Bernard, and Germain in 1955[302] who reported a case of femoral head necrosis in a patient with gouty arthritis. Since this was an

TABLE XXII

NECROSIS OF THE FEMORAL HEAD AND GOUT

Authors	Year	No. of Cases of Necrosis	No. of Cases of Clinical Gout
De Seze Welfling Lequesne	1960	30	3
Massias Chatelin Coste	1962	50	6 (2 also steroid)
Hunder Worthington Bickel	1968	101	4
McCollum Mathews Pickett	1968	68	17
Louyot Gaucher	1970	52	4
Zinn	1971	48	2
Our Series	1974	136	13
Total.................		485	49

isolated case, the association could have been considered fortuitous. Moreover, the infrequency of hip involvement in patients with gout (whether directly related to gout or with an osteonecrosis) was confirmed in all statistical reports concerning gout. The incidents varied from 0% (Scudamore, reported by Rotes Querol and Munoz Gomez[376]) to 6.6%[396]. Nonetheless, Rotes Querol and Munoz Gomez reported 12 clinical radiological observations of great interest. They described three types of "gouty hips." The first type (five cases) corresponds to acute gouty arthritis. In two cases, which were x-rayed at the time of the crisis, the authors documented a marked, diffuse osteoporosis involving the femoral head on the symptomatic side. Moreover, this osteoporosis was completely reversible. The second type (six cases) presented with painful limitation of movement of the hip, clinically simulating arthrosis, although the roentgenograph remains normal or near normal. The third type presented with progressive destruction of the femoral heads and acetabular protrusion. One cannot help but speculate that vascular abnormalities were already present in the femoral heads described above. Only the functional exploration of bone could have aided in further delineating the problem.

Over the past several years, reports of definite and advanced necrosis of the femoral head associated with clinical gout and hyperuricemia have increased to the point that hyperuricemia is now considered as one of the etiologic factors, or at least epidemiologic

TABLE XXIII

NECROSIS OF THE FEMORAL HEAD AND HYPERURICEMIA

Authors	Years	No. of Cases of Necrosis	No. of Cases With Hyperuricemia	Mean Uric Acid Level
De Séze Welfling Lequesne	1960	13	7 (3 with clinical gout)	
Serre Simon	1962	20	5 (no clinical gout)	
Louyot Gaucher	1962	30	6 (no clinical gout)	6.1
McCollum Mathews Picket	1968	68	27 (17 with clinical gout)	
Louyot Gaucher	1970	52	10 (4 with clinical gout)	
Zinn	1974	37		6.37 Control 4.9
Our Series	1975	136	22	7.7

factors, in bone necrosis. DeSéze[394,398] and Lequesne et al.[272,278] can be credited with initially recognizing the evidence for this association. Three aspects of this association require elaboration: the incidence of bone necrosis associated with gout and hyperuricemia, the type of gout within the association and the mechanism of osteonecrosis associated with hyperuricemia.

Frequency Of Clinical Gout And Hyperuricemia In INFH

Table XXII shows that clinical gout is infrequently observed in association with INFH with the exception of the series reported by McCollum et al.[287,288]. In the Mayo Clinic series[217], there was a 4% incidence, which is not significant since the same percentage can be found in any group of patients with articular complaints. In the reported series, the incidence varies from 4% to 25% with an average of approximately 10%. The association between hyperuricemia and INFH seems much more significant (Table XXIII) since all series reported an association between 16% and 39%. This is an abnormal incidence, irrespective of sex and age, since, in a normal population, hyperuricemia is found in only 5.7% of individuals.

Types Of Gout Associated With INFH

In our opinion, the relatively benign characteristic of clinical gout associated with necrosis of the femoral head has not been sufficiently emphasized. Personally, we have never seen tophaceous gout and have only seen one case of chronic polyarticular gout associated with bone necrosis . Most of our patients had had only a small number of acute crises, which were easily treated, and had had symptoms for only a few years. Hofmeister and Brandt[206] noted that only two of their nine patients with gout-associated INFH (with the presence of urate crystals in the capsule of the hip) had suffered typical gouty crises. The others had latent gout.

Illustrative Case 33. - Mr. MES..., a 43-year-old butcher, was examined initially in January, 1975, with a history of pain in the left hip for six months. The discomfort was experienced in the groin, with an acute onset. He also was experiencing similar pain in the right hip of a few days duration. The pain was acute, and walking tolerance was limited to 500 meters. Passive movement of the right hip was normal while moderate restriction in movement of the left hip was observed. The left hip showed Stage III INFH, and the right hip was radiologically normal. IMP was elevated bilaterally (right, 57 mm Hg; left, 65 mm Hg). This patient had gout with a typical crisis three years earlier but did not have abnormal lipoprotein levels. In February, 1975, a core biopsy was performed on the right, confirming Stage I necrosis. A cup arthroplasty was carried out on the left with a good functional result ten months later.

Pathophysiology Of Gout - And Hyperuricemia-Related INFH

At the present time, there is no well-established link between gout, hyperuricemia, and INFH. However, some facts are available, and their presentation may lead to further research into pathogenetic mechanisms. The main questions revolve around whether the gout is a direct cause of the necrosis or simply acts as an associated pathology. There is some clinical evidence favoring a direct cause-and-effect relationship, particularly in those rare instances when the surgeon and the pathologist discover urate crystal deposits in the affected articular structures. One of the most interesting observations is that of Hunder, Worthington, and Bickel[217] who reported the case of a 74-year-old man with Stage IV INFH evolving over a four-year period. Several months before total hip replacement, he had a typical gouty attack. At surgery, the surgeon noted that the cartilage of the femoral head and the neighboring synovial membrane were covered by white crystalline deposits identified as monosodium urate crystals. The blood uric acid level was 8.9 mg%. McCollum et al.[289] discovered intrasynovial uric acid crystals in 12 of their 68 cases with INFH. Eight of these 12 were afflicted with clinical manifestations of gout. Hofmeister and Brandt[206] report six similar cases. However, to our knowledge, no observations of urate deposits within the necrotic bone have been reported. It is difficult to understand the exact relationship between cartilaginous and synovial urate deposits and bone necrosis. Perhaps they are secondary to the necrosis which would lower the tissue pH.

The second concept concerns the possibility that gout or hyperuricemia produces secondary pathological changes, which then, in the proper setting, produce bone ischemia. It has long been recognized that there is a relationship between gout and lipid metabolism. Recent work documents the frequency of lipoprotein abnormalities in gout and hyperuricemic patients as compared to control groups[114] Mielants, Veys, and Weerdt[314-316] have shown that the abnormalities are essentially within the triglyceride fraction. In two separate series, they showed that triglyceride levels in patients with gout were more than double those of an equal number of controls.

From these fundamental observations, one can formulate two hypotheses. The first hypothesis would involve the concept that abnormal fat metabolism leads to an increased incidence in atherosclerotic lesions which, theoretically, would involve the vessels feeding the upper end of the femur. In favor of this first hypothesis are the works of Bourde[58] and Jouve et al.[235]. Both of these authors found a statistically significant increased incidence of hyperuricemia in patients with atherosclerosis. Jouve et al.[235] compared 86 patients with atherosclerosis with 86 controls. Seventy percent of the patient population had hyperuricemia of greater than 6.0 mg% compared to 29% of controls. Twenty-nine percent had a uricemia greater than 7.0 mg% compared to 9% of controls. Bourde found similar results in his review of 200 cases of chronic arteriopathy, including documenting the existence of a syndrome of acute, thrombosing, gouty arteritis in this series. Kramer, Perilstein, and Medeiros[258] found hyperuricemia in 20.3% of 271 patients with atherosclerosis.

The second hypothesis is derived from that of Jones[231], concerning fat embolism of bone. According to this author, the osteonecrosis of the femoral head could be produced by repeated fatty microemboli from a focus of fat deposits within the liver. This exists in some alcoholic patients and after corticosteroid treatment. Neither fatty livers nor fat emboli to bone have ever been demonstrated in patients with gout who are non-drinkers or who have not been treated with cortisone. However, Rondier et al.[367] seem to have statistically demonstrated a relationship between the abnormal fat levels and hyperuricemia[367]. According to Gibson and Graham[181], the elevation in triglycerides in gouty patients is related to associated obesity. These latter authors have not been able to establish a relationship between the level of triglycerides and an abnormality in liver metabolism.

BONE NECROSIS OF VENOUS ORIGIN

The significant abnormalities in the venous drainage of bone as demonstrated by intraosseus venography at the earliest inception of ischemia, stimulates speculation that alterations in this portion of the vascular tree can initiate ischemia and necrosis of bone in man. Serre and Simon in 1961[389], as well as Ruffie et al. in 1962[375], documented the frequency, and even the constancy, of stasis and intramedullary hypertension in the tronchanteric region in patients afflicted with INFH. They proposed a venous pathogenetic mechanism as the origin of "primary" osteonecrosis. The proposed sequence of events would be stasis, increased IMP, sinusoidal and arteriolar compression, ischemia, and necrosis. We have confirmed these fundamental observations and compared them with the histological findings in all stages of INFH, particularly the preradiological stage. However, it should be acknowledged that

TABLE XXIV

GROUP ONE – 15 Patients With Evidence of Significant Pre-existing Thrombophlebitis

	Sex	Age	Side	Radio-logic Stage	IMP	Intra-osseous Veno-graphy	Core Biopsy	Clinical History	Clinical Sign Of Venous Insuffi-ciency	Venography Of The Deep Venous System
						FUNCTIONAL EXPLORATION			SIGNS OF PRE-EXISTING PHLEBITIS	
MAR	M	73	R	II	not done	not done	necrosis type 4	2 episodes of phlebitis	++	not done
POL	M	46	L	I	50	stasus at 24 h	necrosis type 3	open fracture of the leg	1+	obliteration of the femoral vein
PAI	F	66	R	I	25	stasus reflux	necrosis type 3	superficial phlebitis	1+	valvular insufficiency in the common femoral tree
CHE	F	68	L	I	80	stasus reflux	necrosis type 2	immobolization for one year	1+	partial obliteration femoral vein
CHA	F	56	R	I	12	stasus	necrosis type 2	leg ulcerations	2+	venous obstruction
			G=L	isch. cox	8	stasus	necrosis type 3			
LAP	M	41	L	I	35/65	stasus reflux	necrosis type 3	femoral diaphyseal fracture	1+	femoral vein thrombosis
GIR	F	34	R	I	20/40	stasus at 6 h	necrosis type 1	patella dislocation treated by cast	1+	venous obstruction
BIE *	M	72	R	III	42 (troch) not done 85 (fem head)	not done	necrosis type 3	repeated episodes v. cava thrombosis	3+	not done
BUG	F	69	L	II	20	stasus reflux	necrosis type 4	recurrent edema-probable phlebities	1+	obliteration common femoral vein
MON **	M	42	R	II	30	stasus reflux	necrosis type 4	saphenous vein ligation for varices	2+	obliteration of the circumflex and ischiatic veins
LAM	M	63	L	III	16	stasus	necrosis type 3		1+	femoral vein thrombosis
LAU ***	F	33	L	I	37	stasus reflux	necrosis type 4	multiple episodes of phlebitis	1+	
MAS	F	67	L	I	23/60	stasus reflux	necrosis type 4	oophorectomy followed by edema	1+	
HER	M	46	R	I	36/54	stasus	necrosis type 3	plaster immobolization for osteo-myelitis	1+	ischiatic thrombosis
			L	I	30/34	reflux				
RAY	M	36	L	I	47	stasus	necrosis type 3	severe sprain left ankle cast	1+	thrombosis main vein of the posterior neck

* Mr. Bie–this patient received Triamcinolone 8 mg x 45 days 7 years earlier
** Mr. Mon–the patient is also obese and a chronic alcoholic
***Ms. Lau–also has Buerger's disease

intramedullary stasis alone is not necessarily synonymous with venous pathology. Shobinger[385] has demonstrated that it can have either a capillary or an arterial origin. Furthermore, intramedullary stasis does not always lead to necrosis. Finally, most experimental works attempting to produce bone necrosis from venous lesions have not been successful. The pathogenetic link between intraosseus stasis of venous origin and bone necrosis can only be made if patients with unquestionable chronic venous circulatory problems either can be demonstrated to have an associated bone necrosis[369] or if experimental techniques can be developed which reproduce the pathological findings of bone necrosis[188]. In this ̄ection, we will present our clinical material which supports this concept as one pathogenetic ̠echanism of bone necrosis. Our experimental ̠ ̣ ̣k will be presented in Chapter IX.

Clinical Material

To our knowledge, there are no statistically valid analytic studies concerning a relationship between chronic venous circulatory problems and osteonecrosis. The bone abnormalities which are often observed in chronic venous disease and thought to be secondary to venous stasis are often of the osteogenic type and not the osteonecrotic type. It is also impossible to establish the incidence of chronic venous circulatory problems in published series of osteonecrosis. We have come to the conclusion that these problems have not always been systematically evaluated. However, in the work of Louyot et al.[286] in 150 cases of INFH where 20 patients were female, four had definite venous circulatory problems in the lower extremities and in the pelvis. In three other cases, the necrosis occurred 10 to 30 days following delivery.

In our own clinical experience, we have encountered 21 cases in which a strong correlation seems to exist between venous pathology and the INFH. Six of these had the clinical onset of disease coincidental with delivery or near the end of pregnancy. The other 15 patients have their clinical associations summarized in Table XXIV.

Illustrative Case 34. - Mr. MAR..., a 73-year-old white male, had a clear-cut history of phlebitis of the right lower extremity. The first episode was in 1915, following typhoid fever, and the second, in 1962, after a fracture of the medial malleolus. Since the second episode, he had chronic edema, induration, and discomfort of the right foot and leg with the typical stasis dermatitis. In early 1964, he noted the onset of right groin pain during ambulation. Physical exam showed some restriction of movement of the right hip with flexion limited to 115° and internal rotation to 15°. X-rays, at that time, did not show any joint line changes or deformities of the femoral head, although there were significant changes in the bony trabecular pattern in both the femoral head and neck. This consisted of thickening and irregularity of the trabeculae in the weight-bearing area mixed with areas of osteoporosis and two rounded cystic lesions with bordered sclerotic margins at the femoral head-neck junction (the sclerotic cyst of Phemister). Based upon radiographic evidence, the patient was thought to have Stage II INFH.

Bone necrosis was confirmed by histologic examination of the specimen removed at core biopsy on May 25, 1964. In the proximal portion of the specimen, the marrow was almost entirely necrotic over a 2 cm-long area with only a few hemorrhagic, edematous areas which remained viable. Newly formed bone covered the surface of many old, necrotic trabeculae (Type 4). The core biopsy procedure was followed with a third episode of thrombophlebitis in the right leg, which responded to anticoagulation with heparin. Postoperatively, the patient's hip pain was considerably improved. This patient was followed for three years following core decompression, after which he died suddenly of an irreversible cardiovascular collapse. The autopsy demonstrated massive embolism of the pulmonary artery. A section through the femoral head showed that the core tract was filled with marrow tissue, showing mixed hematopoiesis and fatty marrow (Fig. 122).

Illustrative Case 35. - —Mr. POL..., a 46-year-old white male, sustained an open fracture of the left tibia in July, 1955, treated by internal fixation and complicated in the postoperative period by a chronic infection lasting six months. He was immobilized for nearly one year and underwent several surgical procedures for debridement. Since the time of the fracture and subsequent surgery, he maintained chronic edema of the leg and foot. In December, 1964, he had the onset of left hip pain exacerbated by walking

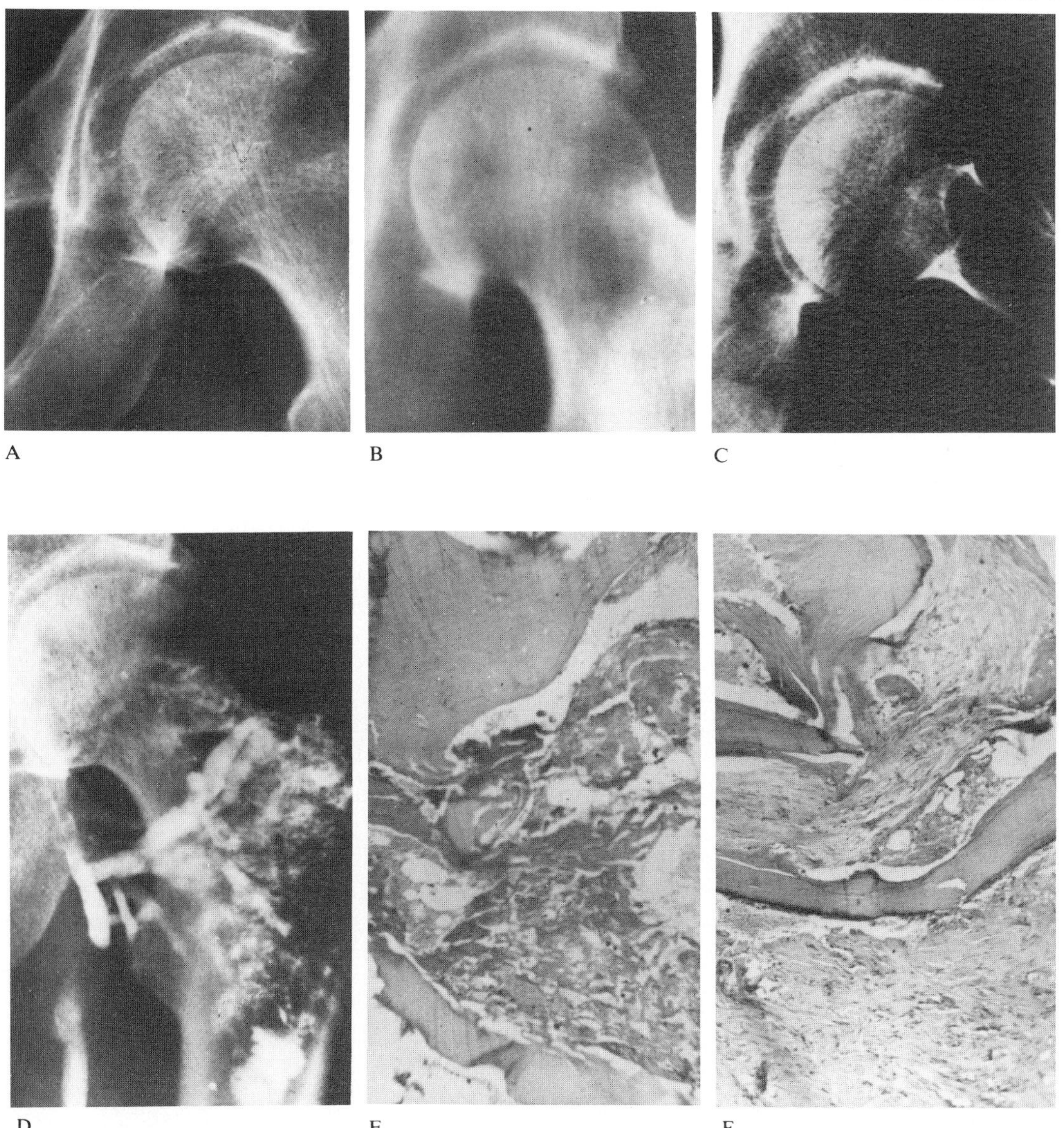

Fig. 115.—Case 35. A, B, C: Normal appearance of the left femoral head on the AP, tomogram and lateral view. D: Phlebography revealing stasis, which persisted for more than 24 hours. E: Granular necrosis of the marrow. F: Area of dense medullary fibrosis.

and by coughing. Physical examination in February, 1965, showed slight but definite limitation of movement of the left hip with discomfort at the extremes of movement, and particularly internal rotation. X-rays demonstrated only spotty demineralization of the femoral head with a perfectly spherical head both on AP and frog-leg views as well as tomographs (Stage I). The hemodynamic exploration of the left trochanter (5-5-65) demonstrated gross circulatory abnormalities. The IMP was significantly elevated at 50 mm Hg, while pertrochanteric venography showed diaphyseal reflux and considerable intramedullary stasis, which was still present 24 hours later (Fig. 115). Moreover, some of the drainage veins were not visible, with the gluteal vein, the posterior vein of the neck, and even the femoral vein itself not being visualized for ten minutes following the injection as demonstrated by cineangiographic studies of the progression of the contrast medium. It could be concluded from this study that the femoral

TABLE XXV
GROUP TWO
Six Patients With Necrosis Beginning During Or Soon After Pregnancy

Name	Sex	Age	Side	Stage	Pressure	Venogram	Histologic Type	Onset Related To Delivery	Signs During Pregnancy Or At Onset
RIG	F	40	R	I	20/35	stasis reflux	necrosis type 3	immediate	pitting edema rt. leg (1st preg.)
AUS*	F	39	L	III	25	stasis	necrosis type 3	immediate post partum	phlebitis, hip pain 3 weeks later
HUC**	F	37	L	IV	12	stasis reflux	necrosis type 2	several days after	twin pregnancy with massive lower extremity edema
BOY	F	21	L	III	28/33	stasis absent circumflex	necrosis type 3		onset of symptoms at 6 months after 20 kg. wt. gain mild albuminuria
PALA	F		bilat	III			necrosis type 2		symptoms began in 6 mo. of preg.
MUN	F	33	R	I	20/45	stasis	necrosis type 2	several days after delivery	lower extremity edema 11 kg. wt. gain occasional rt. hip pain

* Mrs. AUS—the right hip was also painful, it showed limitation of movement. The x-ray was normal although the pressure was 47 mm Hg in the femoral head. A core biopsy was not done.

** Mrs. HUC—the opposite hip showed similar x-ray changes although less mark than on the left side.

vein was obliterated by phlebitis.

Core biopsy was carried out on November 21, 1965, (ten years following the leg fracture). The specimen showed extensive medullary and trabecular necrosis (Type 3) and areas of dense fibrosis. The patient was seen in follow-up 12 years following the core decompression. He was asymptomatic with full, painless range of movement and a radiologically normal femoral head. A second hemodynamic exploration was carried out in the left trochanteric region on February 25, 1966. The pressure was normal at 18 mm Hg. Venographic drainage was not normal, but reflux and stasis were less than pre-operatively. The core channel was demonstrated.

Bone Necrosis Associated With Pregnancy

Table XXV gives the basic clinical information on six cases of which the following is an illustrative example.

Illustrative Case 36. - Mrs. RIG..., a 40-year-old woman, experienced persistent edema of the right lower extremity during her first pregnancy at age 39. The edema was associated with large varicosities. The delivery was normal, but on the day after delivery, she complained of right groin pain with painful limitation of movement of the hip. Six weeks after delivery, at the time of our first examination (November 16, 1966), there was painful limitation of movement with internal rotation reproducing groin pain. An x-ray of the pelvis showed that both femoral heads were radiologically normal. The hemo-dynamic exploration on the right showed two important abnormalities—the stress test was positive (baseline pressure of 20 mm Hg increased to 35 mm Hg after injection of saline), and venography showed metaphyseal stasis and diaphyseal reflux. A core biopsy was carried out on November 23, 1966, and showed both evidence of trabecular necrosis and marrow abnormalities, including stasis, fibrosis, and fat necrosis. At nine-year follow-up, the patient was asymptomatic with full, painless range of movement of the hip and had resumed her full activities as a hairdresser.

Criteria Favoring A Post-Phlebitic Venous Origin Of Femoral Head Necrosis

Although it may be difficult in any specific case to prove an association between femoral head necrosis and thrombophlebitis, a number of associations may lend strong support to the hypothesis of a causal relationship. Many times, the past history includes clear-cut evidence of thrombophlebitis with pain, swelling, and increased temperature of a single extremity frequently following injury or surgery. In the more recent past, phlebitis suspected at an early stage is immediately treated so that the natural clinical history is foreshortened or abbreviated and the diagnosis, in retrospect, is less certain. In some cases of complex fracture, the edema is assumed to be associated with a phlebitis, although it is not always possible to be certain. Nonetheless, the known high incidence of venous complication following fractures lends probability to the association.

Clinical signs of post-phlebitic, chronic venous insufficiency range from pitting edema at the end of the day to post-phlebitic ulcers and varicosities. According to Proche[351], the most characteristic and frequent signs in decreasing order of frequency include: a.) small, superficial lower-leg ulcers with well-defined margins in the middle of pigmented dermatitis located most commonly at the end of a dilated saphenous vein, b.) pigmented stasis dermatitis with varicosities, and c.) edema of one or both lower extremities associated with varicosities. Some of our patients have had recurrent episodes of clinical phlebitis in the same extremities.

On plain x-rays of the lower extremity, one may see cortical periosteal changes, particularly in the vicinity of the leg ulcers. Such changes are testimony of extensive venous abnormalities which also affect the bone in the region. Venography is the definitive radiographic study when the history suggests an old episode of thrombophlebitis. This is done by injecting the saphenous vein at the foot, which will usually visualize the deep venous network from the tibial to the femoral veins. If there has been thrombophlebitis of the large, deep trunks, three abnormalities may be seen: a.) the anatomic sequelae on the deep network, particularly the persistence of thrombosed portions, altered or narrowed trunks, irregularity of the tibialis, popliteal, or iliac vein, b.) filling defects or morphologic changes of the superficial network continuing in its substitutional role and, also, filling from the deep network because of insufficiency or valvular destruction of the communicating veins, and c.) functional changes in the deep network, which may fill in retrograde fashion because the thrombosed veins have recanalized but not recovered

their destroyed valves.

Injection through the vein, from the foot, or in the femoral or iliac veins in the groin is not the only means of obtaining a venogram. Transosseous venography has already been discussed at length in the early diagnosis of ischemia or necrosis of bone but also permits the visualization of lesions remaining after phlebitis of the circumflex or iliofemoral veins.

DYSPLASIAS AND BONE NECROSIS

Dysplasias are mentioned as an etiologic factor in most statistical analyses of osteonecrosis (Coste et al.[9]—34%, Serre and Simon[391]—40%, Merle d'Aubigne et al.[308]—52%, Vignon et al.[453]—5.3%, our personal series—16.1%). Even though most authors note this apparent association, they do not site the dysplasia as a real factor in the necrosis. Nonetheless, most will agree without any discussion that there is a cause-and-effect relationship between dysplasia and arthrosis. There appear to be two reasons for this paradox: Firstly, cartilage degeneration is probably more common and generally earlier than that of bone necrosis; secondly, many necroses, which do not end in the formation of a sequestrum, remain unrecognized because the sclerocystic changes of arthrosis and necrosis are nonspecific. By using solely radiographic criteria to reach a diagnosis, many necroses are missed.

When all the arthroses are subjected to functional exploration of bone, as we have done, one becomes convinced that, in addition to a certain number of true and pure arthroses, there are also mixed forms where the two primary conditions, that of a circulatory disorder of bone and a degenerative condition of cartilage, are associated. It is not usually possible to say which has been first, perhaps they are simultaneous[155].

However, to prove a pathogenetic relationship between dysplasia and osteonecrosis, the best evidence appears to be demonstration of osteonecrosis in a dysplastic joint without joint space narrowing. Most will agree that a normal joint space is the best evidence of cartilage integrity. In an earlier section, we reported 11 cases of necrosis, of which nine patients correspond to these criteria. In five cases, where the x-ray was completely normal (Stage I), the diagnosis was made by the functional exploration of bone and the histologic evidence on the core specimen. In four other cases (three in Stage II and one in Stage III), the radiographic picture was very suggestive of INFH, and the diagnosis was confirmed by the biopsy. Of the remaining two patients, one had sequestrum formation (Stage III), and the other had sclerosis with cysts (Stage II) which were clinically

TABLE XXVI – Dysplasias Without Joint Line Narrowing

Case	Sex	Age	Side	Prior-treatment	Dysplasia	Narrow-ing Wing	Trabec-ulae	Stage	Troch. Press.	Head Press.	Phlebog-raphy	Biopsy	OPERAT.	RESULT
1. FOU	F	28	L	0	A.I.	0	N	I		7 Base ↗ 12	Stasis	Type 2	Shelf+ Core	Excell. at 2 yr.)
2. MUL	M	30	R	0	A.I.	0	Sequestrum	III	Not carried out because of the pathognomonic appearance of the x-ray.				None	Medical follow-up
3. POU (fig. 1,2)	M	25	L	Vaso-dilator	Coxa Valga	0	N	I	27 ↗ 47		Reflux Stasis	Type 1,2	Core	Excell. at 2 yr.
4. BLA (fig. 3)	M	24	R		A.I.	0	Multi-cystic changes	III	N (outside sequest.)			Type 4	Core	Excell.
5. LAU	F	29	R	Sympath for Buergers Disease	Coxa Valga	0	N	I	29 ↗ 60	30 ↗ 60	++ (pos. scan)	Type 4	Core	Excell.
			L		Coxa Valga	0	N	I	37			Type 4	Core	Excell.
6. MON	F	30		Shelf (7 mon.)	A.I.	0	N	I	35		N	Type 2,3	Core	Excell. at 5 yr.
7. PEL	F	24	R	Shelf (7 yr.)	A.I.	0	Cysts in the head & acetab.	II	45			Type 3	Core	Excell. at 2 yr.
			L	Shelf (6 yr.)	A.I.	0	Cysts	II	30 ↗ 40	40	Stasis	Type 2	Core	Excell. at 2 yr.
8. SEL	M	51	L	Osteotomy (4yr.) Shelf (2 yr.)	A.I.	0	Sclerosis & cysts	II	28 ↗ 48	3		Type 2,3	Core	Excell. at 2 yr.
9. SAR	M	25	L	Shelf (7 yr.)	A.I.	0	Sclerosis & cysts	II						Medical follow-up

A.I. = Acetabular Insufficiency
N = Normal

well tolerated; hence, there was no biopsy. It is interesting to note that, of the nine core decompressions carried out, four cases showed Type 3 pathologic changes, i.e., total necrosis of the marrow and trabeculae. Two of these were present in patients with Stage I disease. In addition, four patients from this series had previously had a shelf arthroplasty without success. Only after the decompression did the hip become painless. The clinical points on these nine patients are summarized in Table XXVI. We have also reported 27 cases of necrosis in 24 patients in which the dysplasia and necrosis were also associated with joint line narrowing. In those instances, the cartilage involvement was more severe. In this latter group, it should be emphasized that the superolateral narrowing, typical of the classical arthrosis from dysplasia, was present in only ten of the 17 cases. When the joint line narrowing is medial or global, it is more suggestive of an associated ischemic condition.

In these two groups, increased IMP has proven to be a very reliable sign. The importance of the stress test should also be emphasized since, in ten cases with a normal baseline pressure, the stress test provoked an abnormal pressure response. Venography is also important since, in two cases with normal IMP in the intertrochanteric region, the venogram documented circulatory derangement.

We feel that the demonstration of osteonecrosis with both hemodynamic abnormalities and biopsy confirmation in the presence of a normally maintained joint space and a dysplastic hip is sufficient to implicate direct responsibility of the dysplasia for the occurrence of necrosis. Five of these Stage I cases have a two-year follow-up, and one case, a five-year follow-up with no alteration in the joint space over the follow-up period. Nonetheless, this proof is not airtight since one should also be able to prove the integrity of the articular cartilage by biochemical or microscopic examination. These observations need to be made in the earliest stages, since we know that

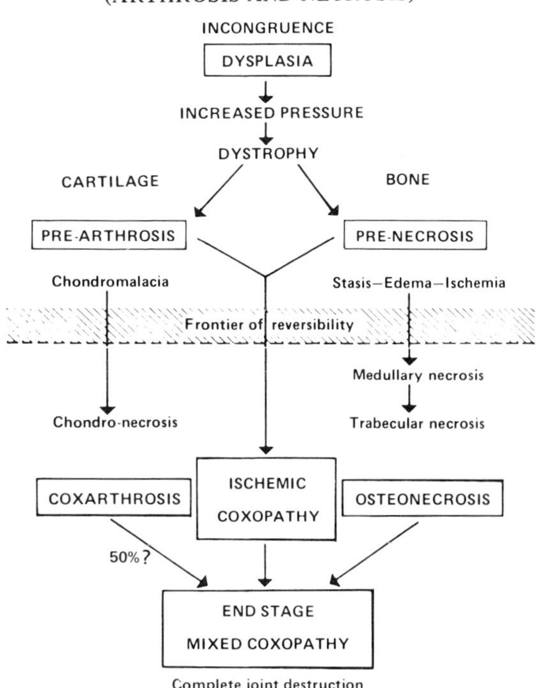

**Dysplasia* could just as well be replaced by *trauma* in this same framework.

osteonecrosis may eventually alter the viability of the articular cartilage. Nevertheless, there appears to be sufficient proof for the practical purposes of the clinician, since in the clinical setting, one must often be content with an approximation of biological proof which cannot always be tested with complete scientific rigor. Table XXVII is an attempt to express the various pathways that a dysplastic hip may take in inducing cartilaginous or bone tissue deterioration. Simple secondary arthrosis by itself cannot explain all of the findings.

Illustrative Case 37. (Fig. 116) - Mrs. COM..., a 41-year-old housewife, was seen by us for the first time in October, 1966. She gave a six-year history of bilateral groin-to-knee pain, greater on the right. Pain was of moderate intensity, with walking limited to a maximum of two kilometers. Movement in both hips was definitely restricted, limited to 90° of flexion. X-rays showed bilateral dysplasia which had been previously undiagnosed (acetabular insufficiency and coxa valga) and a slight flattening of the femoral head contour in the superomedial region

with a small area of cysts surrounded by a zone of sclerosis. Pertrochanteric venography showed a definite stasis (Fig. 116). A core biopsy was carried out on the right on October 14, 1966, showing eosinophilic reticular necrosis of the bone marrow and trabecular necrosis. Improvement in symptoms was only moderate and lasted for one year. The patient was seen again in 1971 with similar clinical and radiographic status to the pre-operative state (Fig. 116).

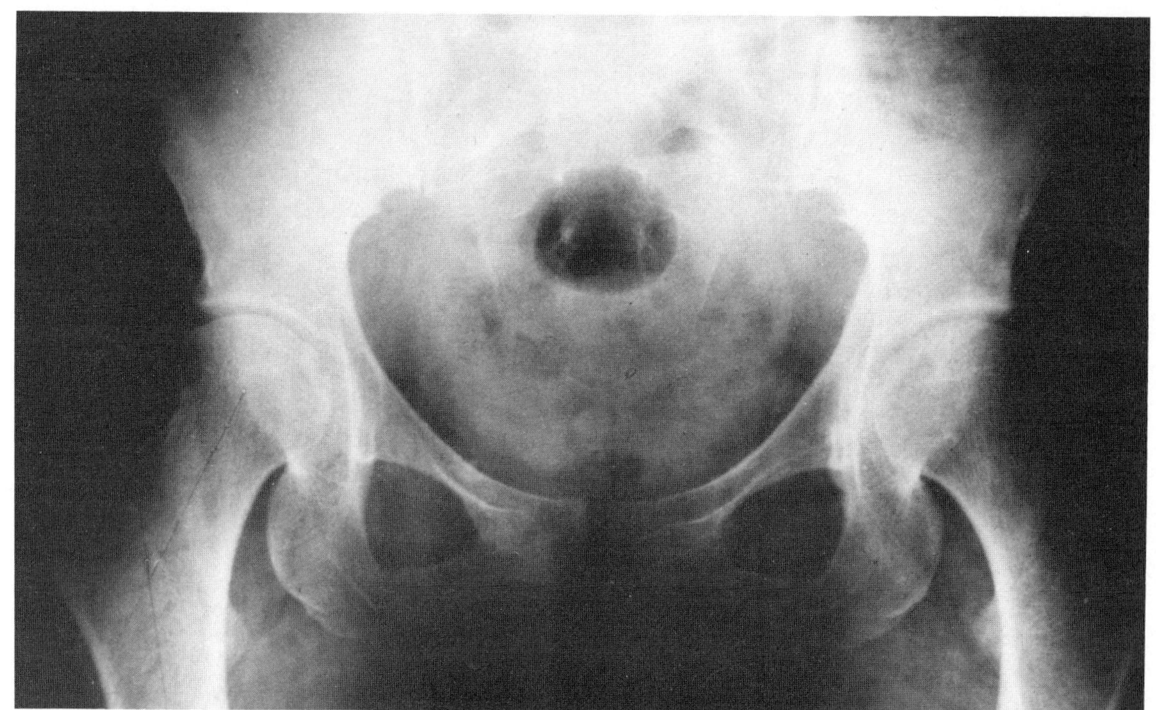

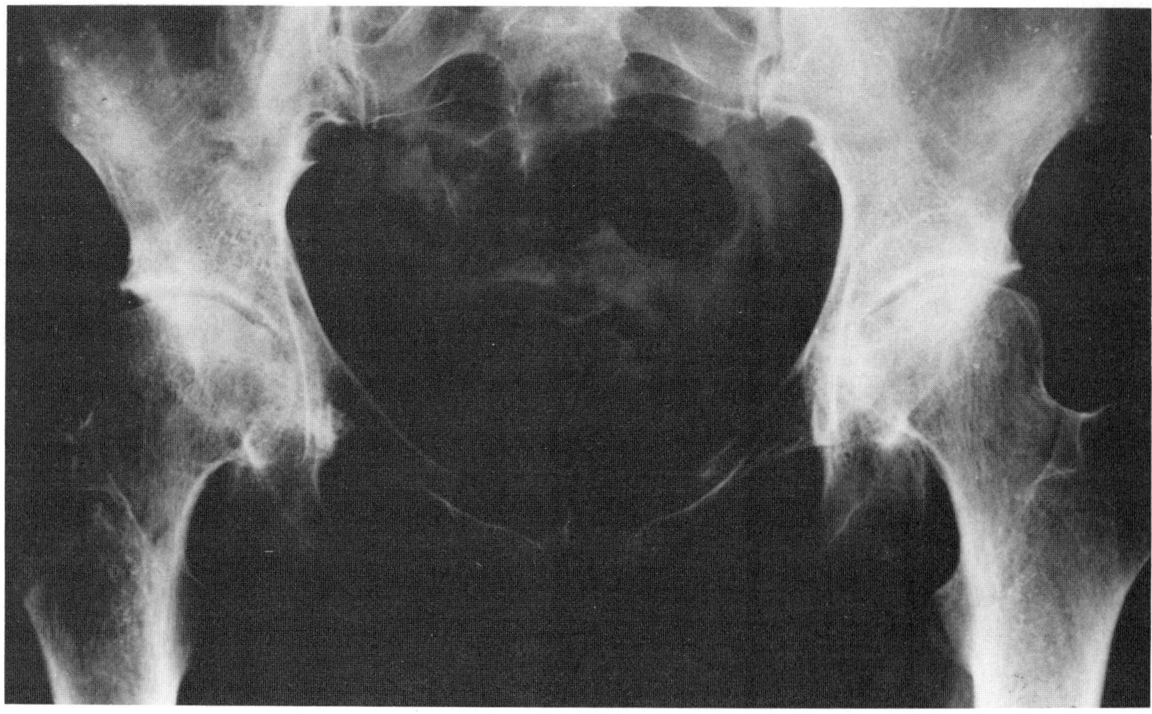

Fig. 116.—Case 37. A: (1960) X-rays taken when the first painful manifestations occured. Coxa valga with a slightly deficient acetabulum. B: (1970) X-rays done four years after core biopsy of the right hip (in October 1966). Slight global jointline narrowing, more marked on the left. Subfoveal flattening. Sclerocystic changes.

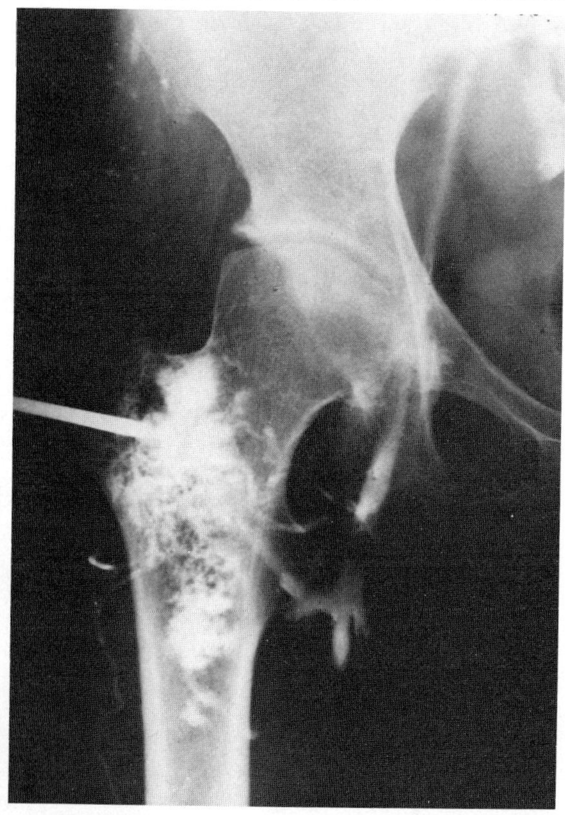

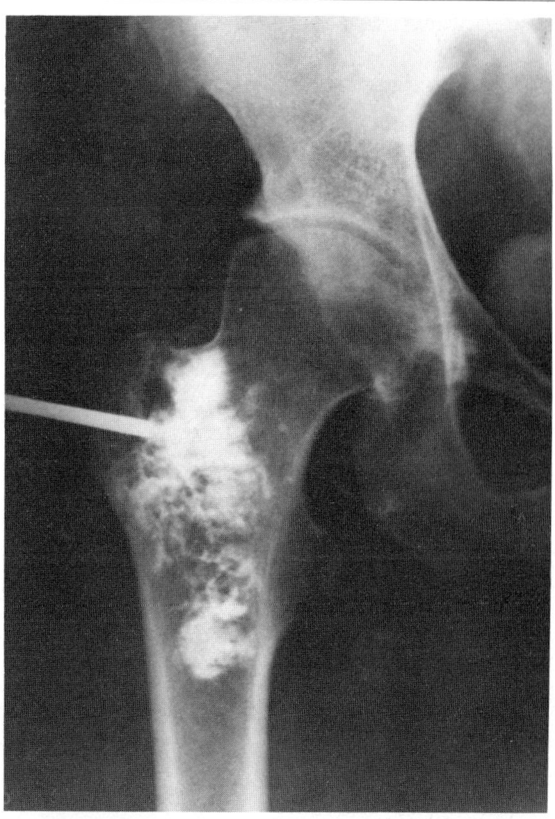

C: Intra-operative phlebography of the right hip (1966) (termination of injection).

D: Stasis 15 minutes later.

Illustrative Case 38. (Fig. 117) - Mr. BLA..., a 24-year-old man, was seen initially in July, 1972, complaining of right groin pain of six years duration. The pain had become constant and was associated with moderate, decreased range of movement. The x-rays showed cystic degeneration in the weight-bearing area of the head with visible collapse on the lateral view. The joint space was increased (Stage III, Fig. 117). IMP was normal both in the neck and in the femoral head. A core biopsy, carried out on July 6, 1972, showed Type 4 necrosis in the cystic area and Type 2 in the rest of the specimen.

Fig. 117.—Case 38. A: AP view shows a slightly deficient acetabulum and cystic changes in the weight-bearing zone of the femoral head. The joint line is preserved. B: Lateral view: flattening with some collapse, joint line widened.

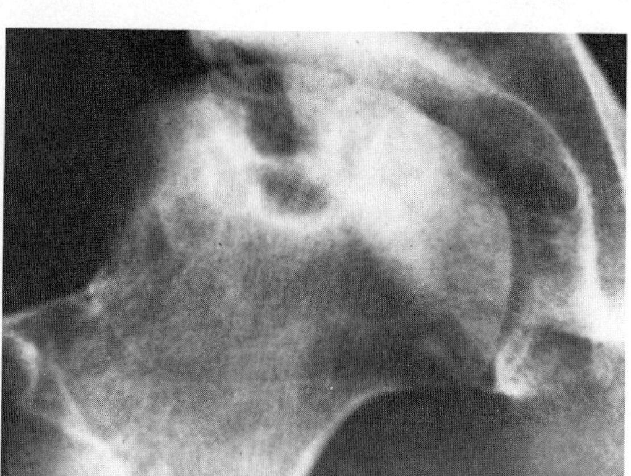

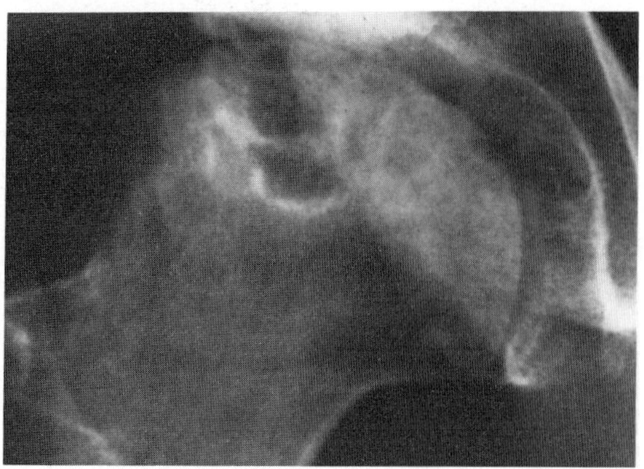

Illustrative Case 39. - Mr. BEN..., a 58-year-old male, sprained his left knee after a fall on cement in 1966. Since the injury, he also had pain in the left hip, which did not prevent him from working. By 1969, the pain in the hip radiated to the knee. Physical examination showed flexion limited to 90° and abduction, to 30°. X-rays revealed superolateral narrowing, sclerotic and cystic lesions of the head, and sclerosis of the roof of the acetabulum with considerable acetabular dysplasia (Fig. 118). Functional exploration of bone carried out in August, 1969, showed a baseline pressure of 15 mm Hg increasing to 50 mm Hg after the injection of 2 ml of saline. Venography failed to visualize the common efferent pathways revealing diaphyseal reflux of the dye and massive stasis. A core biopsy coupled with synovial biopsy showed reactive synovial proliferation and medullary and trabecular necrosis (Type 3). Because of clinical failure and continued pain, a MacMurray type of varus osteotomy was carried out on December, 3, 1970. At the time of the second intervention, IMP of 50 mm Hg was measured in the trochanter, neck, and head. Pressure rose to 70 mm Hg after the stress test. A new core biopsy did not show necrosis but did reveal areas of hemorrhagic change in the marrow. At follow up on July, 21, 1971, the patient was greatly improved as far as pain was concerned and showed increased range of movement as well (flexion - 120°, abduction - 45°). The x-ray at follow-up showed a narrowed joint line and a head which was less dense and better covered than pre-operatively.

Fig. 118.—Case 39. A: (1969) Marked narrowing of the joint line with mirror image sclerosis of the weight-bearing area. B: Intra-operative phlebography: diaphyseal reflux with absence of efferents.

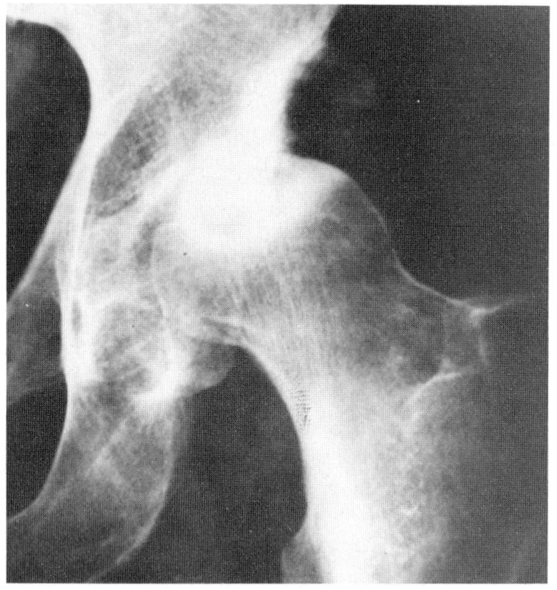

A

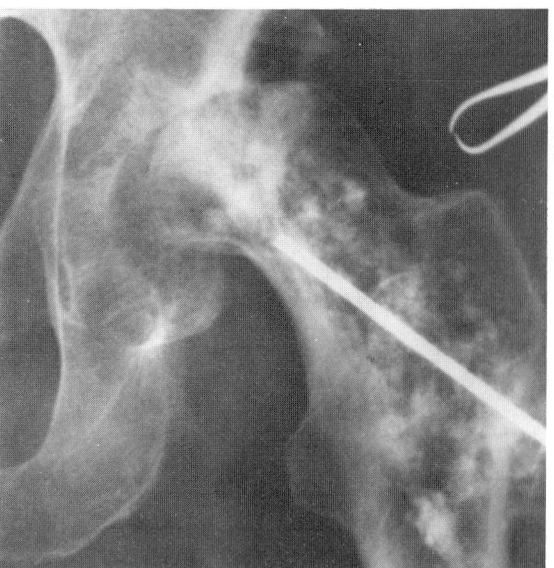

B

Illustrative Case 40. - Mrs. RIP..., a 79-year-old white female, began with radiating pain in the left leg in 1968, which progressed by April, 1969, to pain on weight bearing requiring the use of a single cane. Physical exam showed limitation of movement with flexion restricted to 110°, abduction to 15°, and internal rotation to 10°. The x-rays showed marked joint-line narrowing with loss of head substance and contour and with sclerosis on both sides of the joint. Dysplasia of the acetabulum was evident as well as coxa valga (Fig. 119). Venography was carried out in June, 1969, and demonstrated some reflux and very definite intramedullary stasis. This was followed by a temporary improvement, probably due to the puncturing of the bone for the venography. On October 7, 1969, baseline IMP was measured at 40 mm Hg rising to 66 mm Hg with the stress test. Core biopsy was carried out with a small trephine, and three separate specimens were taken, showing fibrinoid necrosis, marrow fibrosis, and partial trabecular necrosis (Fig. 119B). Following the core biopsy, she had significant reduction in her pain for a year, after which symptoms progressed, necessitating total hip replacement.

Fig. 119.—Case 40. A: Complete destruction and erosion of the whole joint space with sclerosis on both sides of the joint, coxa valga with mild acetabular dysplasia. B: Association of reticular necrosis, fibrosis, and plasmostasis.

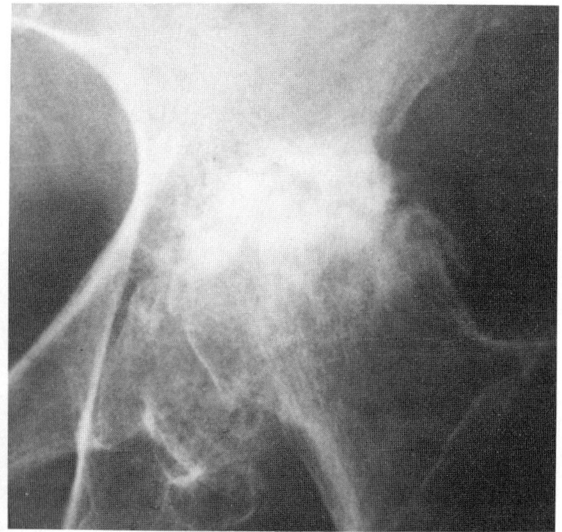

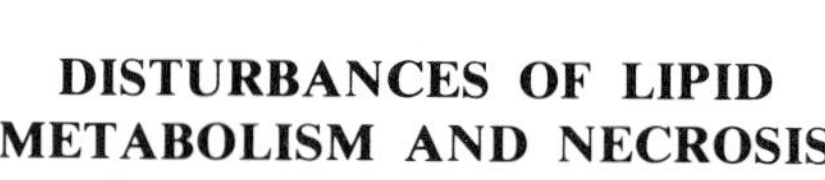

A

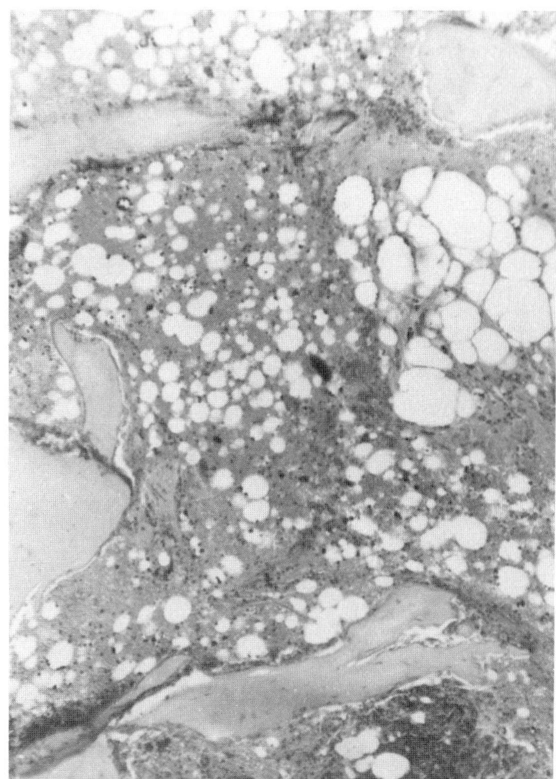

B

DISTURBANCES OF LIPID METABOLISM AND NECROSIS OF THE FEMORAL HEAD

The importance of this section has already been emphasized under the sections dealing with both steroid- and gout-associated necrosis. Moreover, many authors have considered lipid metabolic disturbances as an etiologic factor in alcohol-associated bone necrosis in which the action of alcohol is initially on the liver leading to fatty changes. Fatty changes in the liver are also found in steroid-treated patients. Chronic pancreatitis is also known to lead to necrotic bone lesions through the destructive action of pancreatic lipase.

Jones et al.[234] and Welfling[462,463] have generated a general theory for the pathophysiology of bone necrosis, particularly of the femoral head, which includes fat embolus to bone, resulting from abnormal mechanisms of fat metabolism. The bone necrosis, according to these authors, is the result of repetitive microembolism of the intraosseous vessels by fat globules which originate from a fatty liver. In order to place the role of disturbances in fat metabolism

into proper perspective, in regards to necrosis of the femoral head, the following points need clarification: a.) the nature and incidence of lipoprotein abnormalities in femoral head necrosis, b.) the incidence of alcoholism in femoral head necrosis, c.) the incidence of fatty liver changes in femoral head necrosis, d.) the nature of bone necrosis associated with pancreatitis (and Weber Christian disease), and e.) the eventual role of fat microembolism in the pathophysiology of necrosis of the femoral head.

BONE NECROSIS AND LIPOPROTEIN ABNORMALITIES

To our knowledge, statistics concerning the frequency of bone necrosis in lipoprotein metabolic disturbances have not been reported. Moreover, it can be stated that bone necrosis is not generally considered a predictable complication of lipoprotein disturbances of whatever type even though Pouletty, Cloarec, and Lequesne[350] and DeGennes et al.[79] have reported isolated cases. In spite of this apparent discrepancy, there have been numerous studies of series of cases evaluating lipid levels in patients with known INFH. These reports are summarized in Table XXVIII. The incidence varies from 21 to 81% of the patients showing abnormal lipid levels of one kind or another. Lequesne, Cloarec, and DeSeze[273] were the first to call attention to the relationship of increased levels of triglyceride and pre-beta-lipoprotein in non-traumatic INFH. The abnormalities concerning total lipids and cholesterol were similar to those found in a group of patients with atheromata[278].

BONE NECROSIS AND ALCOHOL EXCESS

The relationships here are particularly difficult to interpret because alcohol excess is so ill defined. What constitutes too much alcohol? Chronic signs of alcohol intoxication, typical facies, and the presence of fatty changes in the liver, proven indirectly by laboratory data or directly by liver biopsy, are all means of arriving at a positive association but are seldom carried out in all patients in any given series. To our knowledge, only one statistical analysis has been done in alcoholics. Schneider and Bick[384] analyzed the radiologic signs of INFH in 202 alcoholics of both sexes and were unable to find an abnormal frequency of necrosis in relation to a control group. On the other hand, we have some data concerning the frequency of alcoholism in patients affected with femoral head necrosis even though the evidence for the diagnosis of alcoholism is not well stated. Table XXIX summarizes the recorded data. From these reports, the percentage of patients giving some evidence of alcohol abuse varies from 10 to 36% of a given series of INFH. Zinn[473] emphasized the difficulty of research in this field and concluded that in the Swiss series the etiologic role of alcoholism cannot be confirmed. However, by taking the overall numbers of the statistics, alcohol abuse appears to be present in 26% of the 344 cases reported. Although we believe that alcohol is an etiologic factor to be considered, and, though proof of intoxication or physical damage due to alcohol is very seldom confirmed in these series, it would be very interesting to know if the hypertriglyceridemia observed in INFH is linked in part or totally with alcohol abuse. Alcoholic beverages are well known to produce hyperlipemia.

BONE NECROSIS AND FATTY LIVER

Fatty liver is considered by some authors as the intermediate lesion between the primary cause of the bone necrosis (cortisone, alcohol, etc.) and the final mechanism of bone necrosis, that of intermittent fat

TABLE XXVIII

DYSLIPOPROTEINEMIA IN PATIENTS WITH INFH

Author Year	Number of Cases in Series	No. Abn.	Abnormalities		
			Cholest.	Triglyc.	Pre-beta
Lequesne et al. 1961	22	18	+		
David Chausse, 1969 (115)	18	10	+	++	
Hartmann, 1971	38	8		+	
Louyot et al. 1971	48	30	+	+	++
Serre et al. 1973	37	17		+	
Tavaux personnels (Baudel), 1975 (37)	32	19		+	+

emboli to bone which eventually results in obstruction of the arteriolar-capillary system of bone. Although it is certain that fatty liver is capable, in rare instances, of producing fat embolism in the lungs, especially after direct contusion of a liver which shows massive cystic fatty degeneration, it is not certain that fatty liver is capable of producing fat embolism to bone. The most important question is, of course, "Is fatty necrosis of the liver commonly encountered in patients affected with INFH?" Classically, fatty liver manifests itself clinically as changes in the facies, grayish sclerae, sallow skin color, and palpable, tender hepatomegaly. In laboratory evaluation, only the BSP is altered in the early stage, transaminased as being raised in the later stages. Alcoholism is responsible for approximately half the cases of fatty liver. Absolute diagnosis must be confirmed by liver biopsy. The search for fatty changes in the liver in patients afflicted by INFH has been done both indirectly with the laboratory and clinical data and directly by biopsy. Hartmann[200] reported 11 abnormal BSP tests in 32 patients with INFH. Velayos et al[451] autopsied ten patients who expired at various times following kidney transplantation, one of whom had INFH. The liver frequently showed fatty changes. Solomon[420] studied 29 cases of INFH in blacks in South Africa who had an iron overload hepatomegaly secondary to heavy beer drinking. He did not find any cases of fatty changes in the liver biopsies carried out on these patients. Gaucher et al[178] carried out 12 liver biopsies in patients with INFH in which they found some evidence of fatty change in all cases, sometimes moderate but usually severe and associated with early cirrhosis in four cases. Simon et al.[418] recently studied ten non-selected patients with INFH in Stage III, half of whom had bilateral involvement. All were men, ranging in age from 31 to 64. One of them was significantly obese, and two had gouty arthritis. Needle biopsy showed a pure fatty degeneration of the liver in eight cases, fibro-fatty changes in one case, and cirrhosis in one case. According to these last two publications, fatty changes in the liver would seem to be a constant finding in INFH. If this were confirmed, it would be an important finding. It should be emphasized, however, that these liver abnormalities were remarkably silent, both clinically and by laboratory examination, in both the series reported by Gaucher et al.[178] and Simon et al.[418].

BONE NECROSIS ASSOCIATED WITH PANCREATITIS OR WEBER-CHRISTIAN DISEASE

Immelman et al.[219] have presented a good review of the considerations in the association of bone necrosis and pancreatitis. Necrotic lesions of bone are probably much more frequent than thought in the course of several kinds of pancreatitis since the bone lesions often go undiagnosed. Scarpelli[383] found evidence of bone necrosis in 10% of 77 patients autopsied following acute pancreatitis. Similar lesions have been described, not only in acute and chronic pancreatitis but also in carcinoma of the pancreas[281]. Occasionally, the clinical picture is one of subacute polyarthralgia, such as one of the cases reported by Immelman. "Fifteen days after laparotomy had demonstrated fatty necrosis of the greater omentum, an 11-year-old girl presented with a clinical picture of polyarthritis, painful effusions of the elbows, wrists, and knees, erythematous, tender, subcutaneous nodules, and fever. This was associated with anemia, leukocytosis, and eosinophilia. Fifteen days after the onset of symptoms, x-rays demonstrated osteolytic lesions of the radius and ulna with periosteal reaction. A subcutaneous nodule was biopsied and showed foci of fatty necrosis surrounded by mixed polynuclear and lymphocytic cellular proliferation." No bone biopsy was carried out, but the radiologic changes disappeared, and the author believed that the bone lesions healed spontaneously.

Not all clinical cases present such an obvious picture. Others may demonstrate the involvement of only a few joints. There are some cases where there are no clinical signs whatsoever. In one case in Immelman's series, the bone lesions were revealed only when the femoral neck spontaneously fractured. X-ray changes usually allow a "probable" diagnosis

TABLE XXIX
INFH AND ALCOHOLISM

Authors	Number In Series of Cases	Alcoholism	
		Number of Cases	*Criteria For Alcoholism*
Massias et al. 1962	50	11	History of abuse
Serre et al. 1962	37	7	History of abuse + 5 cirrhosis
Volle 1963	52	18	Abuse 1.5 liters wine per day
Patterson et al. 1964	52	9	History of abuse (Control population estimate 7 to 10% alcoholics)
McCollum, 1970	68	26	Abuse
Zinn 1971	50	5	History of abuse (Control population 2.5% alcoholics)
Mielants et al. 1975	35	12	History of abuse 2 liters beer per day

to be made, which can be firmly established by biopsy. The reported x-ray changes, consisting of either well-delineated osteolytic lesions or intramedullary sclerotic (calcified) lesions with an irregular outline, are very similar to those seen in caisson disease as reported by Phemister[346]. Pancreatic function itself is not always altered as measured by common methods. Serum lipase was elevated in only one of two cases where it was carried out by Immelman[219].

There are two main hypotheses concerning the mechanism of bone necrosis associated with pancreatitis. In the first hypothesis, bone fat is lysed by enzymes which may either be circulating lipase or by intraosseous embolism of a functioning pancreatic acini that manufacture lipase "in situ." In the second hypothesis, fat microemboli secondary to hyperlipemia block the capillary-sinusoidal system of bone. The bone lesions seen in chronic pancreatitis, carcinoma of the pancreas and during the evolution of Weber-Christian disease are all similar. The systemic forms of the latter disease have been reported by Steinberg[426]. Bismuth et al[52] reported a case and reviewed six cases from the literature. It is possible that the incidence of bony involvement in Weber-Christian disease is more frequent than reported since the lesions may be silent. Weber-Christian disease is known to manifest itself both by episodes of temperature spikes associated with articular, muscular pains and painful nodules in skin folds (gluteal, abdominal) which resorb spontaneously without draining. The bone lesions are frequently located in the fingers and rarely in the knees and hips. They usually take on an irregular lytic appearance, occasionally eroding the inner cortex. Mixed sclerotic lesions and isolated articular lesions with narrowing of the joint space have also been seen. Histologically, the changes are that of fatty necrosis of the marrow with liquefaction of the fatty marrow, appearance of xanthoma, and foam cells associated with medullary fibrosis. These lesions are not very different from those described in idiopathic INFH, although the pathophysiology of bone necrosis associated with Weber-Christian disease is unknown and is thought to be an enzymatic necrosis.

THE ROLE OF FAT MICROEMBOLISM IN THE DEVELOPMENT OF BONE NECROSIS

Histologic demonstration of intraosseous fat emboli is difficult because of the physical characteristics of bone and the quantity of fat already available in the bone marrow in which exogenous fat may not be easily differentiated. The patchy network of embolism, which has been described in the lung and brain[36], has never been observed in bone, although the technical problems of processing bone would make such demonstration difficult. Those who have reported emboli do so on the basis of fat within the lumen of intraosseous vessels. Since normal decalcifying techniques result in extraction of fat from the bone, the technique to demonstrate intraosseous fat requires frozen sections of bone which, technically, must avoid the rupture of the marrow lipocytes. Such rupture of the intraosseous marrow fat could lead to the artifactual filling of the Haversian canals and intraosseous vessels from released cytoplasmic fat. Jones et al[232] have acknowledged the technical difficulties and suggested that some of the smaller fatty droplets which are found in the haversian canal may be too small to represent emboli, being free fat droplets which are artifactually displaced into the canal. However, when the fat is deformed and molded onto the wall of the vessel, which is definitively stained by special stain for reticulin fibers, they feel that this most likely represents a true embolus. Detailed histologic observations are not numerous. Jones reported two separate cases. The first one was that of a 32-year-old man who died suddenly. Autopsy revealed a fatty liver and fat embolism in the pulmonary artery. The right femoral head, which was non-necrotic and otherwise normal, revealed isolated fat and probable intravascular fat within the subchondral capillaries. The second case was that of a 56-year-old alcoholic who had died suddenly. Autopsy revealed the presence of multiple fatty emboli in the hepatic vein in the lungs and the kidneys. There was also necrosis of the right femoral head and a calcified infarction of the lower portion of the femoral diaphysis of the same side. The femoral head and its upper part showed trabeculae without osteocytes and medullary fibrosis which was partially calcified. Fatty globules which were conformed to the vessel walls were found in the Haversian canals adjacent to the "infarcted" region. Jones[234] reported two further cases of cortisone-associated necrosis where intravascular fat globules "seemed" to exist in the femoral head, but few details were provided. Fisher et al[161] reported on one case of a 23-year-old man dying three years after a renal allograft who had been treated with cortisone and azathioprine. At autopsy, there was no evidence of fatty emboli to the soft tissue organs. The liver had moderate fatty changes without the formation of large cysts. Diagnosis of the necrosis of the left femoral head had been made 14 months after the renal allograft. Sectioning of the femoral head was carried out after formal fixation. Frozen sections were stained with "oil red O" and demonstrated fatty globules in the arterioles of many Haversian canals. These globules were clearly intravascular surrounded by a vascular endothelium and were considered to be fat emboli. Neighboring vessels contain blood cells and thin material which was stained with the "oil red O." Cruess has also shown one such case to us. Fisher and Bickel[162] examined 25 femoral heads from 20 patients with steroid-associated INFH. In twelve of the 25 specimens, probable fat embolism was identified in subchondral vessels, however, no detailed description of the histological sections appeared in their paper.

Jones and Sakovich[233] tried to reproduce intraosseous embolism by the injection of Lipiodol into the aorta of the rabbit. During the first five weeks following injection, fatty emboli and, particularly, obstruction by the fat of the subchondral arterioles and capillaries of the femoral head could be histologically demonstrated. After five weeks, these emboli began to break down and became less evident, but autoradiographic signs of necrosis appeared, and histologic lesions of ischemic necrosis were found in both the epiphyseal and metaphyseal regions of the femoral head. These lesions were characterized by disorganization of all the cellular elements of bone, liquefaction of bone marrow fat, coagulation, necrosis, amorphous debris of the bone marrow, separation of the cement lines along the trabeculae with development of microfractures, and sequestration of small fragments of dead bone in the marrow space.

From a clinical point of view, Jones presents two series of cases in which he develops indirect evidence to support the concept of fat embolus as the etiology of the subsequent bone necrosis. The first series consists of 30 cases of INFH in patients in which there was only a strong history of alcohol abuse. Twenty-seven of the 30 patients had hepatomegaly. Nine of these had a needle biopsy of the liver which showed fatty changes in seven instances. The second series consists of 32 cases of femoral head necrosis in patients on large doses of corticosteroids. A systematic search for signs favoring a fat embolism was carried out in 11 patients. Five of these had evidence of lipuria. These indirect arguments are not convincing, particularly those concerning lipuria, which is considered by the biologist as an uncertain parameter to give evidence of fat embolus.

There is certain indirect evidence, as well, to support the conclusion that fat embolus may not be important in the pathogenesis of bone necrosis, particularly the work reported by Hartmann[200] in which over 5000 cases of venous infusion of fat took place without vascular complications. Although Goulon, Barois, Grospuis, and Schortgen[186] described two

cases of fat infusion overload producing a picture similar to post-traumatic embolism with intrapulmonary radiodensities, somnolence, purpura, intravascular hemolysis, and disseminated intravascular coagulation, no mention was made of bone lesions. These accidents would have been produced by lipolysis which would liberate large amounts of nonsaturated fatty acids into the capillaries. This would be toxic for the endothelium and produce a diffuse vasculitis responsible for the pulmonary and cerebral hemorrhagic manifestations.

Lymphangiography is commonly carried out with Lipiodal, resulting in pulmonary microembolism which can be visualized on chest x-ray some time after the lymphangiogram. Hartmann, Noel, and Collard[332] carried out a systematic search for radiologic evidence of bone lesions in 31 cases following lymphangiography without any evidence being found.

From a review of the literature, which is sometimes contradictory, it is difficult to arrive at a satisfactory synthesis of the data. It is likely that there is some link between certain kinds of bone necrosis and metabolic disturbances of fat. The concept that fatty changes in the liver are often, or always, associated with INFH certainly requires confirmation. It should not be forgotten that bone necrosis in all cases involves fatty necrosis of the bone marrow. This is a fundamental concept which we have clearly confirmed but which is seldom mentioned in the discussion of pathophysiology. Although Jones' hypothesis has attractive elements, it lacks solid confirmation. As we and several other authors have stated[154,200], the existence of a few emboli in the subchondral vessels does not account for all of the diffuse necrotic lesions of the femoral head and neck, as we have seen in samples taken at core biopsy or at the time of excision of the femoral head.

As an alternative to the hypothesis that fat embolism is the primary pathophysiologic link between lipid metabolism disturbance and necrosis, the lipid abnormalities observed in the serum could be the consequence and not the cause of the necrosis of bone marrow fat. The fat debris coming from this necrosis could modify lipoprotein in the general circulation. It is also possible that this debris could encroach upon the bone marrow vessels and aggravate the ischemia. The second consideration is that a general alteration of lipid metabolism could create overload lesions in several organs, the bone marrow as well as the liver, without the necessity of embolism per se. This hypothesis is connected with those trying to explain the anatomical, pathological, and clinical picture of post-traumatic fat embolism. Also, lipid overload in the body, and especially triglyceride overload, increases the frequency of arteriosclerosis, and this could induce bone necrosis through large- and medium-vessel disease outside of bone. All of these varying hypotheses require careful consideration in which more data in a larger number of cases may help to interpret some of the pathophysiologic variants in the pathways of bone necrosis.

BONE NECROSIS IN THE CONNECTIVE TISSUE DISEASES

The reported frequency of INFH, as a complication of or association with the connective tissue diseases, varies to the point where a cause-and-effect relationship can be debated. In most instances, it appears to be a complication of corticosteroid therapy. However, the unusual frequency of bone necrosis in systemic lupus erythematosus (SLE) leads most authors to believe that there is a direct link between the two conditions. On the other hand, bone necrosis in rheumatoid arthritis is unusual unless one considers the juxta-articular lytic lesions as included in bone necrosis.

SLE AND BONE NECROSIS

Necrosis of the femoral head associated with SLE was first noted in the literature by Dubois and Cozen[125] in 1960. They commented on the relative frequency of INFH in their series, having only 11 cases in a series of 400 patients with SLE. Eight of the 11 cases were bilateral. Ten of their 11 cases had been treated with corticosteroids, although, in half of these, the doses were very moderate. The existence of a case in which the patient had not received corticosteroids led them to conclude that steroid therapy was not the only responsible factor. Following this initial report, several case reports or small series appeared[35,184,374,415,450]. In 1966, Dubois[124] reported 26 cases of INFH in a series of 520 patients with SLE[124]. Bensasson[47] collected 58 cases from the published literature in which several important features were underlined, including the strong female predominance (90% of SLE patients are women), the young age of the patients (average—36.5 years), the high incidence of bilaterality (87%), and the fact that many patients had multiple joints affected. Ruderman and McCarty's patient[374] had six affected joints. Lightfoot and Lotke[282] appear to hold the world record, reporting 17 foci of bone necrosis in a 28-year-old Puerto Rican man. Their diagnosis, however, was established by radionuclide uptake.

In spite of the extreme rarity of those cases which have not received corticosteroid treatment, most authors search for the pathophysiology of bone necrosis within the context of the lupus itself, in attempting to incriminate the inflammatory arteritis that is part of the pathophysiological substratum of the disease. Siemsen et al[415] and Velayos, Leidholt, and Smyth[451] each reported instances in which vascular lesions consisting of endothelial proliferation, perivascular cellular infiltrate, and thrombosis were present in the resected femoral head of patients with SLE and INFH. These findings were particularly evident intraosseously in the area adjacent to the necrotic zone. Bowie et al[60] put forth the hypothesis that hypercoagulability due to increased production of thromboplastin and in spite of, or perhaps even because of, thrombocytopenia might be another mechanism for the development of bone necrosis. Such a thrombotic microangiopathy is found in thrombotic thrombocytopenic purpura.

NECROSIS OF THE FEMORAL HEAD AND RHEUMATOID ARTHRITIS

Up to now, there has been no formal proof of a link between INFH and rheumatoid arthritis (RA). The cases presented are rare. In fact, it is quite surprising to find so few cases of INFH in a disease in which many cases receive corticosteroid therapy. Hip lesions as they exist in rheumatoid arthritis have a characteristic, radiologic aspect which has been well described by Forestier, Arlet, and Jacqueline[165]. The terminal, destructive lytic lesions of the rheumatoid hip, with loss of both articular cartilage and bone from the femoral epiphysis with protrusio acetabulae, are not at all similar to the radiologic lesions of Stage III, in which the necrosis of bone is associated with both preservation of the articular cartilage and normal contour of the acetabulum.

We agree with DeSeze et al[395] that one is not justified in making a diagnosis of "necrosing coxitis" in RA simply on the basis of rapid, severe destruction of the hip. Histologic proof is required. For this reason, we cannot accept the conclusions of Sutton et al[434], reporting 30 cases of INFH associated with RA nor Streda et al[430], reporting 156 cases of INFH in RA. Glick[183] defined INFH in RA on purely x-ray and clinical grounds, which we believe is of questionable value. He writes, "Sometimes the deformity of the femoral head occurs without destructive lesions of other joints and in the absence of any appreciable previous involvement of the hip. In these cases, standard x-rays are comparable to those of avascular necrosis observed in INFH occurring idiopathically." The same author concludes that there are two types of femoral head necrosis in RA, the first associated with the administration of corticosteroids and the second occurring independently of steroids in long-standing, severe RA with previous destruction of the articular cartilage. We can only emphasize that bone necrosis must be defined histologically.

Bensasson[47] did an excellent critical review of the literature and reported four legitimate cases of INFH among 1500 cases of RA, for an incidence of 3 per 1000. In each of the four cases, there had been prolonged cortisone treatment. In three of these cases, there were additional predisposing factors. In one, a 50-year-old man with seropositive RA of 15 years duration developed INFH in a dysplastic hip. The second case involved a 63-year-old woman who developed INFH after prolonged corticosteroid therapy instituted because of thrombocytopenia. In a third case, a 55-year-old man with RA also had liver cirrhosis. Our own personal cases are also infrequent. The definitive radiologic features of necrosis (Stage III) are very rare in seropositive RA. We have seen only a few cases of histologically evident, diffuse necrosis, either seen on core biopsy or on a femoral head excised for a prosthesis.

Illustrative Case 41. - Mrs. HAN..., a 45-year-old white female with a 12-year history of RA, had been treated with cortisone for only two years prior to being seen and had a dosage of 5 mg of prednisone per day. She was seen initially in 1967, with a six-year history of hip involvement. At the time of initial examination, in addition to the hips, she had painful limitation of movement of her right shoulder, both

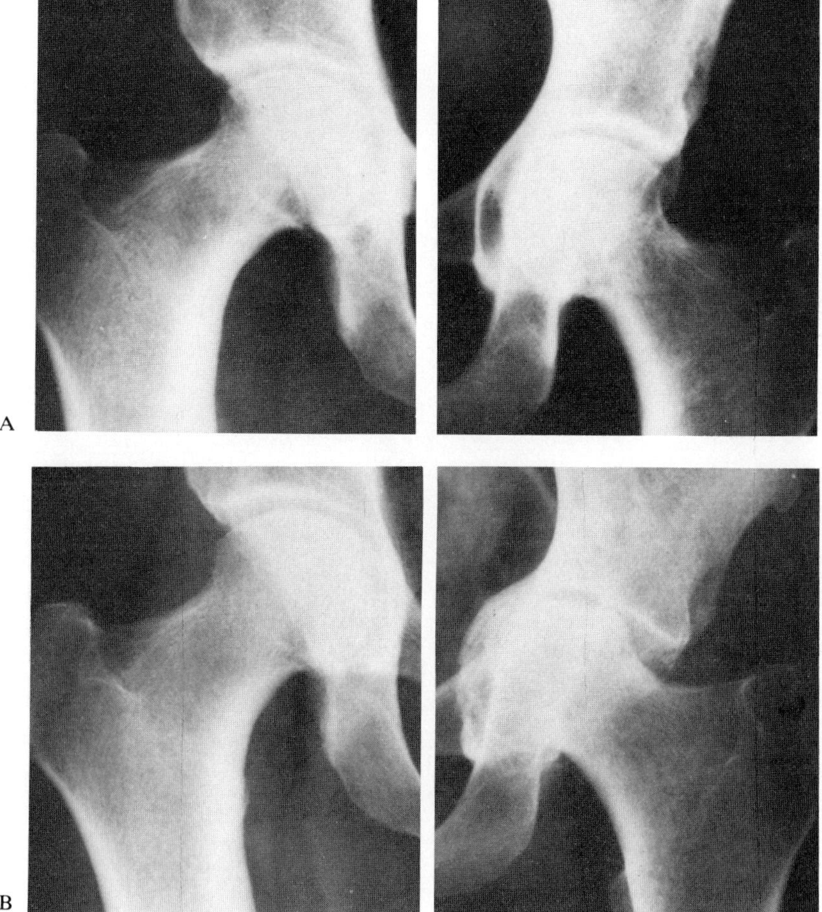

Fig. 120.—Case 41. A: X-rays of the pelvis (1-10-61): bilateral protrusio acetabula. B: X-rays (7-6-63): intrapelvic protrusion of the left hip with joint-line irregularity.

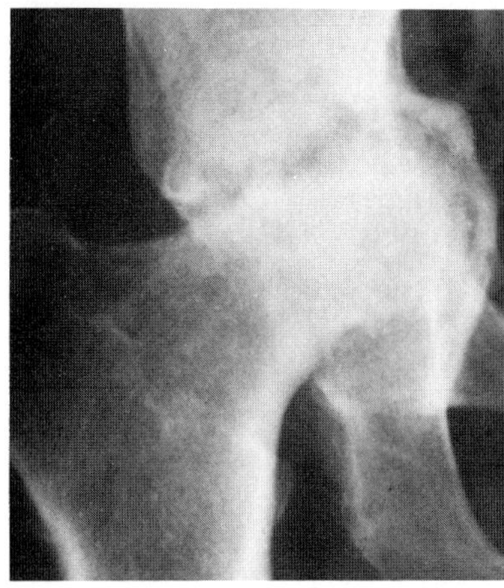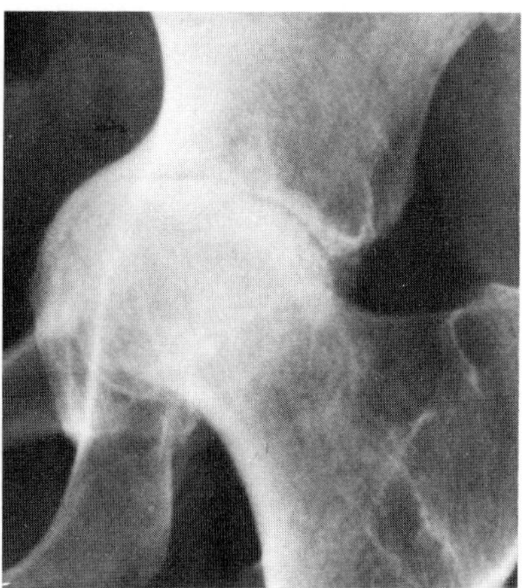

C

Fig. 120 C: X-rays (June 1968) marked protrusion of both femoral heads with destruction of the upper pole of the right hip.

elbows, and both wrists. The hips showed dramatic, painful limitation of movement with only 70° of flexion on the right and 30° of flexion on the left; ambulation was severely restricted. The x-ray showed severe joint line narrowing, protrusio acetabulae, and erosion of the superior pole of the femoral head (Fig. 120). Although IMP at the trochanter was normal, the venogram showed stasis and reflux on both sides. Core biopsy showed diffuse medullary necrosis bilaterally, more marked on the left.

In the review of 136 cases of INFH followed by us, seven patients had an atypical inflammatory arthritis classified as "possible" RA. This incidence is approximately the same as the incidence of elevated sedimentation rate in our series. We have seen that the literature contains some contradictory points of view concerning INFH in RA. We believe, however, that there are several clarifying points which can be made. The first point deals with the role of corticosteroids in the development of bone necrosis. The infrequency of INFH in RA patients receiving cortisone appears, to us, to constitute a powerful argument that the incidence of INFH complicating corticosteroid treatment depends on daily dosage of steroids and that with dosages of less than 10 mg of prednisone per day, INFH does not occur. It is also an argument against the "osteoporotic" theory of INFH since steroid-associated osteoporosis occurs even with small daily doses. One should add that osteoporosis is also a complication of RA which has not been treated by corticosteroids.

Although these considerations are valid in relation to systemically administered steroids, they may not apply to intra-articularly injected steroids. In that instance, the joint lesion is probably on the basis of the direct action of cortisone on the chondrocytes as well as due to the fact that increased use of the joint is possible as the injected joint becomes asymptomatic. A few published reports of the action of local steroids demonstrate a radiologic appearance of joint destruction which is more compatible with a Charcot-type arthropathy than with necrosis.

The second point concerns the histologic lesions which we have seen in femoral heads removed for total hip replacements in patients with RA[307]. These femoral heads are oval, as if progressively worn out by erosion of the superior pole. The articular cartilage is usually absent with the articular surface moderately eburnated over the entire weight-bearing zone. The sclerosis is usually not as thick or as well localized as in osteoarthrosis. Osteophytes are usually moderate or absent. The marrow spaces in these femoral heads show fibrosis, stasis, and cellular infiltrates but no necrosis. We, therefore, feel that INFH is not a common feature of RA.

The third point concerns terminology. It can be said that destroyed bone is dead bone, and, therefore, we can label as necrosis any bone erosion by normal osteoclastic resorption wherein the living bone is partially eroded and resorbed or in cases of proliferative inflammatory disease or a destruction by tumor. If such is to be the definition, then any bone destruction in RA could be called necrosis. We prefer, however, to label such a process as resorption rather than necrosis. Ischemic necrosis of bone, as presented in this monograph, is a primary lesion of bone due to an insufficient blood supply and not produced by "destructive cells," whether they are normally present in bone tissue or foreign to it. In the case of ischemic necrosis, the bone tissue "dies" before any resorption, whereas, in bone erosion, death and resorption are simultaneous.

BONE NECROSIS ASSOCIATED WITH OSTEOPOROSIS AND OSTEOMALACIA

Post-menopausal osteoporosis is very frequent. The reduced physical strength of bone is associated with pathological fractures which are localized to specific regions, including the distal radius, the surgical neck of the humerus, the vertebral bodies, and the femoral neck. In the radius and the humerus, the fractures heal without necrosis of the epiphysis. However, in fracture of the femoral neck, INFH is a frequent complication. Nonetheless, to our knowledge, INFH has not been demonstrated as pre-existing the fracture in usual cases of osteoporosis.

Apart from post-traumatic necrosis, is the usual form of osteoporosis responsible for INFH? Statistically, this is not apparent, since we have seen that INFH is more common in men and is mainly seen between 40 and 60 years of age. There is, however, one etiologic circumstance where the necrosis precedes the fracture of the femoral neck, i.e., in post-irradiation necrosis. The incomplete fracture of the femoral neck has a very peculiar radiologic picture and progression. Such a radiologic picture is also sometimes seen in senile osteoporosis where the incomplete fracture has a good prognosis if the patient can be maintained off weight-bearing for a few months. It is rare for these impacted fractures to develop the typical radiologic picture of INFH, and we do not have either histologic or hemodynamic data which allows us to give a precise account of the cancellous bone in the femoral head and neck of these patients. On the basis of the x-ray and clinical data for which there is seldom any histologic material available, it is, nonetheless, difficult to support the hypothesis of Frost[174] and Vignon and Meunier[454] for whom the bone necrosis is a consequence of repeated microfractures associated with osteoporosis. The latter authors have supported their hypothesis together with Laurent et al.[268] with a study of 35 quantitative biopsies of the iliac crest in patients with osteonecrosis, ten of whom had received cortisone. Thirteen of the 25 non-steroid-associated necroses and seven of ten steroid-associated necroses showed evidence of osteopenia of the iliac crest. According to these authors, the necrosis of the femoral head could originate from a subchondral fatigue fracture or a series of coalescing microfractures which would outline the area that subsequently becomes sequestrum. Traumatic rupture of the capillary microvasculature would effect local ischemia and necrosis so that the sub-sequestrum area would represent a true pseudarthrosis.

Solomon[421] has supported the concept of osteoporosis-linked INFH in his 29 cases of INFH in South African blacks in whom iron over-load hemosiderosis is attributed to excessive consumption of beer which had been placed in iron containers. These patients did not develop fatty changes in their livers but did develop osteoporosis. Solomon believes that the necrosis may be secondary to the osteoporosis.

Osteomalacia is a much rarer condition in which incomplete or pseudofractures are radiologically visible. Some cases of typical INFH (Stage III) have been reported in association with osteomalacia. Jaffres and Cherbury[227] reported osteonecrosis of both the femoral and humeral heads associated with an osteomalacia caused by chronic calcifying pancreatitis with steatorrhea. The Stage II lesions showed dramatic clinical improvement with Vitamin D treatment. May et al.[303] also reported necrosis of both femoral heads associated with osteomalacia produced by lactose intolerance. We have also seen one case of Stage III INFH in a patient with hypophosphatemic osteomalacia.

SUMMARY

In these two chapters on etiology, we have discussed all of the diseases and causes which, by virture of their frequent association with INFH, may be considered as possible etiologic factors, even when the mode of action was not completely elucidated. It is not uncommon that several of these factors may be present in an individual case. Multiple factors may have a cumulative effect which combine to threaten ultimate viability of the tissue. Ischemia begins when, for whatever reason, the blood supply is outstripped by the demands of the tissue. Nonetheless, many cases remain for which no specific cause or association can be found. This void in our understanding should constitute a powerful stimulus for future research.

CHAPTER IX

PATHOGENESIS OF ISCHEMIC
NECROSIS OF THE FEMORAL HEAD

EXPERIMENTAL OSTEONECROSIS

Attempts at producing bone necrosis experimentally are, in a very real sense, a test of pathogenetic mechanisms. The means of producing the necrosis is based upon the authors concept of how such a pathologic condition might have evolved in a clinical setting. In the previous two chapters, we have seen that there are many factors which can lead to bone necrosis. It is, therefore, not surprising that there are many mechanisms which researchers have used in an attempt to produce experimental necrosis.

GENERAL STUDIES ON PATHOPHYSIOLOGY OF BONE BLOOD FLOW

Many of the early studies on bone blood flow involved experiments which were designed to determine the reaction of various segments of bone to complete or partial interruption of the various vascular elements. They were not necessarily attempts to reproduce human disease but more in the manner of attempts to understand the contribution of various parts of the vascular anatomy to the various territorial and histologic elements of the bone.

Interruption of the nutrient artery of the diaphysis produces, above all, necrosis of the bone marrow and incomplete necrosis of the cortex[63,70]. Brookes believes that revascularization of the marrow takes place from the periosteal vessels through enlargement of the intra-cortical canaliculi. Hartmann[199] produced total necrosis of the diaphysis following ligature of the nutrient vessels, a finding which is in

some conflict with previous authors. Several authors have underlined differences according to the age of the animal, where anastomoses between the metaphyseal and epiphyseal vessels diminishes the extent of the necrosis produced by nutrient artery ligation with or without periosteal stripping in the adult animal but results in a more important necrosis in the immature animal[78,164,229,266].

The relative importance of the periosteal blood supply and the nutrient artery supply has also been studied. DeMarneffe[295] found that interrupting the nutrient artery produced discrete lesions in the endosteal third of the compact bone, but, when this was coupled with periosteal stripping, most of the osteocytes through the entire width of cortex showed histologic change. Gallie and Robertson[175] and MacWilliams[293] demonstrated the importance of the periosteal circulation in revascularization of grafts and the associated new bone formation. Attempts to delineate the importance of the nutrient artery in fracture healing has led to discordant results with Houang[208] and Pearse[339] finding that fractures heal in spite of section of the nutrient artery, while several authors found that union was either impeded or prevented by such sectioning[195,229,255,320].

These general experiments lead to several important conclusions concerning bone blood flow. It appears that each specific area of bone has a preferential source of blood flow. The nutrient artery supplies, primarily, the diaphyseal marrow and the endosteal portion of the compact bone. The periosteal vessels nourish the external portion of the cortex, and the metaphyseal arteries are responsible for the articular ends of the long bones. These experiments also show that anastomoses exist between the overlapping systems and, particularly, that more extensive anastomoses are possible under circumstances of need.

METHODS OF EFFECTING VASCULAR CHANGE

Because the proximal femur is the site of several conditions which are suspected to be vascularly determined or which have an important vascular component, much of the experimental work aimed at understanding the pathogenesis of bone necrosis from a variety of causal elements has been directed to the proximal femur. Much of the earlier work was designed to stimulate traumatic interruption to various vascular elements of the proximal femur. Others have tried to produce the more chronic changes which might simulate conditions found in nontraumatic INFH.

Arterial Interruption

Many authors have produced arterial ligation of vessels to the proximal femur in immature animals[81,190,245,256,264,318,333,29,472] with an open epiphysis. The artery of the ligamentum teres is important to the nutrition of the femoral head. Sectioning produces an ischemic lesion of the femoral head with both flattening and coxa vara. Kistler[251] systematically studied the effect of sectioning the multiple points of input to the immature femoral head, showing that the growth plate prevented the development of a collateral circulation when one of the sources was sectioned. Although cutting the artery of the ligamentum teres leads to femoral head necrosis in the immature animal, with subsequent flattening of the femoral head, these arterial lesions do not reproduce the lytic changes which are characteristic of Legg-Calve-Perthes' disease.

Several authors have attempted to determine the time frame for producing evidence of bone necrosis with vascular interruption. This would be, of course, particularly important in clinical circumstances where the interruption would be reversible. Vizkelety et al.[456] produced complete interruption of the circulation to the tails of rats and found that an average of five to six hours of occlusion was necessary to produce bone and bone marrow necrosis. Rosingh et al.[368] produced ischemia of the femoral head by sectioning the artery to the ligamentum teres and placing a tight ligature around the femoral neck with a nylon suture. He observed that the first histologic evidence of ischemia appeared six hours after the production of circulatory interruption. At that time,

the osteocytes began to lose appreciable quantities of DNA. Woodhouse[469] produced circulatory arrest by either intra-articular tamponade or by transection of the neck with torsion of the ligamentum teres to produce arterial occlusion. He concluded that 12 hours of ischemia was necessary to produce bone necrosis. Furthermore, he noted that venous obstruction was more damaging than arterial obstruction.

At the opposite end, several authors have attempted to produce the lesions of osteochondritis of the femoral head by inducing vasodilatation. Bentson[48] and Leriche[279] injected alcohol around the retinacular vessels of the femoral neck. Lemoine[271] transected the principal capsular arteries which produced temporary ischemia followed by hyperemia. These lesions produced rarefaction of bone for these authors. However, others have not been able to reproduce these findings[264,318,364].

Venous Occlusion

Although most authors have studied the effect of manipulation of the arterial side of the vascular tree, some studies have addressed themselves to the venous drainage of bone. As already mentioned, Woodhouse[469] produced extensive necrosis by intra-articular tamponade. Kery et al.[247] produced complete venous block of 4 to 12 hours by tourniquet applied to the tails of rats. Eight hours of venous stasis was sufficient to create extensive necrosis in all of the tissues. The nucleus pulposus was the most sensitive to the circulatory arrest, followed by bone marrow and cartilage. The work of Rutishauser, Rhoner, and Held[378] has been extensively reviewed in an earlier section. The histologic lesions produced by venous stasis were indistinguishable from those produced by arterial and arteriolar blockage. However, repair of the lesions following venous-induced necrosis was much slower than after interruption of the arterial circulation. Gourdou et al.[188] were also able to produce necrotic lesions of the femoral head following ligature of the principal venous pathways of the lower extremity, including the ipsilateral iliac, epigastric and lumbar veins, and the contralateral internal iliac as well as the sacral vein. Bone and bone marrow necroses were observed eight weeks after the surgical intervention. In two cases, the medullary necrosis was associated with distention of the sinusoids and intramedullary new bone formation.

Lesions Produced By Microemboli

Axhausen[31] invoked this mechanism in the pathology of bone infarction in man which he attributed to microbial emboli. Many authors have produced experimental, intra-arterial, emboli-utilizing silver[51], mercury[253], bacteria[223], carbon particles, and killed bacteria[248-250,378]. The fundamental and important work of Rutishauser et al.[378] has been extensively and previously reviewed but cannot be over emphasized. The production of histologically identical lesions by either venous blockage or arteriolar obstruction is of primary importance in the development of any pathogenetic concepts.

The work of Jones and Sakovich[233] has also been previously discussed. The injection of intra-arterial Lipiodol produced necrotic foci, initially in the metaphysis and ultimately in the epiphysis of the rabbit, similar to necrosis produced by other forms of microembolization. The question is not whether microemboli can produce bone necrosis but whether fat embolus is operative in a significant number of human bone necroses, a question which, for us, remains open.

The Effect Of Chronic
Circulatory Derangement

All the above quoted methods use a sudden or complete circulatory arrest by suppression of the arterial supply, the venous return, or of the capillary circulation. It is much more difficult to evaluate the repercussions of a chronic circulatory problem, producing a decrease in blood flow rather than an arrest of circulation, for two reasons. Firstly, as Rutishauser demonstrated[378], the lesions so produced are variable in both their extent and their evolution. Secondly, the creation of the circulatory deficit by ligation of the large arterial or venous vessels very quickly stimulates the development of an important collateral circulation[338]. Thus Benassi[45] does not see any lesions in the bone of a posterior extremity in the ligation of the iliac arteries or veins.

According to MacMaster[290], ligation of the femoral veins produces an acceleration in the repair of fibular fractures. However, Kecke et al.[244] were not able to document any change in the bone. Pearse[339] and Singh[419] asserted that venous stasis accelerates bone growth. For Abdallah[1], the ligation of the inferior vena cava with venous stasis in the posterior portion of the body produces, within a month, a thickening of the diaphyseal wall with proliferation of the periosteum, metaplastic transformation of bone cells into cartilaginous cells, and the development of collateral circulation between periosteal and diaphyseal marrow with enlargement of the channels that are filled with hematopoietic tissue. According to Lilly et al.[283], venous stasis produces an increase of bone formation from the periosteum and bone destruction from the marrow with overall enlargement of the bone and of the medullary canal but without quantitative changes of the bone mass. We have already referred to the important work of Gourdou et al.[188] on the chronic effect of extraosseously ligating the principal venous pathways from the proximal femur.

Evolution And Healing Of
Experimentally Produced Bone Necrosis

Several authors have studied the development of the necrosis and the histologic regeneration at different times following the initial vascular insult[63,164,214,333]. Histologic evidence of necrosis was present following arterial interruption within a few hours or days. Bone marrow changes were more extensive than bone changes, and evidence of reconstruction and repair were usually also evident within a few days and complete within a few months. Foster[164] has produced evidence that the repair process proceeds from peripheral, healthy bone adjacent to the ischemic bone and that this process begins as early as the third day following the onset of ischemia. Beneke[44] supported this concept that peripheral fibrovascular tissue invades the dead bone in a process of resorption and laying down of new bone, with the processes of resorption and reconstruction occurring simultaneously. Although different authors reported modestly different times for the repair and reconstruction from experimentally initiated lesions, all reported revascularization and reconstitution within several weeks or several months at the most[55,96,164,456].

Lesions Of Cartilage Associated
With Experimental Bone Necrosis

Most authors have focused their attention in their experimental work only on bone and bone marrow. Rutishauser et al.[379,380], however, also examined the articular cartilage in their animal models, where they produced bone ischemia either by intra-arterial injection of carbon particles, intramedullary injection of thrombin, or section of the extraosseous vessels. They found pannus encroachment of the articular margins with articular cartilage erosion. The pannus appeared to take its origin from the synovium and the juxta-articular bone tissue. Although they attributed these alterations to the ischemic episodes, the lesions were noted three weeks to one month after the onset of the circulatory interruption. It is possible that the lesions described are due to a fibrovascular proliferative reaction at the margin of the tissue which has been abruptly deprived of its blood supply. Both Beneke[44] and Zahir and Freeman[471] noted thickening of the articular cartilage and alteration in the cells in the deeper layer following surgically produced ischemia of the femoral head in the immature animal. They attributed the articular cartilage thickening to arrest of enchondral ossification. The increased cartilage thickness then impedes nutrition from the synovial fluid to the deep layers, resulting in the abnormalities.

Trueta et al.[446] studied the nutrition of cartilage of the growth plate of the tibia by destruction of the adjacent bone with or without interposition of an inert substance. When the blood supply on the epiphyseal side of the growth plate was interrupted, cartilage necrosis and cessation of growth occurred. Whereas, only cessation of ossification occurred with lesions on the metaphyseal side of the growth plate. Foster[164] also noted that arterial sectioning on the diaphyseal side produced an infarction which was delineated by the growth cartilage which itself did not seem to be affected. Ossification stopped, and the growth plate thickened. However, as the bone healed, ossification recommenced with the growth plate eventually resuming its normal width.

PATHOGENESIS OF HUMAN BONE NECROSIS

There are basically five points in the circulation of bone which could be affected to result in circulatory insufficiency. These can be considered in two groups, extraosseous and intraosseous. Under extraosseous, arterial and venous factors require consideration. Within bone, not only pre- and post-capillary factors are important but also intraosseous, extravascular factors must be considered because bone acts as a closed compartment.

Significant changes in any of these five sectors may not only affect other sectors but may in turn be affected by the change which is initiated, such that a complicated, evolving pattern of change and response may develop in which it is difficult to determine exactly what is primary and what is secondary. We believe that a recognition of this fundamental interdependence of each of these five areas can help to explain the diversity of observations which have been reported concerning the blood supply of both normal and abnormal bone.

EXTRAOSSEOUS ORIGINS OF BONE NECROSIS

It is apparent that any significant long-standing alterations in either afferent or efferent blood flow in the extraosseous vessels can lead to intraosseous ischemia with the tissue alterations, particularly necrosis, which are linked to ischemia.

Arterial Causes Of Bone Necrosis

We have previously reviewed the considerations in post-traumatic INFH, involving interruption of the retinacular epiphyseal arteries. Numerous experimental results have also been reported in the previous section of this chapter and in the chapters on etiology. It is, however, appropriate to review and summarize some of this material. In the experimental situation, ligature of an extraosseous artery produces necrotic lesions, limited to the topographical distribution of the ligated vessel. These lesions are reversible because of the development, sooner or later, of a compensatory collateral circulation. It has been possible to study the effect of chronic arterial changes in the experimental animal and its repercussion on the skeleton. However, considerable human material is also available. The tibiae from patients afflicted with peripheral vascular disease and gangrene show lesions varying both in degree and type, including total necrosis, partial necrosis, fibrosis, edema, evidence of medullary revascularization, and changes in the cortex resulting from expansion of the Haversian canals[75,402]. Although lesions of the femoral head are probably less frequent, they have not been systematically evaluated. We believe that we have proven the existence of necrotic lesions in the femoral head of patients with atherosclerotic and arteritic lesions. These lesions of extraosseous arterial origin may occur in one of three forms: 1.) diffuse and permanent decrease of arterial blood flow as in Buerger's Disease or other diffuse stenosing arteriopathies, 2.) permanent reduction of flow at one or both extremities following arteriosclerotic obliteration of a common iliac artery or at the aortic bifurcation (Leriche Syndrome), and 3.) permanent reduction of blood flow in the epiphysis by obliteration of the epiphyseal-metaphyseal arteries, especially the posterior circumflex artery, which is the main source of blood supply to the upper femoral epiphysis. It should also be noted that necrotic lesions, secondary to atherosclerosis, may result from the distal migration of microemboli arising from the arterial wall themselves or from fragments of atheromatous plaques formed by crystals of cholesterol and fibrin[416].

Venous Causes Of Bone Necrosis

Both the clinical and experimental arguments for a direct extraosseous venous cause of necrosis are less numerous and less certain than for extraosseous arterial causes of bone necrosis. Although it is difficult to produce bone necrosis experimentally by extraosseous venous ligation, we have managed to do this in dogs by extensive venous ligation[188]. To our knowledge, there has been no systematic anatomical/pathological work on the tibiae of patients affected with severe chronic venous circulatory problems. Although the stimulation to periosteal osteogenesis induced by chronic venous stasis is well known, the associated medullary, epiphyseal, and metaphyseal lesions have not been studied. The most poignant argument in favor of the venous origin of some necroses of the femoral head is the intraosseous stasis, nearly constantly seen on venograms in many cases of INFH. Nonetheless, it must be emphasized that intraosseous stasis is not synonymous with extraosseous venous disease and that stasis itself is not synonymous with necrosis. Stasis may be demonstrated when the arterial blood flow is reduced[385], where there is capillary encroachment, or when there is an extraosseous obstacle to the venous drainage of the bone. Stasis is also seen in conditions other than necrosis, specifically in reflex sympathetic dystrophy[140] and Paget's Disease of bone[24].

Clinical signs of chronic venous insufficiency in association with INFH constitute an argument in favor of a direct relationship. Venographic demonstration of obliteration of large extra-osseous trunks (vena cava, iliac, and femoral veins) also suggests the possibility of a direct relationship.

INTRAOSSEOUS CAUSES

This process represents, for us, the most common factor in bone necrosis. Apart from either direct, toxic, cellular necrosis or radionecrosis, the fundamental factor of intraosseous ischemia is a reduction in blood flow in the microvascular tree. Given the remarkable intimacy of the sinusoidal capillary system and the marrow cells, it can easily be seen that what happens to the vascular network will directly influence the marrow. Circulation within this network may be altered by intrinsic factors (obliteration or embolism) or extrinsic factors (compression).

Intrinsic Factors

Fat embolism—This problem has already been extensively discussed in the chapter on etiology. However, direct histological proof of this pathogenesis in cases of necrosis in man has not been convincing. This theory rests, essentially, on the one case of Fisher et al.[161] and four cases reported by Jones[234], two of which are uncertain. Fisher and Bickel[162] observed probable fat emboli in the subchondral vessels in 12 of 25 necrotic femoral heads. There is, however, no proof that this process may be extended to the numerous vessels within the femoral head or that it may not be secondary to liquefaction of the bone marrow, something known to occur with the necrosis.

Gas emboli—This was the initial explanation for barotraumatic necrosis. The pathogenesis has been reviewed by Fournier and Jullien[169], in which they distinguished primary and secondary factors. The primary factor is represented by the formation of nitrogen bubbles following rapid decompression. During a stay in a compressed atmosphere, nitrogen dissolves to a higher degree, both in the blood and the other tissues. Fat and bone marrow have the longest saturation and desaturation time of all tissues. During decompression, if the lowering of the pressure is fairly slow, the nitrogen is normally eliminated via the lungs, with the tissue nitrogen passing into the blood according to the equilibration constants which are specific for each tissue. However, if the decompression is too fast, the nitrogen comes out of solution, forming bubbles both in the blood and in the tissues. This is especially apt to happen in the marrow and in the subcutaneous fat which absorb more nitrogen under the situation of the decompressed atmosphere and which also release the nitrogen more slowly. There are two theories to explain the lesions of bone and bone marrow. In the first, gas emboli form intravascularly, leading to embolic obstruction of the vessels. In the second theory, the bone marrow is mechanically disrupted by the extravascular formation of nitrogen bubbles which also produces an extravascular, intraosseous compression. This affects the microcirculation as well. In all likelihood, both mechanisms are acting together in the determination of the lesions which are typically seen. Other factors may be involved, as well, which could aggravate or trigger the unfavorable reaction. Erythrocyte agglutination could precede the liberation of gas and could be produced by acidification of the tissue through CO_2 excess. Muscular exercise and fatigue which favored the production of CO_2 and accumulation of acid metabolites could also accelerate liberation of the nitrogen gas. Neurovascular factors may also influence bone blood flow with the pain which is significant at the time of decompression, serving to negatively influence circulation via the sympathetic tone. Microlesions of the lateral aspect of the spinal cord have also been described in decompression sickness which explains the associated neurologic signs of radiculopathy and paresthesias. These may also occasion vasomotor disturbances which could negatively affect bone blood flow. Within these pathogenetic explanations for decompression sickness, we again find both intravascular and extravascular, intraosseous aspects which very likely have a synergistic effect in producing bone necrosis.

Red blood cell emboli—The classic example of this mechanism of bone necrosis is in sickle-cell disease. In this condition, most of the direct causes favoring ischemia are present, including anemia, increased blood viscosity during sickling crises, loss of membrane elasticity, changes in the electrical charges in the hemoglobin, a decrease in pH, decrease in pO_2, and rapid destruction of the red blood cells with shortened life span due to hemolysis. The essential characteristic is the occlusion of the microcirculation by sickled cells which obstruct the capillaries and sinusoids. Sickling of the red blood cells is triggered by hypoxia. This polymerization of hemoglobin has two direct consequences. First of all, the oxygen carrying capacity of the blood is reduced to a significant degree by removal from the circulation of a large number of red blood cells. Secondly, the deformed, rigid cells are unable to pass through the microcirculation where they adhere to the vessel wall, eventually completely obstructing the capillary lumen and finally precipitating intravascular thrombosis, leading to extensive areas of stasis and edema. These secondary factors can then lead to intraosseous, extravascular compression of the fine circulatory network.

Intraosseous Extravascular Compression

There are circumstances where the arteriolar capillary lumen may be closed by extrinsic compression or by spasm. The first instance (extrinsic compression) introduces a concept of the intraosseous canal. The metaphyseal-epiphyseal cancellous bone can be considered as a labyrinth of canals or channels within rigid walls which define a non-distensible compartment. All of the physiologic concepts which apply to the various tunnel syndromes (carpal tunnel, tarsal tunnel, etc.) may be applied to bone. Any increase in the volume of one of the constituents (marrow or vessels) will automatically produce a compression of the most vulnerable aspects of the

TABLE XXX

PATHOPHYSIOLOGY OF BONE NECROSIS

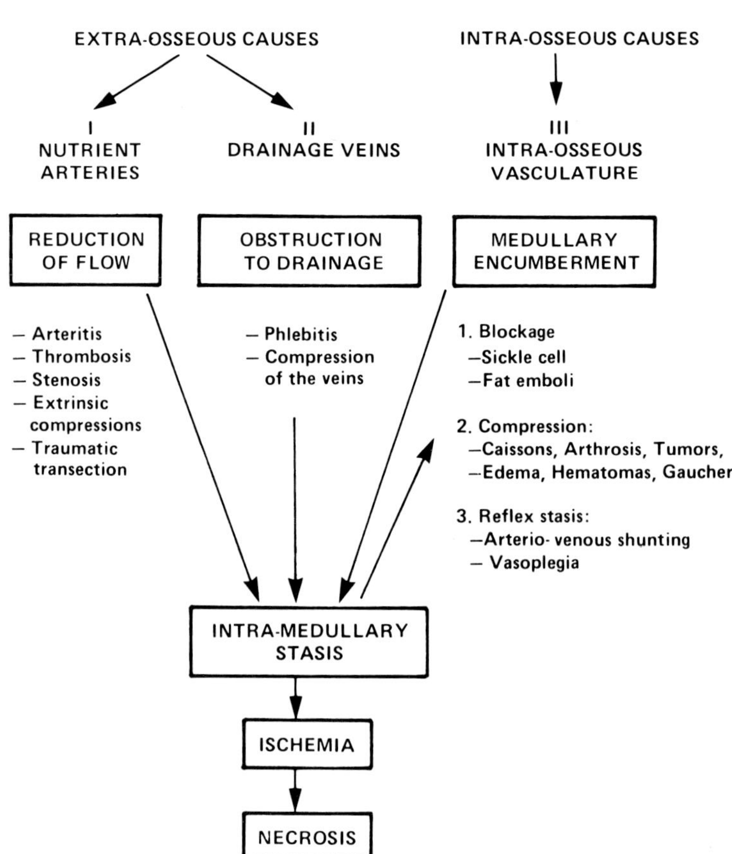

tissue, and in the case of bone, the capillaries and sinusoids. This will produce an obstruction of the microcirculation. It is very probable that this process is operative in conditions with medullary hyperplasia (tumor, abnormalities of fat metabolism, Gaucher's Disease, etc.), intraosseous hematoma (hemophilia, trauma, stress microfracture in osteoporosis), in some arthroses (by thickening of the bone trabeculae which compresses the microcompartment of cancellous marrow), and in venous stasis of whatever origin. Either extraosseous stasis, as we have seen with phlebitis, or intraosseous stasis may produce the same results. The stasis dilates the venules with exudation of plasma, with the development of fibrosis encroaching upon the capillary and intercytic circulation.

The second consideration which may lead to dysfunctioning of the vascular tree consists of vessel spasm. These disorders are poorly understood and are tied into the neurovascular reflex nature of bone blood flow which has been addressed in Chapter II.

Some insight into the nature of these disorders can be obtained from intramedullary pressure measurement and venography. There would seem, theoretically, to be three possibilities. Firstly, there could be a permanent spasm of the intraosseous vessels, which seems to us to be very unlikely. Secondly, a vasomotor paralysis could produce reflex stasis throughout the intraosseous venous plexus. This should be seriously considered since, in the functional exploration of bone, extensive intraosseous stasis has been demonstrated. Thirdly, by reflex closing of precapillary sphincters, arterial blood would be shunted to the venous circulation, bypassing the microcirculation and essentially depriving the tissue of its nutrition. All of these bypassed areas would then undergo ischemic anoxia. Although this hypothesis is very attractive, it remains to be demonstrated.

PATHOPHYSIOLOGY

After review of the hypothetical considerations of

TABLE XXXI

CONSEQUENCES OF MEDULLARY STASIS

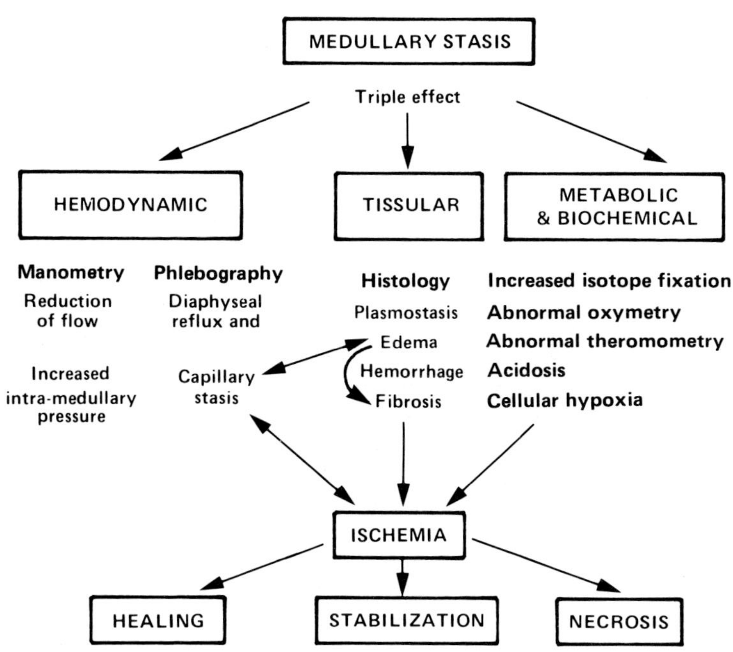

the pathogenesis and all of the specific etiologic considerations, it remains to try to synthesize several main pathophysiological mechanisms. As we have seen, several very different conditions may have a very similar end result. Several of them can trigger similar mechanisms, either simultaneously or successively. On the basis of experience with the functional exploration, it would appear that a common denominator to which all pathological processes converge is represented by intramedullary stasis. Table XXX summarizes the three avenues by which intramedullary stasis may be produced: the nutrient artery pathway, the venous pathway for the extraosseous vascularization, and the intraosseous medullary circulation. From Table XXX, we can also see that each mechanism existing in the various necroses, whatever the starting point, ends in the production of intramedullary stasis.

When the stasis rests on the venous side of the circulation, it appears as a primary phenomenon. On the other hand, it is more difficult to understand the mechanism when the problem begins on the arterial side. Nonetheless, as we have seen, a decrease in arterial flow leads to a slowing of the capillary circulation which is probably the first step in producing intramedullary stasis.

In Table XXXI, the consequences of intramedullary stasis on the various aspects under pathophysiologic consideration are elucidated. As can be seen, ischemia is not synonymous with necrosis. Ischemia is a pathophysiologic concept, and its reversibility is commonly observed in dislocations and fractures of the hip that heal without complication, probably because the ischemia was of moderate, partial, and/or short duration. On the other hand, necrosis is a histopathologic concept that represents the final outcome of unrelenting ischemia. The three parameters which can be measured—hemodynamic, histologic, and metabolic—constitute the basis of the functional exploration. This method, which we have outlined in Chapter III, leaves no areas uncovered but is completely adaptable to a thorough exploration of the processes involved in producing bone ischemia.

CHAPTER X

TREATMENT OF BONE ISCHEMIA AND NECROSIS

MEDICAL TREATMENT

PREVENTION OF NECROSIS

There are certain medical conditions or circumstances where the risk of bone necrosis is high. Each specific pathogenetic association will have individual non-surgical modalities for reducing the risk of necrosis. Often these are empirical, based upon a general understanding of bone circulation and the presumed relationship between the specific underlying "cause" and the subsequent necrosis.

In fractures of the femoral neck that do not require surgical interventions, such as impacted or non-displaced fractures, secondary necrosis is uncommon. A period of protective weight bearing of sufficient duration, three to four months, is necessary, not only to insure consolidation of the fracture, but also to avoid compression of a femoral head which is at risk. Aspiration of the joint at the time of the acute injury is recommended in order to avoid intracapsular tamponade.

Most decompression accidents can be avoided if all decompressions follow the rules which have been established, that is, slow resurfacing with staged decompression.

Each time that corticosteroid treatment is undertaken in moderate or high doses, particularly greater than 20 mg of prednisone equivalent for more than one month, the risk of bone necrosis must be recognized and weighed against the benefits to be derived from this therapy. Only future investigations will tell us if the present practice of alternate-day corticosteroid treatment may further decrease the frequency of bone necrosis as a complication of steroid treatment.

Hyperuricemia and hypertriglyceridemia represent increased risk for atherosclerosis. At the same time, these two abnormalities undoubtedly represent favorable grounds for the development of INFH. This is an additional reason to treat these laboratory findings, even if they are not responsible for clinical symptoms at the time they are discovered.

COMMENTS ON CURING BONE NECROSIS

Is femoral head necrosis curable? We believe that it is, but we cannot yet confirm it. Of course, at Stage III, with fracture and collapse of the weight-bearing zone, healing is impossible. However, as long as the subchondral shell is intact, there is a possibility of healing. The secondary bone lesions of chronic ischemia are complex, as we have already shown. In addition to disseminated foci of necrosis, there are areas of healthy bone and areas of active fibrosis with new bone formation. This last process of repair is probably capable of saving the femoral head, as is commonly observed in experimental pathology where it is difficult to produce progressive definitive necrosis.

When in doubt, one should act as if this healing were possible and treat it and the probable causes of necrosis as soon as possible. This is where early diagnosis and treatment constitute the first line of defense and certainly assure the most likely conditions for success. As we have previously shown, biopsy is always necessary for a formal diagnosis in the early stages, I and II. There are cases, however, where the probability of necrosis is so high that we can decide straight away on treatment. Renal allograft patients are such an instance in which hip pain is practically always a sign of bone necrosis. Furthermore, in those cases with increased radionuclide uptake, increased bone marrow pressure, and increased oxygen saturation in blood aspirated from the greater trochanter, necrosis is almost certain, and determination of treatment can be based upon these findings.

We propose the following medical treatment. The first step is to discontinue weight bearing on the affected hip for at least four to eight weeks. Reduction of alcohol intake and reduction of body weight by dieting constitute important measures. Corticosteroid therapy should be reduced or stopped if at all possible. When not possible due to the systemic disease, daily corticosteroid therapy should be replaced by alternate-day therapy. Hyperuricemia should be reduced to normal levels by allopurinol. Hypertriglyceridemia should be treated by a fat-poor diet.

Vasoactive drugs may play a role in treating early cases of INFH. Although it is difficult to prove the efficacy of so-called peripheral vasodilators, praxilene appears to be useful. Two drugs are of particular interest in the treatment of bone necrosis —Hydergine and Vincamine. Both of these drugs are extensively used in black Africa in the treatment of sickle-cell crises. Roussilhon and Bouyer[370] and Bouyer[59] have demonstrated the efficacy of Hydergine on the painful bone crises of moderate intensity. "The pain decreases within a quarter of an hour of the injection." In very severe crises, they advocate the intravenous route, which apparently shortens the duration of the bone crises. Hydergine may have its effect on the precapillary arterioles. It is also possible that this medication may reduce intramedullary pressure, as we have seen in a few cases. We know from Kabakele[241] that the painful bone crises in sickle-cell disease are usually associated with increased IMP, that is quickly improved by core decompression. We have also had considerable experience with Vincamine, which has the effect of rapidly reducing symptoms in patients who have not responded to either analgesics or anti-inflammatory drugs. Anti-inflammatory drugs may also be used, but their efficacy in bone necrosis, particularly indomethacin, does not seem to be as great as that observed in the inflammatory arthritides or arthrosis.

SURGICAL TREATMENT

This form of treatment is best discussed in its application to bone necrosis by stage (Chapter IV).

STAGE I

X-rays are normal both with regard to the joint space and the bone texture, with the occasional ex-

ception of some non-specific osteoporosis. A diagnosis cannot be made without the functional exploration, even when the bone scan is positive. Bone scanning is non-specific, and we already know that we are dealing with a pathologic hip from the physical examination. In these circumstances, the core biopsy is an essential part of the functional exploration, and it is the first step in treatment. This approach may be criticized as overly aggressive. However, we feel that it is fully justified by the fact that we are only operating on patients who have significant symptoms, either in intensity or in duration. It is true that we may be operating on some patients who would have healed spontaneously. We have seen some cases that showed a clinically favorable evolution after a positive functional exploration which was not followed by biopsy. It was almost certain that these patients did have INFH. However, knowing the natural history of INFH and the guarded functional prognosis, we feel that this surgical intervention (core decompression) is fully justified, the more so because there is no proven curative, conservative medical treatment.

The work of Hungerford[217a] reinforces these concepts. He measured IOP and carried out venography on the radiologically normal, asymptomatic contralateral hip of patients presenting with unilateral INFH. Out of 27 such cases, 10 had normal findings, while 17 were definitely abnormal. Thirteen of these 17 developed symptoms of INFH 18 days to 18 months following evaluation. Positive diagnosis was established by biopsy. Three of the 13 had progressed to Stage III before returning for follow-up. Only one of the patients with a normal evaluation subsequently developed INFH.

Marcus et al[298] have treated 11 early asymptomatic but radiologically evident hips in patients with more advanced disease on the other side by core decompression and tibial strut bone graft (Phemister's operation). Ten hips were satisfactory with a two to four year follow-up. The one failure was associated with a technical error. Although categorical proof of progression of Stage I is not provided by the reports, we believe that they strengthen our belief that all cases must have passed through a Stage I and that most Stage I disease will progress if left untreated.

Core decompression is a benign surgical treatment. We have had no fatalities in over 800 cases. We also know that this procedure is curative for the early stages of necrosis in most instances. To be effective, core decompression must be carried out as early as possible in the course of the disease. We recommend that patients be admitted on a semi-urgent basis. One particular case offers the interesting observation in that discrete, spotty osteoporosis seen on the x-rays at the time of initial consultation changed to early femoral head collapse at the time of scheduled surgery only 15 days later. Carrying out a core decompression accomplishes three specific aims. The specimen obtained at surgery confirms the diagnosis, the pain of which the patient complains is alleviated, and the hemodynamic situation which is created favors healing of the lesion. Not to carry out core decompression under the circumstances where a Stage I INFH is strongly suspected runs the risk that the irreversible lesions of INFH may appear with their ultimate consequences on permanent hip function.

The technique of core decompression has already been described. When the hemodynamic tests are positive, we use an 8 mm trephine and sometimes take a second 6 mm specimen in a separate direction in order to have a better vascularization effect on the cancellous bone of the femoral head.

Results

We are reporting here the results of our first 78 cases of osteonecrosis in Stage I, on which we have sufficient follow-up to demonstrate the effects of core decompression.

Method of Evaluation—We have adapted and simplified the system of Merle D'Aubigne[311] for evaluating our pre- and post-operative clinical findings. In making this adaptation, we have chosen five stages rather than seven and focus particularly on range of movement and pain. Merle D'Aubigne's system, with emphasis on walking ability, is more applicable to advanced stages and arthrosis but is also inapplicable to bilateral cases if one wishes to arrive at a judgement on a single hip. Particularly in the early stages, we also feel that a flexion of 130° rather than 90° constitutes the normal. Table XXXII demonstrates the symptoms corresponding to the degrees of severity, while Table XXXIII represents the pre- and post-operative status of these 78 cases in regards to pain. From this table, we can see that 74 of the 78 cases had significant pain pre-operatively, whereas post-operatively only 13 patients had significant symptoms. Sixty-five of the 78 cases (83.3%) had good or excellent results regarding pain relief from the core decompression. It also should be noted that the ten cases who were rated at Grade 2 pain level post-operatively were all better than their pre-operative situation. Post-operatively, no patients were at Grade 4.

Table XXXIV represents the pre- and post-operative circumstances in regard to limitation of movement. Post-operatively, 62 cases were at Level 0 or 1 compared to 34 cases pre-operatively. These

TABLE XXXII
SYSTEM OF HIP EVALUATION

Pain	Grade	Limitation of Movement	
Rest + Night +	4	NEAR ANKYLOSIS	
Severe with Movement	3	MARKED	FLEX. 60° ± 10° ABD. < 20°
Moderate	2	MODERATE	FLEX. 90° ± 10° ABD. 20° – 30°
Mild	1	MILD	FLEX. 110° ± 10° ABD. 30° – 45°
None	0	NONE	FLEX. ⩾ 130° ± 10° ABD. ⩾ 45°

TABLE XXXIII
EFFECT OF CORE DECOMPRESSION ON PAIN

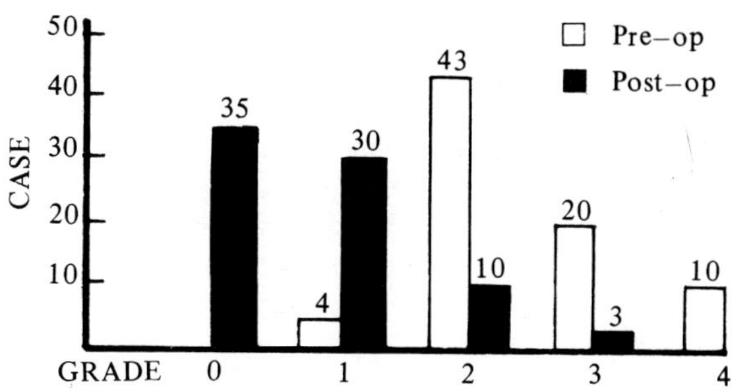

TABLE XXXIV
EFFECT OF CORE DECOMPRESSION ON LIMITATION OF MOVEMENT

results are, perhaps, to be expected at Stage I of the disease since the morphology and bone structure are preserved. The head is round, the cartilage is intact, and restriction of movement is, to a large extent, a simple protective measure in the face of a painful joint. However, the possibility of an adhesive capsulitis may well account for residual stiffness in some cases in spite of complete disappearance of pain. In several cases in which we have done combined synovial, capsule, and bone biopsies, we were surprised to find a thickened, edematous, retracted capsule which could be more than 1 cm thick. This capsulitis would account for the restriction of movement, particularly the reduction in internal rotation that is so often noted on physical examination. The shorter posterior capsule plus the natural tendency of the hip to fall into external rotation would account for a block in internal rotation if the capsule became inflamed. These findings, of course, bring into question the origin of this capsulitis, and we personally feel that, in the absence of other factors, regional ischemia could be responsible for the hypertrophic fibrosis and synovial changes. In some cases where we have seen that the osteoporosis extends beyond the upper end of the femur to involve the acetabulum, we are forced to admit that the vascular problem responsible for the bone ischemia is, in fact, regional and encompasses what we have called the functional articular entity with its integrated vascular network already described.

Radiologic progression following core decompression in Stage I—Although this may seem paradoxical since Stage I is the pre-radiologic stage, it is, however, necessary to follow the x-rays in order to detect failure which may occur in two ways. The disease process may be unaffected by the core decompression so that the typical Stage II findings, and, finally, Stage III radiologic changes develop. In

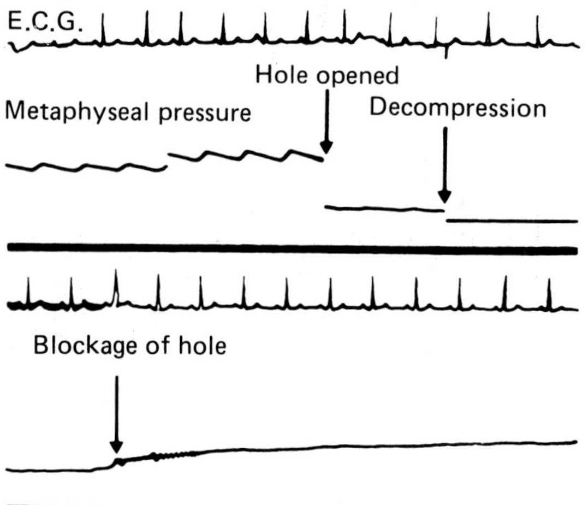

Fig. 121.—Simultaneous tracing of the metaphyseal pressure and an ECG demonstrating the immediate and spectacular effect of the simple cortical window on the intramedullary pressure. The effect of the core is only minimal compared with that of the window. On the lower tracing, it can be seen that the plugging of the window with the finger raises the pressure progressively.

the case of the ischemic coxopathies, the joint space may continue to narrow as a consequence of the effect on the articular cartilage. One case showed partial collapse which could possibly be due to a technical problem since the trephine perforated the articular cartilage during the core decompression. Two cases showed slight joint space narrowing following the core decompression, and, in six cases, some sclerosis developed in the femoral head, suggestive of a Stage II change, although it is possible that these changes were a result of the decompression and not of the disease. Seven of our patients had no relief from the core decompression and, therefore, constitute a complete failure of the treatment method. In one of these patients, the symptoms were associated with a protrusio acetabulae. Three patients had had minor injury to the region. Four of the failures had a particular kind of hip pain which was associated with low back pain. One of these developed after a contusion.

**Mechanism Of Action
Of Core Decompression**

The core decompression does not attack the disease at its etiologic base but rather along the pathophysiologic course. In one sense, its therapy is addressed towards the symptoms of bone necrosis since it does affect a very rapid symptomatic relief. The mechanism of action of the core decompression is complex. By perforating the cortex, the closed bone space is opened, and intraosseous hypertension is immediately relieved, as can be seen in the intramedullary pressure tracing at the time of the cortex penetration (Fig. 121). This decompressive effect would have an immediate, positive effect on circulation. Extending the decompression channel into the femoral neck and femoral head would further contribute to decreasing the "compartment syndrome" much as the incision of the fingertip fat pad decompresses the multicompartment compression of a felon. The cavity which is left with the extraction of the specimen serves as a buffer chamber for adjacent compartments and as a means of evacuating intramedullary stasis.

A well-directed core channel also evacuates some of the necrotic debris. The cutting across of multiple vascular channels and of bone stimulates revascularization much like an intertrochanteric osteotomy. The transection of a myriad of intraosseous vessels stimulates a vasculoneogenesis which affects the entire vasculature of the joint. Since this vasculoneogenesis exists over the entire length of the core channel, it puts the less vascular cephalic portion of the proximal femur into vascular communica-

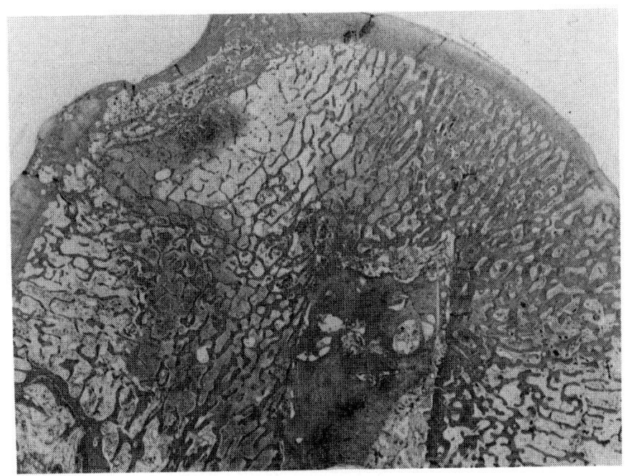
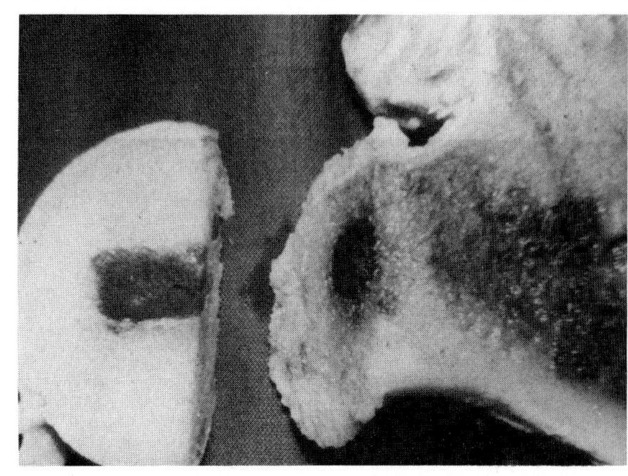

Fig. 122.— A: Microphotography of a section of an excised femoral head two years after forage revealing: the persistence of the forage canal with a sclerotic area at its upper end corresponding to the area with most cartilaginous damage and the filling of the canal by more or less fibrous scar tissue. B: Head of the femur excised three years after the forage. The canal persists and is completely filled with red bone marrow, very rich in young hematopoietic tissue.

tion with the more richly vascularized trochanteric region. This phenomenon can be seen on postoperative venographies. We have also been able to observe, histologically, the evolution of the core channel through the specimens recovered either at autopsy or at total hip replacement at some time following core decompression. We have found several different histologic reactions to the core decompression, including a.) the core channel filled with young, red, hematopoietic marrow with no bone trabeculae (Fig. 122), b.) the channel filled with vascular fibrous tissue, c.) the channel filled with poorly vascularized, fibrous tissue, and d.) the channel totally obliterated by trabecular ossification completely reconstituting normal bone to the point that no trace of the core tract can be seen.

The regional revascularization, which we believe occurs both intra- and extra-osseously, coincides with the transient demineralization phase following the surgery. The transection of multiple vessels can, at a histologic level, be conceptualized as resulting in numerous "minisympathectomies" and that this is responsible for the post-operative vasodilatation.

If we consider the schematic diagram traced in the previous chapter concerning the influence of intraosseous stasis on hemodynamics, tissue, and metabolism, we realize that core decompression effects all of these parameters. Because of its effect on intraosseous stasis, increased intramedullary pressure, and the necrotic debris, the core decompression breaks the vicious cycle which dictates the spontaneous progression of this condition. By early intervention in the first phases of the condition when the changes are still reversible, the core decompression provides the opportunity and time for the body to reverse the pathologic changes. The core decom-

pression can, therefore, be considered as a potentially curative procedure in stimulating the bony response to reverse rather than potentiate the ischemia. Although it is certain that spontaneous healing of bone ischemia can and does exist, the core decompression, nonetheless, is a powerful and effective stimulus towards this healing response.

Antalgic Action Of Core Decompression

Although the reduction in pain is obviously a result of the previously mentioned effects of core decompression, it remains, nonetheless, the most spectacular and remarkable action of the procedure. In over half of the cases, the decrease in pain was immediate, having more or less completely disappeared by the evening of surgery. The antalgic action of the procedure is more marked when rest and night pain were present prior to surgery. Usually, limitation of movement, which was on the basis of protective limitation, is quickly recovered. It is tempting to attribute these changes to the sudden fall in the intramedullary pressure, thereby implying that increased intramedullary pressure is directly responsible for the pain. Indeed, the pain produced by injection of saline for the stress test or contrast medium for venography into ischemic bone shows a striking resemblance to the spontaneous pain described by the patient, again implicating increased pressure as the phenomenon responsible for the symptoms. In spite of this, the actual mechanism for pain must be considerably more complicated since we have recorded high intramedullary pressures in patients without pain. The equation, Increased IMP = Pain, is, therefore, not entirely true. The equation could better be written—Increased IMP + Factor X = Pain. Factor X may or may not be dependent upon the increased IMP. This factor or factors require further elucidation.

At other times, the improvement in pain is less spectacular and occurs gradually over a period of several days and may not be complete. Although the overall level of pain is generally much improved, it may return with physical effort or fatigue. It is plausible for the post-operative, regional hypervascularization to extend to the vascular unity of the joint and specifically to the soft tissue parts, capsule, and synovium. One can understand, then, that in cases of ischemic capsulitis, the regression of the lesions is slower and less certain. In summary then, the results of core decompression have been dramatic but are not constant. The partial or total failures can rarely be explained on the basis of technical failures. We have, therefore, to think that they are often due to the spontaneous potential evolution of the disease. We know very little about that except with some specific etiologies such as in the renal allograft group where the general severity of the necrosis is well known. Nevertheless, although the evolution is not predictable, it remains very favorable after core decompression for the so-called idiopathic necroses.

Long-Term Follow-Up Of Core Decompression In The Pre-Collapse Stages Of INFH (I andII)

In our series of 131 cases done five or more years ago, we have follow-up in 108 cases of Stage I and II INFH treated by core decompression. Twenty-three cases were lost to follow-up in the first five years. Five died from a disease unrelated to the bone necrosis, and 18 had been reviewed from one to three years following the decompression but have subsequently been lost to follow-up. At the time of last review in those cases, 15 had good or excellent results, and three were unsatisfactory.

Ninety-nine patients with 108 affected hips in Stage I and II were available for review. Twenty-seven of the 99 patients had bilateral INFH, but only nine of these were in the pre-collapse stages. There were 55 men and 44 women, 57 right hips and 51 left hips. Sixty-nine of the cases were in Stage I, and 39, in Stage II. Overall results have been evaluated according to clinical criteria and radiologic progression. Very good results were graded either O or 1 in both limitation of movement and pain (Table XXXII). Good results had no greater grade than 2 on either pain or limitation of movement, while Grades 3 and 4 in either pain or movement would constitute failure. The follow-up range was from a minimum of five years to a maximum of 15 years with a mean follow-up of 7.9 years.

The clinical results according to stage are seen in Table XXXV. Ninety-nine of the 108 cases showed a good or very good result (91.7%).

LONG–TERM FOLLOW–UP OF CORE DECOMPRESSION IN THE PRE–COLLAPSE STAGES OF INFH (I + II)

TABLE XXXV
CLINICAL RESULTS OF CORE DECOMPRESSION IN STAGE I + II

	Stage I	*Stage II*	*TOTAL*
Very Good	48	17	65
Good	17	17	34
Failure	4	5	9
TOTAL	69	39	108

TABLE XXXVI
RADIOLOGICAL STATUS FOLLOWING CORE DECOMPRESSION FOR INFH IN STAGE I & II

	Stage I	*Stage II*	*TOTAL*
Unchanged	60	25	85
Some Progression	7	10	17
Progress to Stage III	2	4	6
TOTAL	69	39	108

TABLE XXXVII
LONG–TERM CLINICAL AND RADIOLOGIC RESULTS OF CORE DECOMPRESSION IN STAGE I AND II INFH

No. of Cases	*Good and Very Good*	
	Clinical	*Radiological*
Stage I 69	65 (94.2%)	60 (86.9%)
Stage II 39	34 (87.1%)	25 (64.1%)
TOTAL 108	99 (91.6%)	85 (78.4%)

Radiologic status following core decompression is shown in Table XXXVI and has been satisfactory in 85 cases. There was some evidence of radiologic deterioration in 23 of the 108 cases (21.5%), whereas the clinical failure rate was only 8.3%. Radiologic deterioration can include a progressive narrowing of the joint space (17 cases) which was seen in seven cases in Stage I and ten cases in Stage II, or a collapse of the femoral head seen in six cases (two in Stage I and four in Stage II). By grouping the good and very good results on both the clinical and radiologic bases, we can see the overall effect of core decompression in Stage I and II in INFH (Table XXXVII). Even though there was evidence of x-ray progression in 21.6% of the cases, only six (5.5%) progressed to collapse of the femoral head with this mean follow-up of 7.9 years.

STAGE II

In Stage II, the outlines of the femoral head and the joint space remain normal. However, the bone texture may show cysts or sclerosis or a mixture of both. In early Stage II, the diagnosis may be suspected but cannot be confirmed on the basis of the x-ray alone. In these early cases, the functional exploration with core biopsy is indispensable. The surgical results of core decompression in earlier Stage II have been incorporated into the previous section. However, in late Stage II, that is in those cases in which the outline of the sequestrum can be clearly seen even though there is no collapse of the femoral head as yet, the results of core decompression are less satisfactory. We believe that more aggressive surgery is necessary to avoid the completion of the sequestrum which becomes irreversible. At this stage, the cartilage is still preserved and, we believe, deserves to be saved if possible. There is also a transitional stage between Stage II and Stage III which behaves more like Stage III and requires more aggressive treatment. It is important to carefully review x-rays of good quality in both the AP and frog-leg position in order to accurately arrive at the staging if it is to have prognostic and therapeutic significance. The transitional stage is signified by the development of a crescent sign or slight superior or anterosuperior flattening without collapse. This latter development can best be seen on the frog-leg view of the femoral head.

Pedicle Graft

After having tried all of the possible techniques of muscle pedicle bone graft with all of the accessible muscles (tensor fascia lata, gluteus medius), we have finally settled on the use of the direct head of the rectus femoris. This technique was perfected by Cuzacq in our clinic and seems, to us, to be the most direct, rapid, and efficacious method[452].

Technique—The hip is approached via the anterior Smith-Petersen incision with the patient in the supine position on an operating table suitable for use with an image intensifier. The direct head of the rectus femoris is isolated and the anterior inferior iliac spine, including its intrapelvic portion, is exposed. A bone graft 2 cm wide and 5 to 6 cm long, including both cortices of the iliac, is removed with the attached insertion of the rectus femoris. The bone graft is a direct extension of the tendinous portion of the muscle and is directed slightly superiorly. The hip capsule is opened anteriorly in a T-shaped incision. Femoral neck retractors are inserted intracapsularly to expose the anterior aspect of the femoral neck. By flexing and externally rotating the lower extremity, the lateral part of the articular cartilage of the femoral head can be examined and biopsied if desired. A rectangular window, approximately 1.5 to 2 cm wide and 3 cm long in the axis of the neck, is removed from the anterior portion of the femoral neck beginning at the margin of the articular cartilage of the head. Through this opening, necrotic and sequestered bone is excised with a curette or a drill if the bone is too dense. This is done under fluoroscopic control. A standard core decompression is also carried out through a separate, short, midlateral incision just distal to the prominence of the greater trochanter. When the curettage is complete, the cavity is rinsed with saline, and the graft is tightly fitted through the window in the neck into the cavity, inserting it well inside the head up to and including the distal portion. The remainder of the cavity is filled with cancellous bone. In general, impacting the graft into the head provides satisfactory stability, but, when this is in question, it can be held in place by a suture through the two margins of the window and over the graft. The capsule is closed, paying particular attention not to strangulate the muscular pedicle. The wound is closed over a suction drain.

Post-operatively, the patient is maintained in balanced suspension with skeletal traction through the tibial tubercle for 15 days. Active mobilization of the limb is begun as soon as the post-operative pain has subsided. Bedrest is continued for another two weeks out of traction. Protective weight bearing with two crutches is continued for another two months. Weight bearing is permitted after three months if the x-rays are satisfactory.

There are several advantages of this technique over others, particularly those that use the posterior approach as Judet has advocated for pseudarthrosis of the femoral neck. The supine position facilitates anesthesia. The anterior approach facilitates exposure of the anterior neck, which is the most logical access into that area of the femoral head which is most commonly involved. The rectus femoris, because of its proximity to the femoral head and, more particularly, to the anterolateral aspect of the femoral head, presents the ideal pedicle source. Moreover, the massive bone graft can be adapted to need. Also, the muscle is not under tension when the bone graft is in position in the femoral head. Curettage of the femoral head is done under direct vision supplemented by image intensifier control. Because of the normal femoral neck anteversion, access to the anterolateral area is not technically difficult.

Results—We have carried out 18 such pedicle grafts using this technique with 11 good or excellent results and seven fair results. This small series included both Stage II and Stage III cases, and all seven fair results had sequestrum formation evidenced on the x-ray with evidence of early collapse. It is probable that this particular surgical intervention is ideally suited for the transition between Stage II and Stage III, where the sequestrum formation may be evidenced, but the epiphyseal outline is in continuity.

STAGE III

When the epiphyseal outline is no longer intact, even though joint space is preserved, the necrosis has evolved beyond the stage of reversibility. Even if the condition could be arrested, there would remain a change in the gross morphology of the femoral head, the degree of which will determine the ultimate, functional prognosis. The surgeon must choose from the entire therapeutic range which encompasses all of the surgical interventions which have been proposed for the treatment of osteonecrosis. These include core decompression, pedicle bone graft, osteotomy, arthroplasty (cup, surface replacement, or total hip replacement), and even arthrodesis. Core decompression and pedicle bone graft have been reviewed for Stages I and II[149]. When the lesion has reached Stage III, we frequently add multiple tenotomies similar to the Voss "hanging hip" procedure and continue the protective weight bearing for a long period of time.

Arthrodesis does not seem to be a logical solution since the acetabulum in Stage III is unaffected, and the necrosis in the femoral head leads to a high incidence of pseudarthrosis. For these reasons, arthrodesis has been virtually abandoned. Total hip replacement will be reviewed in reference to Stage IV lesions.

Femoral head replacement of the Austin-Moore type seems, at first, to be the most satisfactory solution since it replaces the necrotic femoral head while preserving the normal acetabulum. Therefore, from the theoretical point of view, it would seem justified. However, the late, functional results have left much to be desired. Aubriot[30] reported a statistical follow-up of 60 patients afflicted with INFH with 78 operated hips, 68 with an Austin-Moore prosthesis (cemented in seven cases), and ten by an acrylic femoral head replacement. Pain relief was rated as good or excellent on 67% of the cases. However, of the 46 cases followed for more than three years, only 41% had good or very good results. In these 46 cases, the joint space before surgery was normal in 13, narrowed in 21, and absent in 12 cases. Of the 13 normal cases, only five remained so after three years.

Although there is not a strict correlation between radiologic and functional results, it does appear that the main factor influencing the unsatisfactory results arose from secondary degeneration of the acetabulum. Therefore, we believe that only two operations at our present state of knowledge are specifically applicable to Stage III. These are osteotomy and cup arthroplasty.

Osteotomy

The most extensive experience in France was recently published by Kerboul, Thomine, Postel, and Merle D'Aubigne[246]. The principal aim of surgery is to reposition that portion of the superolateral segment of the femoral head which is not affected by the sequestrum into the weight-bearing position through an intertrochanteric osteotomy. The extent of the necrosis is calculated by adding the two angles of the necrotic segment measured on the AP and lateral x-rays respectively. If the total is greater than 200°, the involvement can be labeled "severe" (47% of the cases). If it is less than 160°, the area of involvement is "small" (15% of the cases). The remaining 38% of the cases fall in an intermediate zone.

The repositioning osteotomy is carried out by removing an appropriate wedge from the intertrochanteric region[27] either in the transverse plane[6] or through an oblique osteotomy[59]. The purpose of all of the techniques is to remove the sequestered area from the weight-bearing zone.

Results—In this series, 76 patients, ranging in age from 33 to 63 years, had 112 hips involved with INFH. Ninety-three osteotomies were carried out. Although 68% of the cases were operated on during the first year of symptoms, there was already some collapse of the femoral head in 87% of the cases. Table XXXVIII shows that there is some deterioration of the clinical result with time, as might be ex-

TABLE XXXVIII

RESULTS OF INTERTROCHANTERIC OSTEOTOMY FOR STAGE III INFH

Relief of Pain		*Preservation of Functional Capacity*
After 1 Year	89%	60%
After 5 Years	59%	47%
After 6 Years	47%	32%

pected. Radiologic results parallel the clinical evaluation with 58% of the involved hips stabilizing. Thirty-three percent showed evidence of revascularization of the involved segment, while 25% remained unchanged. Forty-two percent of the cases showed secondary, continuing collapse with 90% demonstrating evidence of secondary arthrosis. The overall results represent 40% failures (15% immediate, 7% early, and 18% late) and 60% good results remaining painless after five years. The authors emphasized that the necrotic zone must be of such a dimension and localization that it can be repositioned out of the weight-bearing area. In this series, only 45% of the cases fulfilled these criteria. However, in all cases where it was possible to remove the sequestrum from the weight-bearing area, there was complete disappearance of pain. In those cases, it was necessary that there remained a large, lateral and posterior segment not involved in the sequestrum formation.

A similar study was reported by Cartier[82,83] in which 35 cases of varus osteotomy for INFH were followed up for a minimum of one year. He suggested that the degree of varus displacement was important since in those cases with more than 15° of varus repositioning, 91% had good or very good results, while only 65% had this level of success with a varus displacement of less than 15°. He also emphasized that a sufficient lateral wall of normal appearing bone was necessary. Cystic changes or osteoporosis involving the lateral area of the femoral head carried a poor prognosis.

Cup Arthroplasty

The cup arthroplasties reported here are different from the cup arthroplasty popularized by Smith-Petersen in that the cup is tightly fitted over the femoral head and protects the necrotic sequestrum, transferring weight bearing to the healthy parts of the femoral head that are not involved in the sequestration.

Technique—Thomine[436] cups are available in six sizes from 40 to 50 mm at 2 mm increments. The appropriate size cup is chosen after measuring the acetabulum and checking the congruence with the cup in the acetabulum. The head is then carefully and progressively reamed preserving as much of the lateral margin of the head as possible. The cup is tightly fitted over the reamed surface and impacted in place. The margin of the cup is oriented strictly perpendicular to the axis of the femoral neck.

Results—Sixty-five patients with 80 hips, all of whom presented some degree of collapse, were followed for one to six years. Pain relief was complete in 75% of the cases and partial in 10%. Fifteen percent were rated as failures. The overall results, taking into consideration pain, movement, and function, gave 66.25% good and very good results, 16.25% partial improvement, and 17.5% failure. In analyzing their results, the authors noted that, in two-thirds of the cases, there was some migration of the cup with a varus migration in 57%, valgus migration in 6%. There was no correlation between direction of migration and the functional status or subsequent subluxation of the cup (nine cases). Evidence of resorption of the femoral neck was present in 83% of the cases. Twenty-five cases showed changes in the acetabulum, and two cases showed post-surgical heterotopic new bone formation.

The authors concluded that the main cause of failure consisted of progression of the necrosis with collapse of bone under the cup. If one separates out those cases in which more than a 20° arch of the weight-bearing segment is preserved, then good results were obtained in 88% of these cases. It would appear that the limitations of this surgical intervention and the indications are similar to those that we have just described for osteotomy.

Discussion

The results of osteotomies and cup arthroplasties are only moderately satisfactory, taking into account that late deteriorations increase with time. Some authors have suggested that improvement in technique using a different cup arthroplasty, such as that described by Luck, may give better results. Gerard[180] reported 97.5% good and very good results on 24 hips followed up for more than one year following such a cup arthroplasty. However, perhaps over emphasis on technique leads us away from the biological determinants which may be more important than mechanical factors in the final functional long-term results. Secondary arthroses and continuation of the necrotic process are the most probable factors involved in the secondary decompensations seen in most series. Unfortunately, it is not possible to radiologically follow the progress of the necrosis under a cup arthroplasty. In some cases, the functional exploration with decompression constitutes an invaluable means of diagnosis and has allowed us, in some cases, to improve painful cups.

Selection of the appropriate surgical procedure in Stage III represents probably the most difficult decision regarding treatment in INFH. All of the surgical procedures which have previously been reviewed may have a role in treatment. Many factors need to be taken into account, including the age, sex, and profession of the patient, the status of the opposite hip, lumbosacral joints, and knees, the underlying disease condition and life expectancy of the patient, as well as the level of clinical symptoms and degree of radiologic progression in the affected hip.

The extent and location of the sequestrum are important in choosing a procedure which preserves the femoral head. If there is a good, lateral margin of the femoral head, the indications for osteotomy or Thomine cup are strengthened. We prefer the osteotomy for several reasons. Hip dislocation and section of the ligamentum teres are avoided. Both of these procedures deprive the already ischemic head of a portion of its blood supply. Varus osteotomy results in effective decompression of the gluteus medius. We believe that it is a good practice to include tenotomy of the adductors and even of the psoas at the time of osteotomy. Moreover, we recommend systematic core decompression through the osteotomy cut as an added stimulus to revascularization of the femoral head.

On the other hand, if the sequestrum is superolateral or affecting the entire superior pole of the femoral head, osteotomy is contraindicated. In such a case, the cup arthroplasty described by Luck may be more advantageously used since sufficient lateral femoral head margin is less important. We feel that the extent of the sequestrum formation towards the center of the head is also important, although it is seldom mentioned by other authors. A superficial sequestrum in the form of an egg shell or as a narrow band without collapse is best treated, in our opinion, with a pedicle bone graft since the cartilage may be preserved. On the other hand, a deep sequestrum reaching the center of the head signals impending morphologic failure of the bone leaving only the lower third of the head separated from the sclerotic arch. In such cases, it is obvious that, in spite of preservation of the joint line, long-term preservation of the functional capacity of the femoral head cannot be anticipated. Prosthetic replacement becomes indicated when symptoms demand it unless a poor,

general status precludes it. In that case, a core decompression could provide palliation, particularly if it is associated with tenotomy and prolonged, protective weight bearing. The long-term results of femoral head replacement suggest that total hip replacement is the procedure of choice. Considerable progress would seem to be possible in this field. We have been experimenting with a type of femoral head replacement prosthesis which absorbs shock-loading with the hope of improving the longterm mechanical survival of the acetabular cartilage. However, results are too early to be reported as yet.

The nearer the patient is to 60 years of age, the more likely a total hip replacement would be the procedure of choice. If the complaint is mainly one of pain, the sequestrum is small, and the general medical condition necessitates a surgery of short duration, a core decompression can provide significant pain relief. If the hip is very stiff and there are other pathological sites (opposite hip, knees, etc.), there will be a tendency to prefer total hip replacement. In the face of failure of a previous surgical procedure, whether it be core decompression, pedicle bone graft, osteotomy, or cup, total hip replacement becomes the last recourse.

STAGE IV

This stage represents the end of the line when the sequestrum and superior weight-bearing portion of the femoral head have collapsed, associated with dramatic reduction in the joint line. In this case, arthrosis merges with necrosis. Joint function is destroyed with only limited, painful movement remaining. In this advanced stage of disease, there is only one reasonable solution—total hip replacement. The results are those of total hip replacement in general. The nature of the condition no longer plays a role in the end results, since the contact zone between the prosthesis, cement, and bone are usually located in healthy tissue. In that case, prognosis is dependent mainly on technique. Our results are similar to those contained in arthrosis with good and excellent results in about 90% of the cases.

MEDICAL-LEGAL CONSIDERATIONS

The medical-legal repercussions of post-traumatic osteonecrosis deserve considerable attention and must be classified and determined on better scientific grounds then is usually done. In cases of fracture of the femoral neck, the acetabulum, or dislocation of the hip, the cause-and-effect relationship with a subsequent osteonecrosis is easily established and accepted. There is no discussion when the x-rays are abnormal, but it is another thing when the pictures are less specific or when it is a question of Stage I disease with painful limitation of movement of the affected hip but no suggestive radiologic signs. In these cases, the functional exploration of bone is of great assistance in solving the problem.

Although there are no difficulties in establishing a causal relationship when the necrosis quickly follows the traumatic episode, the expert may raise doubts when there is a significant symptom-free interval between the resolution of the immediate effects of the accident and the subsequent diagnosis of osteonecrosis. Also, a long duration of relatively benign or non-specific symptoms may put the cause-and-effect relationship into question. In relationship to the first point, there is also a tendency to minimize certain clinical signs and residual radiologic abnormalities. This interval is frequently, not truly, asymptomatic, particularly if that categorization is based upon a cursory examination and erroneous interpretation of non-specific symptoms. The acceptable interval cannot be fixed on scientific bases. It should be recalled that a latent period of 20 years between exposure to compressed air (caisson disease) and osteonecrosis has been officially accepted in establishing a causal relationship.

With the epidemiologic knowledge that we now have on the anatomic evolution of the lesion, we believe that an interval of five years with no clinical or radiologic signs during this period could constitute a good discriminatory element in rejecting the responsibility of injury. On the other hand, if during this interval, the patient has experienced symptoms, restriction of movement, restriction of work, or demonstration of specific signs on periodic, radiologic evaluation, we do not hesitate to establish a cause-and-effect relationship with the antecedent trauma, even if there has been a ten-year interval between the injury and the time of review.

Unquestionably, there are difficult and debatable cases. More and more of these involve minor injury, particularly contusions without x-ray evidence of bone lesions. Several points should be emphasized. In his initial report, the practitioner should carefully note all areas affected by the injury. The recording of "multiple contusions" is not satisfactory. Contusions are frequently overlooked in comatose and polytraumatized patients because the contusion is initially of little importance in a patient with several lesions. However, any detail to substantiate contusion of a joint is of great interest. Superficial wounds, hematoma, ecchymosis in the gluteal or trochanteric regions, and anything in the clinical history that could incriminate an indirect contusion or a twisting injury to the hip should be recorded.

Dashboard injury with or without x-ray evidence of bony injury to the knee, a lateral blow to the trochanter, and falling on the feet from a significant vertical height are all clinical associations which we have seen with osteonecrosis of the hip. It is obvious that if nothing is noted on the initial report, even though the clinical history suggests a mechanism of trauma to the affected hip, it will be difficult to establish the reality of an association between the hip injury and the necrosis.

For the hip which presents with a normal x-ray but painful limitation of movement, the establishment of the diagnosis of osteonecrosis depends upon the functional exploration. In the appropriate patient, tomogram of the femoral head and the functional exploration of bone should both be employed.

Permanent total disability in relation to the osteonecroses can be reasonably assessed at the following rates: 25-35% for necrosis at Stage III and IV, 15-25% for necrosis at Stage II, and 10-15% for necrosis in Stage I. The severity of the radiologic lesion and the functional disability play a role in disability determination. The patient and compensation carriers need to be advised of the possibility of a progression of the disease requiring upgrading of the percent of the disability.

CONCLUSIONS

We have arrived at the end of the road. However, finishing a book represents opening new avenues since it raises more questions than it answers. In medical research, there is never an end. There are certain halting places where one stops to meditate, assimilate, and to subsequently start again a little richer. This was our goal. We have tried to break out of a concept of bone pathology which we feel to be too mechanistic. We consider that dogmatic attitudes, basing the diagnosis and therapeutic indications on the x-ray picture alone, are "passé." Following such an attitude leads us to study only secondary and late stages of bone disease. We must free bone pathology from its calcific prison.

We have adopted a more dynamic concept of this pathology and have tried to give back to the marrow and vascular tissues (the soft tissues of bone) their pre-eminence. They are, at the same time, the source of trophic changes in bone and the origin of internal remodeling; they are also responsible for the initial process in mulitiple-disease states. Since these soft tissues completely escape the usual radiologic investigations, a new method of exploration had to be developed. After 15 years of continuous work as a team, we have been able to present this new method of diagnosis, which we have christened the functional exploration of bone. The intraosseous circulation is, in fact, the support of the life and function of the osteoarticular system. The functional exploration of bone probes it in all its aspects. Application of these techniques to human pathology has lead us to confront the classic data (clinical, biological, and radiologic) with the functional exploration data of bone (hemodynamic, histologic). Although we have essentially limited our field of investigation in this monograph to the femoral head, we have published other works on its application to other joints, including the knee[156], shoulder, wrist, foot, and to other diseases like Paget's disease[24] and arthrosis. We believe that our efforts have been rewarded by results which have wide repercussions in many fields in Orthopaedics. The application of the functional exploration of bone has resulted in several advances including:

1. demonstration that classification systems based solely on radiologic criteria are unsatisfactory and lead to only late diagnoses.

2. better understanding of pathogenetic and pathophysiological mechanisms.

3. the establishment of an early diagnosis which permits studying and treating early phases in the disease. The technique has virtually defined the pre-radiologic stage of INFH.

4. the greater applicability of non-surgical therapeutic measures applied at an earlier and perhaps more reversible phase of the lesions. The possibility of prophylactic treatment can already be visualized.

In summary, we would like this monograph to represent an introduction to the ischemic pathology of bone.

BIBLIOGRAPHY

[1] ABDALLA (A.B.), HARRISON (R.G.). — Observations on the reaction of tubular bone to venous stasis. *J. Anat. (Londres)*, 1966, *100*, 627.

[2] ADER (J.L.), GERAL (J.P.), ARLET (J.). — Modifications de la pression médullaire osseuse chez le chien par section des nerfs frénateurs. *Rev. Rhum.* 1973, *42*, 333.

[3] AHLBÄCK (S.), BAUER (G.C.H.), BOHNE (W.H.) — Spontaneous osteonecrosis of the knee. *Arthritis Rheum.* 1968, *11*, 705.

[4] AMAKO (Tamikasu). — Bone and joint lesions in decompression sickness. « R », 1973, *3*, 637.

[5] ANDERSON (W.D.). — Studies of the lymphatic pathways of bone and bone marrow. *J. Bone Joint Surg.* 1960, *42 A*, 716.

[6] ANDERSON (cité par CRUTHLOW).

[7] ARFI (S.), HENRARD (J.C.), PAOLAGGI (J.B.). — L'ostéonécrose aseptique de la corticothérapie. *Nouv. Presse Méd.* 1974, *2*, 1719.

[8] ARFI (S.), MOREAU (F.), HEUCLIN (C.), KREISS (H.), PAOLAGGI (J.B.), AUQUIER (L.). — L'ostéonécrose aseptique de la transplantation rénale. *Rev. Rhum.* 1975, *42*, 167.

[9] ARLET (J.), FICAT (P.). — Forage-biopsie de la tête fémorale dans l'ostéonécrose primitive ; observations histopathologiques portant sur huit cas. *Rev. Rhum.* 1964, *31*, 257.

[10] ARLET (J.), FICAT (P.), SEBBAG (D.). — Intérêt de la mesure de la pression intra-médullaire dans le massif trochantérien chez l'homme, en particulier pour le diagnostic de l'ostéonécrose fémoro-capitale. *Rev. Rhum.* 1968, *35*, 250.

[11] ARLET (J.), FICAT (P.), LARTIGUE (G.). — Mode de début de l'ostéonécrose fémoro-capitale primitive. Etude de 20 observations histologiquement prouvées par le forage-biopsie. *Rev. Rhum.* 1968, *35*, 235.

[12] ARLET (J.), FICAT (P.), PUJOL (M.), LARTIGUE (G.), LATORZEFF (S.). — Ischémie et nécrose de la tête fémorale après traumatisme sans fracture. *Rhumatologie* (Aix-les-Bains), 1973, *25*, 159.

[13] ARLET (J.), FICAT (P.). — Diagnostic de l'ostéonécrose fémoro-capitale au stade I. *Rev. Chir. Orthop.* 1968, *54*, 637.

[14] ARLET (J.), FICAT (P.), DURROUX (R.). — Enseignement de la biopsie couplée (os + synoviale) dans le diagnostic des coxopathies rhumatismales. *Rev. Rhum.* 1970, *37*, 3.

[14a] ARLET (J.), FICAT (P.), DURROUX (R.), THEALLIER (J.P.), MAZIÉRES (B.), BOUTEILLER (G.) — Histopathologie des lésions osseuses dans 9 cas d'algo-dystrophie de la hanche. *Rev. Rhum.* 1978, *45(12)*, 691–698.

[15] ARLET (J.). — Pertrochanteric phlebography in necrosis of the femoral head in the initial stage, in « *Idiopathic ischemic necrosis of the femoral head in adults* ». Edited by W.M. Zinn, G. Thieme Publishers (Stuttgart), 1971, p. 152.

[16] ARLET (J.), FICAT (P.), DURROUX (R.), GOURDOU (J.F.). — Observations anatomo-cliniques de coxites rhumatismales isolées. *Rev. Rhum.* 1971, *38*, 107.

[17] ARLET (J.), FICAT (P.). — Biopsy drilling as a means of early diagnosis, in « *Idiopathic ischemic necrosis of the femoral head in adults*. Edited by W.M. Zinn, G. Thieme Publishers (Stuttgart), 1971, p. 74.

[18] ARLET (J.), FICAT (P.), DURROUX (R.), GOURDOU (J.F.). — Formes anatomo-cliniques (radiologiques et étiologiques) de l'ischémie chronique et de l'ostéonécrose, dite primitive de l'épiphyse fémorale supérieure. *Rev. Rhum.* 1971, *38*, 41.

[19] ARLET (J.), FICAT (P.), GÉDÉON (A.), CAUSSANEL (J.P.). — Nécrose et ischémie de la tête fémorale au cours des artérites oblitératives des membres inférieurs. (A propos de 5 observations). *Rev. Rhum.* 1972, *89*, 523.

[20] ARLET (J.), FICAT (P.), LARTIGUE (G.), TRAN (M.A.). — Recherches cliniques sur la pression intra-osseuse dans la métaphyse et l'épiphyse fémorales supérieures chez l'homme. *Rev. Rhum.* 1972, *39*, 717.

[21] ARLET (J.). — *La pression intra-médullaire comme méthode d'exploration de la circulation intra-osseuse.* Compte rendu du 1er Symposium International sur la Circulation osseuse, Toulouse, 1973, p. 111, Editions INSERM, Paris, 1973.

[22] ARLET (J), DURROUX (R.). — *Diagnostic histologique précoce de l'ostéonécrose aseptique de la tête fémorale par le forage-biopsie.* Compte rendu du 1er Symposium International sur la circulation osseuse, Toulouse, 1973, p. 293, Editions INSERM, Paris 1973.

[23] ARLET (J.), PUJOL (M.), TRAN (M.A.). — Premiers résultats d'une étude gazométrique du sang osseux trochantérien dans les coxopathies. *Rev. Rhum.* 1973, *40*, 515.

[24] ARLET (J.), MAZIÈRES (B.). — La circulation dans l'os pagétique. *Rev. Rhum.* 1975, *42*, 643.

[25] ARLET (J.), PUJOL (M.), MAZIÈRES (B.), CHARPIOT (J.P.). — La coxopatia pagetica : estudio de 100 cases. Datos clinicos, radiologicos y emodinamicos. *Rev. Esp. Rheum.* 1975, *2*, 61.

[26] ARNOLDI (C.C.), LEMPERG (R.K.), LINDERHOLM (H.). — Immediate effects of osteotomy on the intra-

medullary pressure of the femoral head and neck in patients with degenerative osteoarthritis. *Acta Orthop. Scand.* 1971, *42*, 357.

[27] ARNOLDI (C.C.), LINDERHOLM (H.). — Fractures of the femoral neck. I. Vascular disturbances in different types of fractures, assesed by measurements of intraosseous pressure. *Clin. Orthopaedics* 1972, *84*, 116.

[28] ARNOLDI (C.C.), LEMPERG (R.K.), LINDERHOLM (H.). Intraosseous hypertension and pain in the knee. *J. Bone Joint Surg.* 1975, *3*, 360.

[29] ARNOLDI (C.C.), LINDERHOLM (H.), MUSSBICHLER (H.). — Venous engorgement and intraosseous hypertension in osteoarthritis of the hip. *J. Bone Joint Surg.* 1972, *54B*, 409.

[30] AUBRIOT (J.H.). — Traitement par prothèses fémorales métalliques des ostéonécroses aseptiques primitives fémorales. *Rev. Chir. Orthop.* 1973, *59*, Suppl. n° 1, 81-89.

[31] AXHAUSEN (G.). — Über anämische infarkte am knochensystem und ihre bedeutung für die lehre den primaren epiphyseonekrosen. *Arch. f. Klin. Chir.* 1928, *151*, 72.

[32] AZUMA (H.). — Intraosseous pressure as a measure of hemodynamic changes in the bone marrow. *Angiology* 1964, *15*, 396.

[33] BACLESSE (F.). — Fractures du col fémoral observées après la radiothérapie dans les cancers du col utérin. *Bull. Cancer.* 1955, *42*, 141.

[34] BAILEY (G.L.), GRIFFITH (H.L.), MOCELIN (A.J.), GUNOY (P.H.), HAMPERS (C.L.), MERILL (J.P.). — Avascular necrosis of the femoral head on patients on chronic hemodialysis. *Trans. Am. Soc. for Artificial Internal Organe* 1972, 401.

[35] BAGANZ (H.M.), BAILEY (W.L.). — Systemic lupus erythematosus complicated by avascular necrosis of the hip. *Delaware M.J.*, 1961, *33*, 34.

[36] BALIUS JULI (R.), RUBIO ROIG (J.), COROMINAS (A.), PIULACHS (P.). — Embolismo pulmonar graso postraumatico. Estudio anatomopathologico y bioquimico. *Medicina clinica* 1972, *59*, 120.

[37] BAUDEL (F.). — Exploration lipidique de 60 coxopathies. *Thèse Médecine, Toulouse* 1975.

[38] BAUER (G.C.H.), CARLSSON (A.), LINDQUIST (B.). — Evaluation of accretion, resorption and exchange reactions in the skeleton. Konghga Fysiografsks Sällkapets i lund Forhandlingeer, 1955, 25.

[39] BAUER (G.C.H.), RAY (R.D.). — Kinetics of strontium metabolism in man. *J. Bone Joint Surg.* 1958, *40A*, 171.

[40] BAUER (G.C.H.), SMITH (E.M.). — 85 sr scintimetry in osteoarthritis of the knee. *J. Nucl. Med.* 1969, *10*, 109.

[41] BAUER (G.C.H.). — The use of radionucleids in orthopedics. *J. Bone Joint Surg.* 1968, *50A*, 1681.

[42] BAUER (G.C.H.). — Diagnostic and treatment of gonarthrosis (osteoarthritis of the knee). Sicot, XIᵉ Congrès, Mexico, octobre 1969, p. 369, Imprimerie des Sciences, S.A., Bruxelles, 1970.

[43] BAUX (R.), POULHES (J.). — La phlébographie pelvienne. *J. Radiol. et Electrol.* 1950, *31*, 7.

[44] BENEKE (G.), DEUTSCHELE (N.). — Frühveranderungen in der proximalen Femurepiphyse nach experimenteller Blut Kreislauf störung. *Virchow's Arch. Acta path. Anath.*, 1968, *344/2*, 125.

[45] BENNASSI (E.). — Lo suiluppo e trofismo dello scheletto degli arti in rapporto alla allacciutura dei vasi principali. *Arch. Ital. Chir.* 1931, *28*, 49.

[46] BENASSY (J.). — *Phlébographie dans les coxarthroses.* Compte rendu du Iᵉʳ Symposium International sur la circulation osseuse. Toulouse, 1973, p. 177. Editions INSERM, Paris, 1973.

[47] BENSASSON (M.). — L'ostéonécrose aseptique de la tête fémorale au cours des rhumatismes inflammatoires et de la goutte. Revue de la littérature et étude de 29 observations de la clinique rhumatologique de l'Hôpital Lariboisière. *Thèse Médecine, Paris,* 1969.

[48] BENTSON (P.G.K.). — A new theory about the pathogenesis of coxa plana and other manifestations of local dyschondroplasy. *Brit. J. Radiol.* 1926, *31*, 439.

[49] BÉRARD (A.). — Mémoire sur le rapport qui existe entre la direction des conduits nourriciers des os longs et l'ordre suivant lequel les épiphyses se soudent au corps de l'os. *Arch. Gén. Méd.* 1835, 2ᵉ série, *7*, 176-183.

[50] BERGMAN (E.). — Experimentelle untersuchungen über druck-wirkung in der knochenmarkhöhle. *Arch. f. Klin. Chir.* 1927, *145*, 568.

[51] BERGMAN (E.). — Theorisches, klinisches und experimentelles zur frage der aseptichen knochennecrose. *Deutsch Ztschr. f. Chir.* 1927, *206*, 18.

[52] BISMUTH (V.), DUPERRAT (B.), GAQUIÈRE (A.), BARD (M.), BOURDON (R.). — Maladie de Weber-Christian à détermination mésentérique et osseuse. *Ann. Radiol.* 1964, *7*, 197.

[53] BLOCH-MICHEL (H.), BENOIST (M.), MANGIN (A.). — Une nouvelle complication de la corticothérapie, l'ostéonécrose aseptique. *Bull. Soc. Méd. Hôp. Paris* 1961, *77*, 1026.

[54] BLOOMENTHAL (D.E.), OLSON (R.W.), NECHELES (H.). — Studies on the bone marrow cavity of the dog : fat embolism and marrow pressure. *Gynec. Obstet.*, 1952, *94*, 215.

[55] BONFIGLIO (M.). — Aseptic necrosis of the femoral head in dogs. Effect of drilling and bone grafting. *Surg. Gynec. Obstét.* 1954, *98*, 591.

[56] BONFIGLIO (M.), VOKE (E.M.). — Aseptic necrosis of the femoral head and non union of the femoral neck. Effect of treatment by drilling and bone grafting (Phemister technique). *J. Bone Joint Surg.* 1968, *50A*, 48.

[57] BOUISSOU (H.), DURROUX (R.). — Les modifications ischémiques du tissu osseux. *Sem. Hôp. Arch. Anat. Pathol.* 1972, *20A*, 99.

[58] BOURDE (C.). — L'hyperuricémie des artériopathies des membres. Bilan de 15 années d'observation. Etude statistique de 200 cas. *Angeiologie* 1971, *14*, 1599.

[59] BOUYER (C.L.). — Traitement des crises douloureuses de la drépanocytose par un vaso-dilatateur artériolaire. *Ann. Soc. Belge Med. Trop.* 1968, *48*, 597.

[60] BOWIE (E.J.W.), THOMPSON (J.H.), PASCUZZI (C.A.), OWEN (C.A.). — Thrombosis in systemic lupus erythematosus despite circulating anti-coagulants. *Coll. Pap. Mayo Clin.* 1963, *55*, 222.

[61] BOYD (H.B.), ZILVERSMIT (D.B.), CALANDRUCCIO (R.A.). — The use of radio active phosphorus to determine the viability of the head of the femur. *J. Bone Joint Surg.* 1955, *37A*, 260.

[62] BOYD (H.B.), CALANDRUCCIO (R.A.). — Further observations on the use of radio active phosphorus (P. 32) to determine the viability of the head of the femur. Correlation of clinical and experimental data in 130 patients with fracture of the femoral neck. *J. Bone Joint Surg.* 1963, *45A*, 445.

[63] BRAGDON (H.), FOSTER (L.), SOSSMAN (M.C.). — Experimental infarction of bone and marrow. *Amer. J. Pathol.* 1949, *25*, 709.

[64] BRANEMARK (P.I.). — Vital microscopy of bone marrow in rabbit. *Scand. J. Clin. Lab. Invest.* 1959 *2, sup.* 38, 5.

[65] BRANEMARK (P.I.). — *Bone marrow. Microvascular structure and function. Advances in microcirculation.* Vol. I. Karger, Bäle, New York, 1968.

[66] BROOKES (M.). — Femoral growth after occlusion of the principal nutrient canal in day-old rabbits. *J. Bone Joint Surg.* 1957, *39B*, 563.

[67] BROOKES (M.), HARRISON (R.G.). — The vascularization of the rabbit femur and tibio fibula. *J. Anath.* 1957, *91*, 61.

[68] BROOKES (M.). — The vascular architecture of tubular bone in the rat. *Anat. Rec.* 1958, *132*, 25.

[69] BROOKS (M.). — The vascular reaction of tubular bone to ischemia in peripheral occlusive vascular disease. *J. Bone Joint Surg.* 1960, *42B*, 110.

[70] BROOKES (M.). — Sequelae of experimental partial ischemia in long bones of the rabbit. *J. Anat.* 1960, *94*, 552.

[71] BROOKES (M.), ELKIN (A.C.), HARRISON (R.G.), HEALD (C.B.). — A new concept of capillary circulation in bone cortex. Some clinical applications. *Lancet* 1961, *1*, 1078.

[72] BROOKES (M.). — Red cell volumes and vascular patterns in long bones. *Acta Anat.* 1965, *62*, 35.

[73] BROOKES (M.). — The vascular factors in osteoarthritis. *Surg. Gynecol. Obstet.* 1966, *123*, 1255.

[74] BROOKES (M.), HELAL (B.). — Primary osteoarthritis, venous engorgement and osteogenesis. *J. Bone Joint Surg.* 1968, *50B*, 493.

[75] BROOKES (M.). — *The blood supply of bone.* Butterworths and Co, London 1971.

[76] BROOKES (M.), SINGH (M.). — Bone blood pH and gas tensions after femoral vein ligation. *Surg. Gynecol. Obstet.* 1972, *135*, 873.

[77] BROWN-GRANT (K.), CUMMING (J.D.). — A study of the capillary blood flow through bone marrow by the radio isotopic depot clearance technique. *J. Physiol. London* 1962, *162*, 21.

[78] BRUNSCHWIG (A.). — Experimental infarction of bone marrow. *Proc. Soc. Exp. Biol. Med.* 1930, *27*, 1049.

[79] BUDGE (A.). — Die lymphwarzein der knochen. *Arch. f. Mikroskopische anatomie*, 1877, *13*, 87.

[80] BURKHARDT (R.). — Communication orale.

[81] BURROWS (H.J.). — Coxa plana with special reference to its pathology and kinship. *Brit. J. Surg.*, 1941, *29*, 23.

[82] CARTIER (P.H.). — L'ostéotomie de varisation dans la nécrose idiopathique de la tête fémorale. *Thèse Médecine, Paris* 1970.

[83] CARTIER (P.H.), HAUTIER (S.), LEMOINE (A.). — L'ostéotomie de varisation dans la nécrose idiopathique de la tête fémorale. *Ann. Chir.* 1972, *26*, 483.

[84] CASTRO (F. de). — Quelques observations sur l'intervention du système nerveux autonome dans l'ossification-innervation du tissu osseux et de la moelle osseuse. *Trav. Lab. Tech. Univ. Madrid*, 1930, *26*, 215.

[85] CATTO (M.). — Avascular necrosis of the femoral head after transcervical fracture. *J. Bone Joint Surg.* 1965, *47B*, 749.

[86] CAUCHOIX (J.), DEBURGE (A.), HANTIC (S.), HERIPRET (C.). — Prévision de l'ostéonécrose céphalique dans les fractures du col du fémur. Etude radio-isotopique. IIe Congrès International SICOT, Mexico 1969.

[87] CHANDLER (F.A.). — Coronary disease of the hip. *J. Internat. coll. Surgeons* 1948, *11*, 34.

[88] CHARNLEY (J.), BLOCKEY (N.J.), PURSER (D.W.). — The treatment of displaced fractures of the neck of the femur by compression. *J. Bone Joint Surg.* 1957, *39B*, 45.

[89] CHEWITZ (O.), HEVESY (G.C.). — Radio active indicators in the study of phosphorus metabolism in rats. *Nature* 1935, *136*, 754.

[90] CHIRAY (M.L.), JUSTIN-BESANÇON (R.), BENDA (R.), DEBRAY (C.), LACOUR (M.). — Influence des injections intra-médullaires osseuses sur la pression artérielle du chien. *Ann. Méd. Paris* 1940, *46*, 267.

[91] CHUNG (S.M.K.), RALSTON (E.L.). — Necrosis of the femoral head associated with sickle-cell anemia and its genetic variants. A review of the litterature and study on thirteen cases. *J. Bone Joint Surg.* 1969, *51A*, 33.

[92] CLAMENS (J.). — Le réticulosarcome osseux. Un diagnostic difficile à propos de 4 observations. *Thèse Médecine, Toulouse*, 1975.

[93] COCKSHOTT (W.P.). — Haemoglobin S.C. disease. *J. Faculty Radiol.* 1958, *9*, 211.

[94] COHN (J.), HARRIS (W.H.). — The three dimensional anatomy of the haversian system. *J. Bone Joint Surg.* 1958, *40A*, 419.

[95] COLLARD (M.), COLLARD (P.). — Etude micro-angiographique de l'ischémie céphalique fémorale. *J. Radiol. Electrol. Med. Nucl.* 1972, *53*, 797.

[96] COOLBAUGH (C.C.). — Effects of reduced blood supply on bone. *Amer. J. Physiol.* 1952, *169*, 26.

[97] COOPER (R.R.). — Nerves in cortical bones. *Sciences* 1968, *160*, 327.

[98] COPP (D.H.), SHIM (S.S.). — Extraction ratio and bone clearance of Sr 85 as a measure of effective bone blood flow. *Circ. Res.* 1965, *16*, 461.

[99] COSTE (F.), MASSIAS (P.), CHAFI-ZADEH. — Ostéonécrose primitive de la tête fémorale et malformation congénitale de la hanche. *Rev. Rhum.* 1962, *29*, 575.

[100] COSTE (F.), VERSPICK (R.), GUIRAUDON (C.). — Coxites et coxarthroses : coxarthrose « usante ». *Sem. Hôp. Paris* 1963, *39*, 2108.

[101] COSTE (F.), MERLE D'AUBIGNÉ (R.), POSTEL (M.), MASSIAS (P.), GUEGUEN (J.), GRELLAT (P.). — Evolution de l'ostéonécrose primitive de la tête fémorale et perspectives thérapeutiques. *Presse Méd.* 1965, *73*, 263.

[102] COUTELIER (L.). — Recherche sur la guérison des fractures. *Thèse d'agrégation* 1969, Editions Arscia, S.A., Bruxelles 1969.

[103] CRUESS (R.L.), BLENNERHASSETT (J.), MACDONALD (F.R.), MAC LEAN (L.D.), DOSSETOR (J.). — Aseptic necrosis following renal transplantation. *J. Bone Joint Surg.* 1968, *50A*, 1577.

[104] CRUTCHLOW (W.). — Sr. 85 scintimetry of the hip in osteoarthritis and osteonecrosis. *Amer. J. Roentgenth, radiumth. Nucl. Med.* 1970, *109*, 803.

[105] CUMMING (J.D.). — A method for studying the rate of blood flow through the bone marrow of a rabbit's femur. *J. Physiol. London* 1960, *152*, 39.

[106] CUMMING (J.D.). — A study of blood flow through bone marrow by a method of venous effluent collection *J. Physiol. London* 1962, *162*, 13.

[107] CUMMING (J.D.), NUTT (M.E.). — Bone marrow blood flow and cardiac output in the rabbit. *J. Physiol. London* 1962, *162*, 30.

[108] CURTISS (P.H.), KINCAID (W.E.). — Transitory demineralisation of the hip in pregnancy. A report of three cases. *J. Bone Joint Surg.* 1959, *41A*, 1327.

[109] CUTHBERTSON (E.), GILFILLAN (R.S.). — Spontaneous and induced variations in bone marrow pressures in the dog. *Angiology* 1964, *15*, 145.

[110] CUTHBERTSON (E.), SIRIS (E.), GILFILLAN (R.S.). — The femoral diaphyseal medullary sinus as a venous collateral channel in the dog. *J. Bone Joint Surg.* 1965, *47A*, 965.

[111] DAHL (B.). — Nouvelles recherches sur l'effet inhibiteur des rayons de Röntgen. *Acta Radiol.* 1937, *18*, 565.

[112] DALBY (R.G.), JACOB (H.W.), MILLER (N.F.). — Fracture of femoral neck following pelvic irradiation. *Amer. J. Obstet. Gynecol.* 1936, *32*, 50.

[113] DANIELSON (L.B.), DYMLING (J.F.), HERIPRET (G.). — Coarthrosis in man studied with external counting of Sr and Ca. *Clin. Orthop.* 1963, *31*, 184.

[114] DARLINGTON (L.G.), SCOTT (J.T.). — Plasma lipids level in gout. *Ann. Rheum. Dis.* 1972, *31*, 487.

[115] DAVID-CHAUSSE (J.), VARNOUX (L.). — Résultats de l'exploration du métabolisme lipidique chez 18 malades atteints de nécrose primitive de la tête fémorale. *Bordeaux Méd.* 1969, *2*, 1741.

[116] DAYROSE (J.). — Nécrose de la tête fémorale après traumatismes mineurs. *Thèse Médecine, Bordeaux,* 1957.

[117] DEBEYRE (J.), KENESI (C.), BOUCKER (C.). — Trois observations de fractures cervico-capitales spontanées, complications de la nécrose primitive de la tête fémorale. *Rev. Rhum.* 1960, *36*, 23.

[118] DECOULX (P.). — Fractures-luxations de la hanche et leur traitement précoce. *Rev. Chir. Orthop.* 1959, *45*, 496.

[119] DEGEILH/ (G.). — Analyse statistique d'une population de 181 ostéonécroses fémoro-capitales. *Thèse Médecine, Toulouse* 1975.

[120] DELOUCHE (G.), BRUNET (M.), GUÉRIN (P.), GEST (J.). — Les lésions osseuses de la radiothérapie intensive des cancers gynécologiques. *Ann. Radiol.* 1970, *13*, 793.

[121] DIAS-AMADO (L.E.). — L'irrigation de la diaphyse de l'os pré-haversien. *Arch. port. Sci. Biol.* 1947, suppl. 9, 150.

[122] DOAN (C.A.). — The capillaries of the bone marrow of the adult pigeon. *Bull. Johns Hopk. Hosp.* 1922. *33*, 222.

[123] DRINKER (C.K.), DRINKER (K.R.). — A method for maintaining an artificial circulation through the tibia of a dog with a demonstration of the vasomotor control of the marrow. *Amer. J. Physiol.* 1916, *40*, 514.

[124] DUBOIS (E.L.). — *Lupus erythematosus. A review of the current status of discoïd and systemic LE and their variants.* Mc Grawhill Book Company Ed., 1 vol., 479 p., 1966, New York.

[125] DUBOIS (E.L.), COZEN (L.). — Avascular aseptic bone necrosis associated with systemic lupus erythematosus. *J. Amer. Med. Ass.* 1960, *174*, 966.

[126] DUCUING (J.), MARQUES (P.), BAUX (R.), PAILLE (J.), VOISIN (R.). — Physiologie de la circulation osseuse. *J. Radiol.* 1951, *32*, 16.

[127] DUCUING (J.), MARQUES (P.), BAUX (R.), PAILLE (J.), VOISIN (R.). — Les différentes voies d'exploration pelvienne par la phlébographie. *J. Radiol. Electrol.* 1951, *32*, 713.

[128] DUPARC (J.), FROT (B.). — Fracture du col fémoral après irradiation pelvienne. *Rev. Chir. Orthop.* 1971, *57*, 227.

[129] DURIEZ (J.), CAUCHOIX (J.). — Le rôle des ostéocytes dans la résorption du tissu osseux. *Presse Méd.* 1967, *75*, 1297.

[130] DURROUX (R.), ARLET (J.). — Critique des signes histologiques de nécrose osseuse. *Rhumatologie* 1971, *23*, 309.

[131] EBERLE (H.). — Die intra ossäre Femurkopfvenographie bei schenkelhalsfrakturen und Hüftgelenksluxationen. *Radiol. Clin. Biol.* 1967, *36*, 277.

[132] EBERLE (H.). — Venographic differences in traumatic hip affections and in idiopathic femoral head necrosis. In « *Idiopathic ischemic necrosis of the femoral head in adults* », p. 162. Edited by W.M. Zinn, G. Thieme publisher, Stuttgart 1971.

[133] EBERLE (H.). — Situation et différence de la phlébographie osseuse de la tête du fémur en cas de fractures, luxations de la hanche, nécroses idiopathiques et coxarthroses. Compte rendu du Ier Symposium International sur la Circulation osseuse, Toulouse 1973, p. 167, Editions INSERM, Paris 1973.

[134] ECOIFFIER (J.), PROT (D.), GRIFFIER (R.), CATACH (D.). — Etude du réseau veineux dans les os longs du lapin. *Rev. Chir. Orthop.* 1957, *43*, 29.

[135] EDHOLM (O.G.), HOWARTH (S.), MC MICHAEL (J.). — Heart failure and bone blood flow in osteitis deformans. *Clin. Sc. London* 1945, *5*, 249.

[136] EISINGER (J.B.), VALENTE (J.P.), DELL-ANNO (R.), RECORDIER (A.M.). — La pression intra-médullaire sternale et iliaque. Compte rendu du Ier Symposium International sur la Circulation Osseuse, Toulouse 1973, p. 151. Editions INSERM, Paris 1973.

[137] ENRIA (G.), FERRERO (R.). — La flebographia degli arti per via ossea. *Chirurgia Milan* 1950, *5*, 289.

[138] EWING (J.). — Radiation osteitis. *Acta Radiol.* 1926, *6*, 399.

[139] FÉRY (A.). — La vascularisation osseuse. *Thèse Médecine, Nancy,* 1972, 321 p., dont 118 de bibliographie.

[140] FICAT (P.), ARLET (J.), LARTIGUE (G.), PUJOL (M.), TRAN (M.A.). — Algodystrophie réflexe post-traumatique. Etude hémodynamique et anatomo-pathologique. *Rev. Chir. Orthop.* 1973, *59*, 401.

[141] FICAT (P.). — L'articulation, entité fonctionnelle. *Rev. Méd. Toulouse,* 1966, *2*, 719.

[142] FICAT (P.). — L'articulation, entité fonctionnelle. *Rev. Méd. Toulouse,* 1966, *3*, 347.

[143] FICAT (P.), ARLET (J.). — Diagnostic de l'ostéonécrose fémoro-capitale primitive au stade I (stade pré-radiologique). *Rev. Chir. Orthop.* 1968, *54*, 637.

[144] FICAT (P.), UTHEZA (G.). — Le forage-biopsie de la hanche. *Rev. Méd. Toulouse* 1968, *4*, 223.

[145] FICAT (P.), ARLET (J.), PUJOL (P.), VIDAL (R.). — Traumatisme, dystrophie réflexe et ostéonécrose de la tête fémorale. *Ann. Chir.* 1971, *25*, 911.

[146] FICAT (P.), ARLET (J.), VIDAL (R.), RICCI (A.), FOURNIAL (J.C.). — Résultats thérapeutiques du forage-biopsie dans les ostéonécroses fémoro-capitales primitives (100 cas). *Rev. Rhum.* 1971, *38*, 269.

[147] FICAT (P.). — Résultats du forage-biopsie dans les ostéonécroses de la hanche. *J. Belge Rhum. Méd. Phys.* 1972, *27*, 204.

[148] FICAT (P.), ARLET (J.). — Coxopathies ischémiques. *Rev. Chir. Orthop.* 1972, *58*, 563.

[149] FICAT (P.). — Opérations palliatives dans les ostéonécroses évoluées. *Rev. Chir. Orthop.* 1973, *59*, suppl. I, 48.

[150] FICAT (P.). — Phlébographie trans-osseuse. Compte rendu du Ier Symposium International sur la Circulation osseuse. Toulouse 1973, p. 157. Editions INSERM, Paris 1973.

[151] FICAT (P.), ARLET (J.). — Stade pré-radiologique de l'ostéonécrose fémoro-capitale. Possibilités diagnostiques et thérapeutiques. *Rev. Chir. Orthop.* 1973, *59*, suppl. 1, 26.

[152] FICAT (P.), ARLET (J.), LARTIGUE (G.), PUJOL (M.), TRAN (M.A.). — Exploration de la circulation intra-osseuse, exploration fonctionnelle médullaire. *Sem. Hôp. Paris* 1973, *49*, 587.

[153] FICAT (P.). — Diagnostic précoce de l'ostéonécrose drépanocytaire. *Médecine d'Afrique Noire* 1974, *21*, 959. Premières Journées Médicales de Yaoundé.

[154] FICAT (P.). — Arthrose et nécrose ou le double visage de la dystrophie dégénérative ostéo-articulaire. *Rev. Chir. Orthop.* 1974, *60*, 123.

[155] FICAT (P.), ARLET (J.). — Dysplasies, coxarthroses et ostéonécroses. *Sem. Hôp. Paris* 1974, *50*, 567.

[156] FICAT (P.), ARLET (J.), MAZIÈRES (B.). — Ostéochondrite disséquante et ostéonécrose de l'extrémité inférieure du fémur. Intérêt de l'exploration fonctionnelle. *Sem. Hôp. Paris* 1975, *51*, 1907.

[157] FICAT (P.). — Evolution du diagnostic en pathologie ostéo-articulaire. *J. Radiol. Electrol.* 1975, *56*, 355.

[158] FICAT (P.), ARLET (J.). — Arthrosis : new diagnostic procedures. *Acta Orthop. Scand.* 1975, *46*, 329.

[159] FIDERER (D.). — Le rôle des traumatismes mineurs dans le déclenchement des ischémies et nécroses de la tête fémorale. A propos de 18 cas. *Thèse Médecine, Toulouse* 1972.

[160] FILIPPI (G.). — Contributo allo studio della osteocondrite dissecante. *Chirg. Org. Mov.* 1931, *16*, 35.

[161] FISCHER (D.E.), BICKEL (W.H.), HOLLEY (K.E.). — Histologic demonstration of fat embolism in aseptic necrosis associated with hypercortisonism. *Mayo Clin. Proc.* 1969, *44*, 252.

[162] FISCHER (D.D.), BICKEL (W.H.). — Corticosteroid induced avascular necrosis. *J. Bone Joint Surg.* 1971, *53A*, 859.

[163] FOA (P.P.). — Studies on the innervation of the bone marrow. *Univ. Hosp. Bull.* 1943, *9*, 19.

[164] FOSTER (L.N.), KELLY (R.P.), WATIS (W.M.). — Experimental infarction of bone and bone marrow. Sequelae of severance of the nutrial artery and stripping of periosteum. *J. Bone Joint Surg.* 1951, *33A*, 396.

[165] FORESTIER (J.), ARLET (J.), JACQUELINE (F.). — L'atteinte de la hanche dans la P.C.E. de l'adulte. Evolution clinique et radiologique. *Rev. Rhum.* 1951, *18*, 304.

[166] FORGUE (A.). — Etude gazométrique du sang osseux trochantérien dans les coxopathies. *Thèse Médecine, Toulouse,* 1975.

[167] FOURNIAL (J.C.). — Résultats thérapeutiques du forage-biopsie dans les ostéonécroses fémoro-capitales primitives (à propos de 100 cas). *Thèse Médecine, Toulouse* 1971.

[168] FOURNIE (A.), AYROLLE (C.). — La phlébographie per-trochantérienne de la hanche. *Ann. Radiol.* 1962, *5*, 523.

[169] FOURNIER (A.M.), JULLIEN (G.). — *La maladie ostéo-articulaire des caissons.* Paris, Masson et Cie, 1965. 158 p.

[170] FREDERICKSON (J.M.), HONOUR (S.A.), COPP (D.H.). — Measurement of initial bone clearance of Ca 45 from blood in the rat. *Fed. Proc.* 1955, *14*, 49.

[171] FREUND (E.). — Osteochondritis dissecans of the head of the femur. Partial idiopathic aseptic necrosis of the femoral head. *Arch. Surg.* 1939, *39*, 323.

[172] FROST (H.M.). — In vivo « osteocyte death ». *J. Bone Joint Surg.* 1960, *42A*, 138.

[173] FREDRICKSON (D.S.), SLOAN (H.R.). — Glucosyl ceramide lipidosis : Gaucher's disease. In « *The Metabolic basis of inherited disease* », Mc Graw Hill Book Cie, New York, 1972.

[174] FROST (H.M.). — *The etiodynamics of aseptic necrosis of the femoral head.* Proceeding of the conference on aseptic necrosis of the femoral head St Louis 1964, 393.

[175] GALLIE (W.E.), ROBERTSON (D.E.). — The repair of bone. *Brit. J. Surg.* 1919, *7*, 211.

[176] GASCO GOMEZ DE MEMBRILLERA (J.). — Necrosis aseptica parcelar idiopatica de la cabeza femoral. *Rev. Esp. Cir. Osteoart.* 1970, *5*, 285.

[177] GAUCHER (A.). — L'étiologie, le terrain biologique et la pathogénie de l'ostéonécrose aseptique de la tête fémorale chez l'adulte (à propos de 32 nouvelles observations). *Ann. Méd. Nancy* 1971, *10*, 23.

[178] GAUCHER (A.), HURIET (C.), ROBERT (J.), NAOUN (A.), KESSLER (Mme), STRAUB (J.). — Les ostéonécroses des transplantés rénaux. Intérêt de la scintigraphie dans leur dépistage. *Rev. Rhum.* 1974, *41*, 759.

[179] GENNES (J.L. de), SAPORTA (L.), COSTE (F.), TOURAINE (R.). — Stéatonécrose osseuse associée à une hyperlipémie non dépendante des graisses. *Bull. Soc. Méd. Hôp. Paris* 1966, *117*, 1211.

[180] GÉRARD (Y.). — Nécroses idiopathiques de la tête fémorale. Traitement par cupules à appui cylindrique. *Rev. Chir. Orthop.* 1973, 59, suppl. 1, 74.

[181] GIBSON (J.), GRAHAM (R.). — Gout and hyperlipidemia. *Ann. Rhum. Dis.* 1974, *33*, 298.

[182] GILLET (M.), DAVID CHAUSSE (J.), BASSE-CATHALINAT (B.), BLANQUET (P.). — *Exploration des ostéonécroses par les radio-isotopes.* Compte rendu du 1er Symposium International sur la Circulation Osseuse, Toulouse 1973, Editions INSERM, Paris 1973.

[183] GLICK (E.N.). — Avascular necrosis of the femoral head in rheumatoid arthritis. In « *Idiopathic ischemic necrose of the femoral head in adults* », p. 168. Edited by W.M. Zinn, G. Thieme Publishers, Stuttgart 1971.

[184] GOLDIE (I.), TIBEIN (G.), SCHELLER (S.). — Systemic lupus erythematosus and aseptic bone necrosis. A discussion based on one case treated with corticoides. *Acta Med. Scand.* 1967, *182*, 55.

[185] GOOD (A.E.). — Bilateral aseptic necrosis of femur following a 16 days course of corticotrophin. *J. Amer. Med. Ass.* 1974, *228*, 497.

[186] GOULON (M.), BAROIS (A.), GROSPUIS (S.), SCHORTGEN (G.). — Embolie graisseuse après perfusions répétées d'émulsions lipidiques. *Nouv. Pres. Méd.* 1974, *23*, 13.

[187] GOURDOU (J.F.). — Exploration fonctionnelle de la hanche chez l'adulte dans le diagnostic de l'ostéonécrose post-traumatique. *Thèse Médecine, Toulouse* 1973.

[188] GOURDOU (J.F.), DANET (A.), GUIRAUD (R.), DURROUX (R.), FICAT (P.), ARLET (J.). — Nécrose expérimentale de la tête fémorale d'origine veineuse chez le chien. *Rev. Rhum.* 1974, *41*, 739.

[189] GRABER-DUVERNAY. — Forage de la hanche dans la coxarthrose. *J. Méd. Lyon* 1932, *304*.

[190] GRAHAM (R.V.). — Experimental considerations in Perthe's disease (Division of ligamentum teres). *Med. J. Australia* 1930, *1*, 207.

[191] GROS (M.). — La disposition des nerfs des os. *Bull. Soc. Anat. Paris* 1846, *21*, 369.

[192] GUIRAUD (R.), BESSOU (P.), ARLET (J.), MILLET (H.). — *Apports de l'exploration au strontium 87 m dans le diagnostic précoce des ostéonécroses aseptiques de la tête fémorale.* Compte rendu du Ier Symposium International sur la Circulation Osseuse, p. 217. Toulouse 1973. Editions INSERM, Paris 1973.

[193] GUIRAUDON (C.), COSTE (F.), MASSIAS (P.). — A propos de 34 cas de coxopathies destructives. *Rev. Rhum.* 1970, *37*, 67.

[194] HAENISCH (F.). — Tagung der Vereinigung. *Nord West Deutscher Z. Chir.* 1926, *52*, 999.

[195] HALDEMAN (K.O.). — The role of the periosteum in healing of fractures. Experimental study. *Arch. Surg.* 1932, *24*, 440.

[196] HARRINGTON (K.D.), MURRAY (W.R.), DOUNTZ (S.L.), BELZER (F.O.). — Avascular necrosis of bone after renal transplantation. *J. Bone Joint Surg.* 1971, *53A*, 203.

[197] HARRIS (H.M.). — *Bone growth in health and disease.* Oxford Univ. Press. London, 1933.

[198] HARRISSON (H.M.H.). — A preliminary report of avascular essay in prognosis of the fractured femoral neck. *J. Bone Joint Surg.* 1962, *44B*, 858.

[199] HARTMANN (F.). — Nekrose herbeigeführt durch verstopfung des foramen nütritium. *Virc. Arch. F. Path. Physiol. u. f. Klin. Med.* 1855, *8*, 114.

[200] HARTMANN (G.). — The possible role of fat embolism in idiopathic ischemic necrosis of the femoral head. In « *Idiopathic ischemic necrosis of the femoral head in a adults* », p. 140. Edited by W.M. Zinn, G. Thieme Publishers, Stuttgart, 1971.

[201] HELD (D.), THRON (H.L.). — Etudes de la circulation de l'os. I. La pression tissulaire de la moelle. *Arch. Sc. Physiol.* 1962, *16*, 167.

[202] HERNBORG (J.). — Elimination of Na 131 I from the head and the neck of the femur in unaffected and osteoarthritic hip joints. *Arthritis Rheum.* 1969, *12*, 30.

[203] HERZIG (E.), ROOT (W.S.). — Relations of sympathic nervous system to blood pressure of bone marrow. *Amer. J. Physiol.* 1959, *196*, 1053.

[204] HIPP (E.). — Zur idiopathischen Huftkopfnekrose. *Zeitschrift für orthopädie* 1966, *101*, 398.

[205] HIPP (E.). — *Angiographic studies in idiopathic osteonecrosis of the femoral head.* Compte rendu du Ier Symposium International sur la Circulation Osseuse, Toulouse 1973, p. 189. Editions INSERM, Paris 1973.

[206] HOFMEISTER (F.), BRANDT (H.). — Die Lokalisation der Gicht im Hüftgelenk. *Arch. Orthop. Unfall Chir.* 1972, *73*, 267.

[207] HOLDSWORTH (F.W.). — Epiphyseal growth : speculations on the nature of Perthes' disease. *Ann. R. Coll. Surg.* 1966, 39, 1.

[208] HOUANG (K). — Le rôle des artères nourricières des os longs dans la formation du cal et de la calcification de la cavité médullaire. *Press Méd.* 1934, *42*, 2074.

[209] HUET (P.), HUGUIER (J.). — Le rôle probable de la stase capillaire réflexe en chirurgie générale. *J. Chir.* 1946, *62*, 184.

[210] HULTH (A.). — Intra-osseous venographies of medial fractures of femoral neck : residual vascularity of head fragment in different types of fractures and its relation to prognosis. *Acta Chir. Scand.* 1956, suppl. 214.

[211] HULTH (A.). — Femoral head phlebography, a method of predicting vialidity. *J. Bone Joint Surg.* 1958, *40A*, 844.

[212] HULTH (A.). — Femoral head venography in the prognosis of fractures of the femoral neck. *Acta Chir. Scand.* 1962, *123*, 287.

[213] HULTH (A.). — Prediction of the viability of the femoral head in femoral neck fractures. A survey of different predicting methods. *Acta Chir. Scand.* 1965, *119*, 72.

[214] HUGGINS (C.), WIEGE (E.). — The effect on the bone marrow of disruption of the nutrient artery and vein. *Ann. Surg.* 1939, *110*, 940.

[215] HUGHES (E.C.), SCHUMACHER (H.R.), SPARBARO (J.L.). — Bilateral avascular necrosis of the hip following Leriche Syndrome. *J. Bone Joint Surg.* 1971, *53A*, 380.

[216] HUNDER (G.G.), KELLY (P.J.). — Roentgenologic transient osteoporosis of the hip. A. Clinical syndrome ? *Ann. Intern. Med.* 1968, *68*, 539.

[217] HUNDER (G.G.), WORTHINGTON (J.W.), BICKEL (W.H.). — Avascular necrosis of the femoral head in a patient with gout. *J. Amer. Med. Ass.* 1968, *203*, 47.

[217a] HUNGERFORD (D.S.) — Bone marrow pressure, venography, and core decompression in ischemic necrosis of the femoral head. IN: The Hip: Proceedings of the Seventh Open Scientific Meeting of the Hip Society, pp 184–210. Edited by CB Sledge, CV Mosby Company, St. Louis, Missouri, 1979.

[218] HUNTER (W.). — Of the structure and diseases of articulating cartilage. *Phil. Trans. R. Soc. London* 1743, *42*, 514.

[219] IMMELMAN (E.J.), BANK (S.), KRIGE (H.), MARKS (N.). — Roentgenologic and clinical features of intramedullary fat necrosis in acute and chronic pancreatitis. *Amer. J. Med.* 1964, *36*, 96.

[220] JACQUELINE (F.), RABINOWICZ (T.H.). — *Lésions de la hanche secondaires à la fracture du col du fémur.* Compte rendu du Ier Symposium International sur la Circulation Osseuse, Toulouse 1973, p. 283. Editions INSERM, Paris 1973.

[221] JACQUELINE (F.), RUTISHAUSER (E.). — Idiopathic necrosis of the femoral head. Anatomopathological study. In *Idiopathic ischemic necrosis of the femoral head in adults*, p. 34. Edited by W.M. Zinn, G. Thieme Publishers, Stuttgart 1971.

[222] JACQUELINE (F.). — Communication orale.

[223] JACKSON (L.). — Experimental streptococcal arthritis in rabbits. *J. Infect. Dis.* 1913, *12*, 364.

[224] JAFFE (H.L.), POMERANZ (M.M.). — Changes in the bones of extremities amputated because of arterio vascular disease. *Arch. Surg.* 1934, *29*, 565.

[225] JAFFRES (R.), MERER (P.), NICOLET (L.). — Les ostéoarthrites baro-traumatiques. *Rev. Rhum.* 1955, *22*, 722.

[226] JAFFRES (R.), MERER (P.). — Considérations pathologiques sur l'ostéonécrose aseptique baro-traumatique de la hanche et sur la coxarthrose. *Rev. Rhum.* 1960, *27*, 467.

[227] JAFFRES (R.), CHERBUY (J.). — Un cas d'association d'ostéonécrose de la tête fémorale et de la tête humérale à une ostéomalacie secondaire à une pancréatite chronique. *Rev. Rhum.* 1974, *41*, 57.

[228] JOHANSSON (S.J.). — Prognostic assessment in fractured neck of femur using 131 I and venography. *Acta Chir. Scand.* 1962, *123*, 298.

[229] JOHNSON (R.W.). — A physiological study of the blood supply of the diaphysis. *J. Bone Joint Surg.* 1927, *9*, 153.

[230] JONES (J.P.), ENGELMAN (E.P.), STEINBACH (H.L.), MURRAY (W.R.), RAMBO (O.). — Fat embolisation as a possible mechanism producing avascular necrosis. *Arthritis Rheum.* 1965, *8*, 449.

[231] JONES (J.P.), ENGELMAN (E.P.), NAJARIAN (J.S.). — Systemic fat embolism after renal homotransplantation and treatment with corticosteroids. *N. Engl. J. Med.* 1965, *273*, 1453.

[232] JONES (J.P.), SAKOVICH (L.). — A technique for staining bone fat. *Arthritis Rheum.* 1965, *8*, 448.

[233] JONES (J.P.), SAKOVICH (L.). — Fat embolism of bone : a roentgenographic and histological investigation by use of intra-arterial lipiodol in rabbit. *J. Bone Joint Surg.* 1966, *48A*, 149.

[234] JONES (J.P.). — Alcoholism, hypercortisonism, fat embolism and osseous avascular necrosis. In « *Idio-*

pathic ischemic necrosis of the femoral head in adults », p. 112. Edited by W.M. Zinn, G. Thieme Publishers, Stuttgart 1971.

[235] JOUVE (A.), GÉRARD (R.), VAGUE (P.), ARNOUX (M.). — Les troubles métaboliques dans l'artériosclérose. Métabolisme des glucides et de l'acide urique. *Presse Méd.* 1966, *76,* 1665.

[236] JOWSEY (J.). — Age changes in human bones. *Clin. Orthop.* 1960, *17,* 210.

[237] JUDET (J.), JUDET (R.), LAGRANGE (J.), DUNOYER (J.). — A study of the arterial vascularisation of the femoral neck in the adult. *J. Bone Joint Surg.* 1955, *37A,* 663.

[238] JUDET (R.), LETOURNEL iE.). — *Les fractures du cotyle.* Masson et Cie, Paris 1974.

[239] JUNG (A.), WURTZ (J.P.), RANDRIANORIVO (P.). — Les modifications circulatoires artérielles dans les nécroses aseptiques de la hanche et dans l'épiphysiolyse. *Méd. Acad. Chir.* 1965, *91,* 489.

[240] JUNG (A.), KEHR (P.), HAMID (M.). — *Pathogénie artérielle de l'ostéonécrose primitive de la hanche.* Compte rendu du Ier Symposium International sur la Circulation Osseuse, Toulouse 1973, p. 193. Editions INSERM, Paris 1973.

[241] KABAKELE MBANDAKULU. — Contribution au diagnostic précoce de l'ostéonécrose drépanocytaire. *Thèse d'agrégation, Kinshasa, Zaïre,* 1972.

[242] KALSER (M.H.), IVY (H.K.), PREVSNER (J.), MARBARGER (J.P.), IVY (A.L.). — Changes in bone marrow pressure during exposure to simulated altitude. *J. Aviat. Med.* 1951, *22,* 286.

[243] KANE (W.J.), GRIM (E.). — Blood flow to bone : a quantitative method and its validation. *J. Bone Joint Surg.* 1966, *48A,* 1008.

[244] KECK (W.J.), KELLY (P.J.). — The effect of venous stasis on intraosseous pressure and longitudinal bone growth in the dog. *J. Bone Joint Surg.* 1965, *47A,* 539.

[245] KEMP (H.S.), BOLDERO (J.F.). — Radiological changes in Perthes disease. *Brit. J. Radiol.* 1966, *39,* 744.

[246] KERBOUL (M.), THOMINE (J.), POSTEL (M.), MERLE D'AUBIGNÉ (R.). — The conservative surgical treatment of idiopathic aseptic necrosis of the femoral Head. *J. Bone Joint Surg.* 1974, *56B,* 291.

[247] KERY (L.), VITZKELETY (T.), WOUTERS (H.W.). — Recherches expérimentales à propos de l'effet de la stase veineuse sur l'os, le cartilage et le disque intervertébral. *Rev. Chir. Orthop.* 1971, *57,* 99.

[248] KISTLER (G.H.). — Séquences of experimental bacterial infarction of the femur in rabbits. *Surg. Gynecol. Obstet.* 1935, *60,* 913.

[249] KISTLER (G.H.). — Formation of bone by the periosteum after experimental infarction by embolism of femur in rabbits. *Proc. Soc. Exp. Biol. Med.* 1934, *31,* 1218

[250] KISTLER (G.H.). — Sequences of experimental infarction of the femur in rabbits. *Arch. Surg.* 1934, *29,* 589.

[251] KISTLER (G.H.). — Effects of circulatory disturbances on the structure and healing of bone injuries of the head of the femur in young rabbits. *Arch. Surg.* 1936, *33,* 225.

[252] KITA (R.), WITOSZKA (N.M.), HOPKINS (R.W.), SIMEONE (F.A.). — Bone marrow, pressure and blood flow resistance in experimental hemorrhagic shock. *Amer. J. Surg.,* 1972, *123,* 380.

[253] KOCH (W.). — Ueber embolische knochennecrosen. *Arch. f. Klin., Chir.* 1879, *23,* 3315.

[254] KOK (G.). — Spontaneous fractures of the femoral neck after the intensive irradiation of carcinoma of the uterus. *Acta Radiol.* 1953, *40,* 511.

[255] KOLODNY (A.). — The periosteal blood supply and healing of fractures. *J. .Bone Joint Surg.,* 1923, *5,* 698.

[256] KOLODNY (A.). — The architecture and the blood supply of the head and neck of the femur and their importance in the pathology of fractures of the neck. *J. Bone Joint Surg.* 1925, *7,* 575.

[257] KOTTMEIER (J.L.). — Complications following radiation therapy in carcinoma of the cervix. *Amer. J. Obstet. Gynecol.* 1964, *88,* 854.

[258] KRAMER (D.W.), PERILSTEIN (P.K.), MEDEIROS (A. de). — Metabolic influences in vascular disorders with particular references to cholesterol determinations in comparison with uric acid level. *Angiology* 1958, *9,* 162.

[259] KUNTZ (A.), RICHINS (C.A.). — Innervation of the bone marrow. *J. Comp. Neurol.* 1945, 213.

[260] LAING (P.G.), FERGUSON (A.B.). — Radiosodium clearance rate as indicators of femoral head vascularity. *J. Bone Joint Surg.* 1959, *41 A,* 1409.

[261] LALANNE (C.M.), FAJBISOWICZ (S.). — Complications post-radiothérapiques dans le cancer du col utérin. Comparaison entre la radiothérapie classique et la télécobalthérapie associée à la curiethérapie intracavitaire. *Ann. Radiol.* 1965, *8 ,*697.

[262] LAMACHE (A.), BOUREL (M.), PAILHERET (P.), HOUSSET (J.), LENOIR (P.), BASSET-LACHRONIQUE. — Etudes histologiques et thérapeutiques au cours de la maladie de Gaucher. *Rev. Rhum.* 1956, *23,* 760.

[263] LANGER (K.). — Uber das Gefässystem der Röhrenknochen mit Beiträgen zur Kenntnis des Baues und der Entwicklung des Knochengewebes. *Deut. Akad. Wissen (Wien),* 1876, *36,* 1.

[264] LAPORTE (A.). — Pathogénie des ostéochondrites déformantes de l'enfant. *Bordeaux Chir.* 1933, *4,* 370.

[265] LARSEN (R.M.). — Intramedullary pressure with particular reference to massive diaphyseal bone necrosis. Experimental observations. *Ann. Surg.* 1938, *108,* 127.

[266] LARSON (R.L.), KELLY (P.S.), JANES (S.M.), PETERSON (L.F.A.). — Suppression of the periosteal and nutrient blood supply of the femora of dogs. *Clin. Orthop.* 1961, *21,* 217.

[267] LAURENT (J.). — Etude anatomo-pathologique et pathogénique de la nécrose de la tête fémorale chez l'adulte. *Thèse Médecine, Lyon* 1972.

[268] LAURENT (J.), MEUNIER (P.), COURFRON (P.), EDOUARD (C.), BERNARD (J.), VIGNON (G.). — Recherches sur la pathogénie des nécroses aseptiques de la tête fémorale. *Nouv. Presse Med.* 1973, *2,* 1755.

[269] LEJEUNE (E.), NOEL (G.), FRIES (D.), CREYSSEL (R.), MOREL (P.). — Drépanocytose et ostéonécrose de la hanche. *Rev. Rhum.* 1962, *29,* 564.

[270] LEJEUNE (E.), BOUVIER (M.), QUENEAU (P.), LAHNÈCHE (B.), RUITTON (P.). — *Exploration isotopique des ostéonécroses aseptiques épiphysaires par le Strontium 87 m.* Compte rendu du Ier Symposium International sur la Circulation Osseuse, Toulouse 1973, p. 225. Editions INSERM, Paris 1973.

[271] LEMOINE (A.). — Vascular changes after interference with the blood flow of the femoral head of the rabbit. *J. Bone Joint Surg.* 1957, *39B,* 763.

[272] LEQUESNE (M.), CLOAREC (M.), DE SÈZE (S.). — Le terrain biologique de la nécrose primitive de la tête fémorale, hyperuricémie, hyperlipidémie. Xe Congrès de la Ligue Internationale contre le Rhumatisme, Rome 1961. *Minerva Medica,* Turin 1961.

[273] LEQUESNE (M.). — L'algodystrophie de la hanche. *Presse Méd.* 1968, *76,* 973.

[274] LEQUESNE (M.), AMOUROUX (J.). — La coxarthrose destructrice rapide. *Presse Méd.* 1970, *78,* 1435.

[275] LEQUESNE (M.), CASSAN (P.). — Huit cas de nécrose de la tête fémorale par contusion. Vᵉ Conférence Internationale des maladies rhumatismales, Aix-les-Bains, juin 1972, vol. des Communications, p. 129.

[276] LEQUESNE (M.). — Les formes bien et assez bien tolérées de la nécrose ischémique de la tête fémorale de l'adulte. *Rev. Chir. Orthop.* 1973, *59*, suppl. 1, 43.

[277] LEQUESNE (M.), CAZALS (S.), SÈZE (S. de). — Le devenir fonctionnel de 61 cas de nécrose idiopathique de la tête fémorale. Déductions thérapeutiques. *Revue Rhum.* 1974, *41*, 157.

[278] LEQUESNE (M.), BENSASSON (M.), KAHN (M.F.), SÈZE (S. de). — Goutte, hyperuricémie et ostéonécrose de la tête fémorale. *Rev. Rhum.* 1975, *42*, 177.

[279] LERICHE (R.). — Recherches expérimentales sur le mécanisme de formation de l'ostéochondrite de la hanche. *Lyon Chir.* 1934, *31*, 610.

[280] LERICHE (R.). — *La chirurgie de la douleur.* Masson et Cie, éd., Paris, 1940, 1 vol.

[281] LIÈVRE (J.A.), CAMUS (J.P.), MAY (V.), BÉNICHOU (C.), MARCAIS (J.). — Stéatonécrose disséminée, ostéolyse ostéonécrotique et cancer du pancréas. *Bull. Soc. Méd. Hôp. Paris*, 1964, *115*, 755.

[282] LIGHTFOOT (R.W.), LOTKE (P.A.). — Osteonecrosis of metacarpal heads in systemic lupus erythematosus. Value of radio strontium scintimetry in differential diagnosis. *Arthritis Rheum.* 1972, *15*, 486.

[283] LILLY (A.D.), KELLY (P.J.). — Effects of venous ligation on bone remodeling in the canine tibia. *J. Bone Joint Surg.* 1970, *52A*, 515.

[284] LINDSAY (cité par MOURGUES).

[285] LINTON (P.). — On the different types of intracapsular fractures of the femoral neck. A surgical investigation of origin, Treatment, prognosis and complication in 365 cases. *Acta Chir. Scand.* 1944, suppl. 86.

[286] LOUYOT (P.), GAUCHER (A.), POUREL (J.), MONTET (Y.), TAMISIER (J.N.). — De quelques problèmes posés par l'ostéonécrose aseptique de la tête fémorale. *Rev. Rhum.* 1971, *38*, 201.

[287] MAC COLLUM (D.E.), MATHEWS (R.S.), PICKETT (P.T.). — Gout, hyperuricemia and aseptic necrosis of the femoral head. *Arthritis Rheum.* 1967, *10*, 295.

[288] MAC COLLUM (D.E.), MATHEWS (R.S.), O'NEIL (M.T.). — Aseptic necrosis of the femoral head. Associated diseases and evaluation of treatment. *South Med. J. (U.S.A.)*, 1970, *63*, 241.

[289] MAC COLLUM (D.E.), MATHEWS (R.S.), O'NEIL (M.T.), PICKETT (P.T.). — Gout, Hyperuricemia and aseptis necrosic of the femoral head. In « *Idiopathie ischemic necrosis of the femoral head in adults* », p. 133. Edited by W.M. Zinn, D. Thieme, publishers, Stuttgart 1971.

[290] MAC MASTER (P.E.), ROOME (N.W.). — The effect of sympathectomy and of venous stasis on bone repair. An experimental study. *J. Bone Joint Surg.*, 1934, *16*, 365-371.

[291] MAC PHERSON (A.), SCALES (J.T.), GORDON (L.). — A method of estimating qualitative changes of blood flow in bone. *J. Bone Joint Surg.* 1961, *43B*, 791.

[292] MAC PHERSON (A.), SHAW (N.E.). — Circulation of Bone. *Lancet* 1961, *1*, 1285.

[293] MAC WILLIAMS (C.A). — The periosteum in bone transplantations. *J. Amer. Med. Ass.* 1974, *62*, 346.

[294] MADRIGAL (J.J.), SCHWARTZ (S). — *Oxymétrie de l'os sous-chondral.* Compte rendu Iᵉʳ Symposium international sur la circulation osseuse, Toulouse 1973, p. 247. Edition INSERM, Paris 1973.

[295] MARNEFFE (R. de). — Recherches morphologiques et expérimentales sur la vascularisation osseuse. *Acta Chir. Belg.* 1951. *50*, 568.

[296] MARNEFFE (R. de). — Vascularisation des os. Incidences sur la pathologie de ce tissu. *Revue Rhum.* 1953, *20*, 114.

[297] MARCHI (E. de), SANTACROCE (A.), SOLARINO (G.B.). Su di une peculiare artropathia rarefacente dell' anca. *Arch. Putti* 1966, *21*, 62.

[298] MARCUS (N.D.), ENNEKING (W.F.), MASSAM (R.A.). — The silent hip in idiopathic aseptic necrosis. Treatment by bone grafting. *J. Bone Joint Surg.* 1973, *55A*, 1351.

[299] MARTEL (W.), SITTERLEY (B.H.). — Roentgenologic manifestations of osteonecrosis. *Amer. J. Roentgenol.* 1969, *106*, 509.

[300] MASSIAS (J.), CHATELIN (N.), COSTE (F.). — Données nosologiques sur les ostéonécroses primitives de la tête fémorale (50 cas). *Sem. Hôp.* 1962, *38*, 677.

[301] MATUMOTO (Y), MIZUNO (S.). — Rate of the blood flow in the femoral head. *Med. J. Osaka Univ.* 1966, *16*, 431.

[302] MAUVOISIN (F.), BERNARD (J.), GEMAIN (J.). — Aspects tomographiques des hanches chez un goutteux. *Rev. Rhum.* 1955, *22*, 336.

[303] MAY (V.), ARASTOFF (H.), GLOWINSKI (J.), GRIMBERT (T.) (cité par JAFFRES et CHERBUY).

[304] MAYER (S.), BERREBI (A.), MAYER (G.), OBERLING (F.), WAITZ (R.). — La pression intra-osseuse. I. Premiers résultats. *Pathol. Biol.* 1972, *20*, 757.

[305] MAZABRAUD (A.). — Necrose massive polaire supérieure de la tête fémorale. *Rev. Chir. Orthop.* 1973, 59, suppl. 1, 7.

[306] MEARY (R.), MONAT (Y). — Les coxarthroses post-radiothérapiques. *Rev. Chir. Orthop.* 1970, *56*, 287.

[307] MERIC (G.). — Confrontation anatomo-clinique à propos de 61 coxopathies. *Thèse Médecine Tououse*, 1974.

[308] MERLE D'AUBIGNÉ (R.), RAMADIER (J.O.). — *Traumatismes anciens : rachis, membres inférieurs.* Masson et Cie, Paris, 1959.

[309] MERLE D'AUBIGNÉ (R.), MAZABRAUD (A.), CAHEN (C.). — La nécrose idiopathique de la tête fémorale. Etude anatomo-pathologique et orientations thérapeutiques. *Sem. Hôp. Paris* 1963, *39*, 2773.

[310] MERLE D'AUBIGNÉ (R.), POSTEL (M.), MAZABRAUD (A.), MASSIAS (P.), GUEGEN (J.). — Idiopathic necrosis of the femoral head in adults. *J. Bone Joint Surg.* 1965, *47B*, 612.

[311] MERLE D'AUBIGNÉ (R.). — Cotation chiffrée de la fonction de la hanche. *Rev. Chir. Orthop.* 1970, *56*, 481.

[312] MICHELSEN (K.). — Pressure relationships in the bone marrow vascular bed. *Acta Physiol. Scand.* 1967, *71*, 16.

[313] MICHELSEN (K.). — Hemodynamics of the bone marrow circulation. *Acta physiol. Scand.* 1968, *73*, 264.

[314] MIELANTS (H.), VEYS (E.M.), DE WEERDT (A.). — Gout and its relation to lipid metabolism. I. Serum uric acid lipid and lipoprotein levels in gout. *Ann. Rheumat. Dis.* 1973, *32*, 501.

[315] MIELANTS (H.), VEYS (E.M.), DE WEERDT (A.). — Gout and its relation to lipid metabolism. II. Correlation between uric acid, lipid and lipoprotein levels in gout. *Ann. Rheumat. Dis.* 1973, *32*, 506.

[316] MIELANTS (H.), VEYS (E.M.), DE BUSSERE (A.), Van der JENGHT (J.). — Relations entre la nécrose avasculaire et le métabolisme des lipides et des purines. *Rev. Rhum.* 1975, *42*, 505.

[317] MILES (J.S.). — The use of intramedullary pressures in the early determination of aseptic necrosis of the femoral head. *J. Bone Joint Surg.* 1955, *37A*, 622.

[318] MILTNER (L.S.), HU (C.H.). — Osteochondritis of the head of the femur. An experimental study. *Arch. Surg.* 1933, *27*, 645.

[319] MILLET (J.P.). — Coxopathies ischémiques et nécroses de la tête fémorale chez les artéritiques des membres inférieurs. *Thèse Médecine, Toulouse,* 1974.

[320] MOORE (J.E.), CORBETT (J.F.). — Studies on the function to the periosteum. *Surg. Gynecol. Obstet.* 1914, *19*, 5.

[321] MORSCHER (E.), FRIDRICH (R.). — Detection and pathogenetic significance of venous stasis in idiopathic necrosis of the femoral head. « *Idiopathic ischemic necrosis of the femoral head in adults* ». Edited by W.M. Zinn. G. Thieme Publishers, Stuttgart 1971, p. 158.

[322] MOULONGUET (P.). — Ostéochondrite disséquante de la hanche (Maladie de Konig de la hanche). *Bull. Soc. Chir. Paris* 1932, *58*, 1471.

[323] MOURGUES (G. de), MACHENAUD (A.), FISCHER (L.), COMTET (J.J.). — Fractures du col et nécroses coxofémorales post-radiothérapiques. *Lyon Chirurgical,* 1970, *66*, 241.

[324] MUHEIN (G.), BOHNE (W.H.). — Prognosis in spontaneous osteonecrosis of the knee. *J. Bone Joint Surg.* 1970, *52B*, 605.

[325] MUHEIM (G.), CRUTCHLOW (W.P.). — 18 F and 85 Sr Scintimetry in the study of primary arthropathies. *Brit. J. Radiol.* 1971, *44*, 290.

[326] MUSSBICHLER (H.). — Arterial supply to the head of the femur. *Acta radiol. Stockholm* 1956, *46*, 533.

[327] MUSSBICHLER (H.). — Arteriographic investigation of the hip in adult human subjects. *Acta Orthop. Scand.* 1970, *39*, Sup. 132.

[328] MUSSBICHLER (H.). — Arteriographic findings in necrosis of the head of the femur after medial neck fracture. *Acta Orthop. Scand.* 1970, *41*, 77.

[329] MUSSBICHLER (H.). — Arteriographic findings in patients with degenerative osteo-arthritis of the hip. *Radiology* 1973, *107*, 21.

[330] MURRAY (W.R.). — Hip problems associated with organ transplants. *Clin. Orthop. Relat. Res.* 1973, *90*, 57.

[331] NAJEAN (Y.), CLÉMENT (F.). — Etude de la circulation médullaire chez l'homme par une technique isotopique. *Nouv. Rev. Fr. Hématol.* 1963, *3*, 92.

[332] NOEL (G.), COLLARD (M.). — Actualités médicales. Embolies graisseuses. *P.M.* 1970, *78*, 16-36.

[333] NUSSBAUM (A.). — Demonstration über die erzeugung von Osteochondrites juveniles und experimentellem wege. *Zentralbalt für Chir.* 1923, *50*, 937.

[334] OBERLING (F.), CAZENAVE (J.P.), WAITZ (R.). — Ultrastructure du tissu adipeux de la moelle hématopoïétique normale du lapin. *Path. Biol.* 1972, *20*, 337.

[334 bis] OBERLING (F.), CAZENAVE (J.P.), SICK (H.)., WAITZ (R.). — Les événements micro-vasculaires dans la moelle hématopoïétique au cours des myélo-scléroses expérimentales. *Nouv. Rev. Fr. d'Hémat.* 1973, *13*, 193.

[335] OTTOLENGHI (D.). — Sur les nerfs de la moelle des os. *Arch. Ital. Biol.* 1902, *37*, 73.

[336] PALAZZI (S.). — *Notre position dans le traitement de l'arthrose.* Congrès des Sociétés de la Méditerranée latine et du Moyen-Orient, Madrid, 21-23 avril 1976.

[337] PATTERSON (R.J.), BICKEL (W.H.), DAHLIN (D.C.). — Idiopathic avascular necrosis of the femoral head of the femur. *J. Bone Joint Surg.* 1964, *46A*, 267.

[338] PEARSE (H.E. Jr.). — An experimental study of arterial collateral circulation. *Ann. Surg.* 1928, *88*, 227.

[339] PEARSE (H.E. Jr.), MORTON (J.J.). — The influence of alterations in the circulation on the repair of bone. *J. Bone Joint Surg.* 1931, *13*, 68.

[340] PECK (W.S.). — Fractures of the femoral neck following pelvic irradiation. *Univ. Hosp. Bull.* 1939, *33*.

[341] PETRAKIS (N.L.), MASOUREDIS (S.P.), MILLER (P.). — The local blood flow in human bone marrow in leukemia and neoplastic diseases as determined by the clearance rate of radioidine 131 I. *J. Clin. Invest.* 1953, *32*, 952.

[342] PETRAKIS (N.L.). — Bone marrow pressure in leukemic and non leukemic patients. *J. Clin. Invest.* 1954, *35*, 27.

[343] PHEMISTER (D.B.). — Lesions of bones ad joints resulting from interruption of circulation. *Mt. Sinaï J. Med.* 1949, *15*, 55.

[344] PHEMISTER (D.B.). — Fractures of the neck of the femur. Dislocations of the hip and obscure vascular disturbances producing aseptic necrosis of the head of the femur. *Surg. Gyn. Obstet.* 1934, *59*, 415.

[345] PHEMISTER (D.B.). — Treatment of the necrotic head of the femur in adults. *J. Bone Joint Surg.* 1949, *31A*, 55.

[346] PHEMISTER (D.B.). — Infarctus unique ou multiple des os chez les adultes. Résultats d'une obstruction vasculaire aseptique. *Presse Méd.* 1950, *58*, 1430.

[347] PIETROGRANDE (V.), MASTROMARINO (R.). — Ostéopatie da prolungato trattamento cortisonico. *Ortop. Traumat.* 1957, *25*, 791.

[348] POLSTER (J.). — *Zur Hämodynamik des knochens.* Ferdinand Enke, Verlag, Stuttgart, 1970.

[349] POST (M.), SHOEMAKER (W.C.). — Method for measuring bone metabolism in vivo. *J. Bone Joint Surg.* 1964, *46A*, 111.

[350] POULETTY (J.), POULETTY (M.), CLOAREC (M.), LEQUESNE (M.). — Nécrose primitive de la tête fémorale et hyperlipidémie (à propos d'une observation). *Rhumatologie,* 1963, *15*, 221.

[351] PROCHE (C.). — Phlébites méconnues révélées par leurs complications. *Phlébologie* 1965, Juillet-Septembre.

[352] PUJOL (M.), TRAN (M.A.). — *Etude gazométrique du sang osseux trochantérien dans les coxopathies.* Compte rendu du Ier Symposium International sur la circulation osseuse, Toulouse 1973, p. 251. Editions INSERM, Paris 1973.

[353] RAVAULT (P.P.), WERTHEIMER (P.), LEJEUNE (E.), VOLLE (L.), Mme VANHEIM. — Aspects radiologiques des os et des articulations dans les artérites des membres inférieurs : étude de 1 000 dossiers d'aortographie. *Sem. Hôp. Paris* 1963, *114*, 1123.

[354] RAY (R.D.), AOUAD (R.), GALANTE (J.). — Isotope studies of circulatory dynamics of bone. 9e Congrès International de Chirurgie Orthopédique. Vienne 1963, p. 27.

[355] RAYNAL (L.), LÉVY (L.), LECRON (L.) et COLLARD (M.). — *Exploration fonctionnelle médullaire au niveau de l'extrémité proximale du fémur.* Compte rendu du Ier Symposium International sur la circulation osseuse. Toulouse 1973, p. 131. Ed. INSERM, Paris 1973.

[356] RAYNAL (L.), LÉVY (L.), LECRON (L.). — Etude préliminaire de la température au niveau de l'extrémité proximale du fémur. Compte rendu du Ier Symposium International sur la circulation osseuse. Toulouse, 1973, p. 143. Ed. INSERM, Paris, 1973.

[357] RÉNIER (J.C.), BRÉGEON (C.), BOASSON (M.), BESSON (J.), BILLABERT (C.). — Contribution à la connaissance de l'évolution de l'ostéonécrose primitive de la tête fémorale. Rev. Rhum. 1972, 39, 697.

[358] RICARD (R.), MOLE (L.). — Les fractures cervicales vraies récentes du col du fémur. Rev. Orthop. 1965, 51, 325.

[359] RHINELANDER (F.W.). — The normal microcirculation of diaphyseal cortex and its response to fracture. J. Bone Joint Surg. 1968, 50A, 784.

[360] RICCI (A.). — Relations pression artérielle et pression intra-osseuse. Mémoire pour le C.E.S. de Rhumatologie. Toulouse, 1973.

[361] RICHARDS (G.E.). — Osteochondritis dissecans. Amer. J. Roentgenol 1928, 19, 278.

[362] RIFFAT (G.), LAHNECHE (B.), DHEM (A.). — Exploration par le strontium isotopique. Compte rendu du Ier Symposium sur la circulation osseuse, Toulouse, 1973, p. 233. Editions INSERM, Paris, 1973.

[363] RINDFLEISCH (G.E.). — Ueber knochemark und Blutbildung. Arch. Mikr. Anat. 1880, 17, 1.

[364] ROCKOFF (S.D.), KAYE (H.), ARMSTRONG (J.D.), STANCEL (H.C.). — Effect of Increased bone blood flow on bone metabolism. Preliminary report. Invest. Radiol. 1969, 4, 230.

[365] ROGGE (C.W.L.). — Necrosis of the femoral head occuring in association with corticosteroïd medication Arch. Chir. Neerl. 1972, 24, 152.

[366] ROHNER (A.). — Contribution à l'étude histo-pathologique de la dystrophie de Südeck. Ann. Anat. Path. 1958, 3, n° 477, 511.

[367] RONDIER (J.), TRUFFERT (J.), LE GO (A.), BROUILHET (H.), SAPORTA (L.), DE GENNES (J.L.), DELBARRE (F.). — Goutte et Hyperlipidémies. Eur. J. Clin. Biol. Res. 1970, 15, 959.

[368] ROSINGH (G.H.), JAMES (J.). — Early phases of avascular necrosis of the femoral head in rabbits. J. Bone Joint Surg. 1969, 51B, 165.

[369] ROUANET (A.). — Phlébites, séquelles de phlébite et affections osseuses. Thèse Médecine, Toulouse, 1972.

[370] ROUSSILHON (J.P.), BOUYER (C.L.). — Le traitement des crises douloureuses osseuses de la drépanocytose. L'Afrique Méd. 1968, 64.

[371] ROUX (J.P.), KERBOUL (M.), POSTEL (M.). — Les coxarthroses à évolution rapide. Rev. Chir. Orthop. 1970, 56, 39.

[372] ROUX (H.), GASTAUT (A.), VOVAN (L.), SEDAT (P.), SERRATRICE (G.), RECORDIER (A.M.). — Exploration lipidique d'un groupe d'ostéonécroses. Rev. Rhum. 1974, 41, 393.

[373] RUBIN (P.), PRAHASAWAT (D.). — Characteristic bone lesions in post-irradiated carcinoma of the cervix. Metastase versus osteonecrosis. Radiology, 1961, 76, 703.

[374] RUDERMAN (M.), MC CARTY (D.J.). — Aseptic necrosis in systemics lupus erythematosus. Report of a case involving six joints. Arthritis Rheum. 1964, 7, 709.

[375] RUFFIE (R.), FOURNIE (A.), AYROLLES (Ch.), CUQ (P.). — Résultats de la phlébographie pertrochantérienne dans les ostéonécroses primitives de la tête fémorale chez l'adulte. Rev. Rhum. 1962, 29, 551.

[376] ROTES QUEROL (J.), MUNOZ GOMEZ (J.). — La Gota. Ediciones Toray, S.A., Barcelona, 1968.

[377] RUTISHAUSER (E.), ROUILLER (C.), VEYRAT (R.). — La vascularisation de l'os. Etat actuel de nos connaissances. Rev. Rhum. 1955, 22, 853.

[378] RUTISHAUSER (E.), RHONER (A.), HELD (D.). — Experimentelle Untersuchungen über die wirkung der ischämie auf den knochen und das mark. Virchow's Arch. Path. Anat. 1960, 333, 101.

[379] RUTISHAUSER (E.), TAILLARD (W.). — L'ischémie articulaire en pathologie humaine et expérimentale. La notion de pannus vasculaire. Rev. Chir. Orthop. 1966, 52, 197.

[380] RUTISHAUSER (E.), TAILLARD (W.), FRIEDLY (B.). — Experimental studies or the non-inflammatory vascular pannus. 3 rd Eur. Symp. on Calcified Tissues, Edit. Fleisch. Blackwood and M. Owen. Springer-Verlag, Berlin 1966.

[381] SABIN (F.R.). — Bone Marrow. Physiol. Rev. 1928, 8, 191.

[382] SALTER (R.B.), BELL (M.). — The pathogenesis of deformity in Legg-Perthes disease. An experimental investigation. J. Bone Joint Surg. 1968, 50B, 436.

[383] SCARPELLI (D.G.). — Fat necrosis of bone marrow in acute pancreatitis. Amer. J. Pathol. 1956, 32, 1077.

[384] SCHNEIDER (P.G.), BICK (J.A.). — Spontane Hüftkopfnekrose und trunksucht. Med. Klin. 1971, 66, 1694.

[385] SCHOBINGER (R.A.). — Intraosseous venography. Grune and Stratton. New York, 1960.

[386] SEMB (H.). — Bone marrow Blood flow studied by iodoantipyrine clearance technique. Surg. Gynec. Obstet. 1971, 133, 472.

[387] SEMB (H.). — Effect of vasoactive drugs on the bone marrow blood flow. Act. Orthop. Scand. 1971, 42, 10.

[388] SERRATRICE (G.), EISINGER (J.). — Innervation et circulation osseuse diaphysaire. Rev. Rhum. 1967, 34, 505.

[389] SERRE (H.), SIMON (L.). — Le facteur veineux dans l'ostéonécrose primitive de la tête fémorale chez l'adulte. Atti del X Congreso della lega internazionale contro il reumatismo. Roma, 1961, II. 388. Minerva Medica, Turin, 1961.

[390] SERRE (H.), SIMON (L.). — L'ostéonécrose de la tête fémorale chez l'adulte. I. Aspects symptomatiques. Rev. Rhum. 1962, 29, 527.

[391] SERRE (H.), SIMON (L.). — L'ostéonécrose de la tête fémorale chez l'adulte. II. Etiologie et pathogénie. Rev. Rhum. 1962, 29, 536.

[392] SERRE (H.), SANY (J.), SIMON (L.), FAYOLLE. — Evolution de l'ostéonécrose primitive de la tête fémorale chez l'adulte. Rhumatologie 1973, 25, 121.

[393] SEVITT (S.). — Avascular necrosis and revascularisation or the femoral head after intracapsular fractures. J. Bone Joint Surg. 1964, 46B, 270.

[394] SÈZE (S. de), WELFLING (J.), LEQUESNE (M.). — L'ostéonécrose primitive de la tête fémorale chez l'adulte (ostéochondrite disséquante de la hanche). Etude de 30 cas. Rev. Rhum. 1960, 27, 117.

[395] SÈZE (S. de), LEQUESNE (M.), WELFLING (J.), JURMAND (S.H.), D'ANGLEJEAN (G.). — Images de nécrose ischémique de la tête fémorale au cours des coxites et des coxarthroses. Rev. Rhum. 1962, 29, 554.

[396] SÈZE (S. de), RICKEWAERT (A.). — La goutte. Expansion Scientifique, Paris, 1960.

[397] SÈZE (S. de). — Un signe précoce de nécrose ischémique de la tête fémorale : une zone de condensation arciforme intra-céphalique. Sem. Hôp. Paris 1964, 40, 1080.

[398] SÈZE (S. de). — Ostéonécrose aseptique primitive de la tête fémorale. *J. Belge Rhumatol. Med. Phys.* 1972, *27*, 143.

[399] SHAW (N.E.). — Observations on the intra-medullary blood flow and marrow pressure in bone. *Clin. Sci.* 1963, *24*, 311.

[400] SHAW (N.E.). — Observations on the physiology of the circulation in bones. *Ann. Roy. Coll. Surg. Engl.* 1964, *35*, 214.

[401] SHAW (N.E.). — *The influence of muscle blood flow on the circulation in bones.* Third European Symposium on calcified tissu. Springer-Verlag, Berlin, 1966.

[402] SHERMAN (M. S.), SELAKOVICH (W. G.). — Bone changes in chronic circulatory insufficiency. A histological study. *J. Bone Joint Surg.* 1957, *39A*, 892.

[403] SHERMAN (M.S.). — Pathogenesis of desintegration of the hip in sickle cell anemia. *South. Med. Journal* 1959, *52*, 632.

[404] SHERMAN (M.S.). — The nerves of bone. *J. Bone Joint Surg.* 1963, *45A*, 522.

[405] SHIM (S.S.). — The effect of epinephrine on bone blood flow in dogs and rabbits. *M. Sc. Thesis University of British Columbia,* 1963.

[406] SHIM (S.S.), COPP (D.H.), PATTERSON (F.P.). — An indirect method of bone blood flow measurement based on the bone clearance of a circulatory bone seeking radioisotope. *J. Bone Joint Surg.* 1867, *49A*, 693.

[407] SHIM (S.S.), PATTERSON (F.P.). — A direct method of qualitative study of bone blood circulation. *Surg. Gyn. Obst.* 1967, *125*, 261.

[408] SHIM (S.S.). — Physiology of blood circulation of bone. *J. Bone Joint Surg.* 1968, *50A*, 812.

[409] SHIM (S.S.), MOKKMAVESA (S.), MAC PHERSON (G.D.), SCHWEIGER (J.F.). — Bone and skeletal blood flow in man measured by a radioisotopic method. *Can. J. Surg.* 1971, *14*, 38.

[410] SHIM (S.S.), PATTERSON (F.P.), COOP (D.H.). — Blood flow through different regions of long bone measured by a bone-seeking radioisotope method. *Surg. Gynecol. Obstet.* 1971, *132*, 58.

[411] SHIM (S.S.), HAWK (H.E.), YU (W.Y.). — The relation-ship between blood flow and bone marrow cavity pressure of bone. *Surg. Gynecol. Obstet.* 1972, *135*, 353.

[412] SHIM (S.S.). — *Physiology of bone blood flow.* Compte rendu du Ier Symposium sur la circulation osseuse, Toulouse, 1973. Editions INSERM, Paris, 1973, p. 41.

[413] SICK (H.), OBERLING (F.), CAZENAVE (J.), WAITZ (R.). — La micro-vascularisation de la moelle osseuse du fémur du lapin. *Arch. Anat. Hist. Embr. Norm. Exp.* 1971, *45*, 59.

[414] SIEGLING (J.A.). — Dans la discussion du travail, de CHUNG et RALSTON (voir réf. 107).

[415] SIEMSEN (T.N.), BROOK (J.), MEISTER (L.). — Lupus erythemateux and avascular bone necrosis : a clinical study of three cases and review of the litterature. *Arthritis Rhum.* 1962, *5*, 492.

[416] SILER (T.N.), MATHEWS (W.H.). — Atheromatous embolization to the proximal end or the femur in man and experimental animals. *Can. J. Surg.* 1963, *6*, 511.

[417] SIMON (L.). — Nécrose primitive de la tête fémorale chez l'adulte. *Thèse Médecine, Montpellier,* 1960.

[418] SIMON (L.), BERTRAND (L.), MICHEL (H.), BLOTMAN (F.), CLAUSTRE (J.). — Ostéonécrose, éthylisme et stéatose hépatique. *Rev. Rhum.* 1975, *42*, 103.

[419] SINGH (M.), BROOKES (M.). — Bone growth and blood flow after experimental venous ligation. *J. Anat.* 1971, *108*, 315.

[420] SOLOMON (L.). — Alcohol, steroïds and idiopathic necrosis of the femoral head. *J. Bone Joint Surg.* 1970. *52B*, 175.

[421] SOLOMON (L.). — Aseptic necrosis of the femoral head in iron overload osteoporosis. « R » 1974, *4*, 457.

[422] SPALTEHOLTZ (W.). — *Über das Durchsischtig Machen von manschlichen und tierischen Praparaten Nebst Anhang Über Knochen Farbung.* Leipzig, Hirzel, 1911.

[423] STEIN (A.H.), MORGAN (H.C.), REYNOLDS (F.C.). — Variations in normal bone marrow pressures. *J. Bone Joint. Surg.* 1957, *39A*, 1129.

[424] STEIN (A.H.), MORGAN (H.C.), PORRAS (R.F.). — The effect of pressor and depressor drugs on intramedullary bone marrow pressure. *J. Bone Joint Surg.* 1958, *40A*, 1103.

[425] STEIN (A.H.), WHITE (N.B.). — The effect of adrenalin on the bone blood flow to a long bone. *Surg. Gynecol. Obstet.* 1966, *121*, 55.

[426] STEINBERG (B.). — Systemic nodular panniculitis. *Amer. J. Path.* 1953, T. *29*, 1059.

[427] STEVENS (J.), RAY (R.D.). — An experimental comparaison of living and dead bone in rats. Uptake of radioactives isotopes. *J. Bone Joint. Surg.* 1967, *49B*, 154.

[428] STEWART (W.J.), MILFORD (L.W.). — Fracture dislocation of the hip. An end-result study. *J. Bone Joint. Surg.* 1954, *36A*, 315.

[429] STEWART (W.J.). — Aseptic necrosis of the head of the femur following traumatic dislocation of the hip joint. *J. Bone Joint. Surg.* 1933, *15*, 413.

[430] STREDA (A.), KRALOVA (M.), BREMOVA (A.). — Osteonecrosis of the large joints in rheumatoid arthritis. *Cas. Lek. Ces.* 1966, *105*, 370.

[431] STREDA (A.). — Participation of osteonecrosis in the developpment of severe coxarthrosis. *Acta Univ. Carol. Med. Monogr. Tchocosl.* 1971, *46*, 166.

[432] SUSSE (H.J.), AURIG (G.). — Uber die transossale venographie. *Zentralbl. F. Chir.* 1954, *79*, 596.

[433] SUSSE (H.J.). — Gefahren und technick der osteomyelographie und transossalen venographie. *Fortschr. Geburtsh. Roentgenstrahl.* 1956, *85*, 181.

[434] SUTTON (R.D.), BENEDEK (T.G.), EDMARDS (G.A.). — Aseptic bone necrosis and corticosteroïd therapy. *Arch. Intern. Med.* 1963, *112*, 594.

[435] TANAKA (K.R.), CLIFFORD (G.O.), AXELROD (A.R.). — Sickle cell anemia with aseptic necrosis of the femoral head. *Blood.* 1956, *11*, 998.

[436] THOMINE (J.M.). — L'arthroplastie par cupule ajustée pour nécrose de la tête fémorale. *Rev. Chir. Orthop.* 1973, Suppl. 1, 61.

[437] TILLING (G.). — The vascular anatomy of long bones : a radiological and histological study. *Acta Radiol. Stockh.* 1958, suppl. 161, I. *Thèse Méd. Uppsala* 1958.

[438] TOCANTINS (L.M.), O'NEILL (J.F.). — Infusions of blood and other fluids into the general circulation via the bone marrow : technique and results. *Surg. Gyn. Obstet.* 1944, *73*, 281.

[439] TOCANTINS (L.M.). — Rapid absorption of substances injected into the bone marrow. *Proc. Soc. Exp. Biol. Med.* 1940, *45*, 782.

[440] TRIAS (A.), BOULLERET (J.). — *Rôle de la circulation du périoste dans la circulation de l'os. La circulation osseuse.* Compte rendu du Ier Symposium sur la circulation osseuse. Toulouse, 1973, p. 21. Editions INSERM, Paris 1973.

[441] TRIAS (A.) et FÉRY (A.). — (Communication orale).

[442] TROJAN (E.). — Luxations et fractures-luxations traumatiques de la hanche à l'exception des fractures-luxations avec enfoncement du cotyle. *Rev. Chir. Orthop.* 1959, *45*, 469.

[443] TROTTMAN (N.M.), KELLY (W.D.). — The effect of sympathectomy on blood flow to bone. *J. Amer. Med. Ass.* 1963, *183*, 121.

[444] TRUETA (J.), HARRISSON (M.H.M.). — The normal vascular anatomy of the femoral head in adult men. *J. Bone Joint Surg.* 1953, *35B*, 442.

[445] TRUETA (J.). — The normal vascular anatomy of the femoral head during growth. *J. Bone Joint. Surg.* 1957, *39B*, 358.

[446] TRUETA (J.), TRIAS (A.). — The vascular contribution to osteogenesis. *J. Bone Joint Surg.* 1961, *43B*, 800.

[447] TRUETA (J.), CALADIAS (A.N.). — A study of the blood supply of the long bones. *Surg. Gynecol. Obstet.* 1964, *118*, 485.

[448] TUCKER (F.R.). — The use of radioactive phosphorus in the diagnosis of avascular necrosis of the femoral head. *J. Bone Joint. Surg.* 1950, *32B*, 100.

[449] VARIOT (G.), RÉMY (C.H.). — Sur les nerfs de la moelle des os. *J. Anat.* 1880, *16*, 273.

[450] VASEY (H.). — *Idiopathic necrosis of the femoral heads and systemic lupus erythematosus.* G. Thieme, Publishers, 1971, *170*.

[451] VELAYOS (E.E.), LEIDHOLT (J.B.D.), SMYTH (C.J.). Arthropathy associated with steroïd therapy. *Ann. Intern. Med.* 1966, *64*, 759.

[452] VIEULES (P.J.). — Contribution à l'étude du traitement de l'ostéonécrose de la tête fémorale : le greffon pédiculé antérieur. *Thèse Médecine Toulouse,* 1973.

[453] VIGNON (G.), FALCONNET (M.), CHAPUY (P.). — *Ostéonécroses aseptiques épiphysaires idiopathiques de l'adulte.* Encyclopédie médico-chirurgicale. Appareil locomoteur. 57e Cahier spécialisé, 1970, *41*.

[454] VIGNON (G.), MEUNIER (P.). — Réflexions sur la pathogénie de l'ostéonécrose primitive de la tête fémorale. L'hypothèse de la fracture de fatigue sous-chondrale. *Nouv. Presse Med.* 1973, *2*, 1751.

[455] VITZKELETY (T.), KERY (L.). — Uber den perivasculärem lymphkreislang des knochens. *Anat. Anz.* 1969, *124*, 37.

[456] VIZKELETY (T.), WOUTERS (H.W.). — Recherches expérimentales sur le développement de la nécrose aseptique ischémique de l'os. *Rev. Chir. Orthop.* 1969, *55*, 603.

[457] VIZKELETY (T.). — *Les lymphatiques de l'os.* Compte rendu du Ier Symposium sur la circulation osseuse, Toulouse, 1973, p. 31. Editions INSERM, Paris, 1973.

[458] VOLLE (L.). — L'ostéonécrose idiopathique de la tête fémorale chez l'adulte (à propos de 52 observations). *Thèse Médecine, Lyon,* 1963.

[459] WALSH (D.). — Deep tissue traumatism from roentgen exposure. *Brit. J. Med.* 1897, *II*.

[460] WEINMAN (D.T.), KELLY (P.J.), OWEN (C.A.), ORVIS (A.L.). — Skeletal clearance of Ca 47 and Sr 85 and skeletal blood flow in dogs. *Mayo Clin. Proc.* 1963, *38*, 559.

[461] WEISS (R.), ROOT (W.S.). — Innervation of the vessels of the marrow cavity of certain bones. *Amer. J. Physiol* 1959, *197*, 1255.

[462] WELFLING (J.). — Nécrose aseptique des os. *Thèse Médecine, Paris,* 1951.

[463] WELFLING (J.). — Considérations sur l'étiologie des nécroses dites primitives de la tête fémorale chez l'adulte. *Press. Med.* 1966, *74*, 2091.

[464] WERTHEIMER (P.), FROMENT (R.), DESCOTTES (J.), SITE (J.), WEBER (B.). — Exiguïté artérielle constitutionnelle. Facteur probable de thrombo-artériose du type Buerger. *Press. Med.* 1964, *72*, 2259.

[465] WHITE (N.B.), TER-POGOSSIAN (M.M.), STEIN (A.H.). — A method to determine the rate of blood flow in long bone and selected soft tissues. *Surg. Gynecol. Obstet.* 1964, *119*, 535.

[466] WILKES (C.H.), VISSCHER (M.B.). — Some physiological aspects of bone marrow pressure. *J. Bone Joint. Surg.* 1975, *57A*, 49.

[467] WOODHOUSE (C.F.). — An instrument for the measurement of oxygen tension in bone. *J. Bone Joint. Surg.* 1961, *32A*, 819.

[468] WOODHOUSE (C.F.). — Anoxia of the femoral head. *Surgery* 1962, *52*, 55.

[469] WOODHOUSE (C.F.). — Dynamic influences of vascular occlusion affecting the development of avascular necrosis of the femoral head. *Clin. Orthop.* 1964, *32*, 119.

[470] YOFFEY (J.M.). — Structural peculiarities of the blood vessels of bone marrow. *Bibl. Anat. (Basel),* 1965, *7*, 298.

[471] ZAHIR (A.), FREEMAN (M.A.R.). — Cartilage changes following a single episode of infarction of the capital femoral epiphyses in the dog. *J. Bone Joint. Surg.* 1972, *54A*, 125.

[472] ZEMANSKY (A.P.), LIPPMANN (R.K.). — The importance of the vessels in the round ligament to the head of the femur during the period of growth and their possible relationship to Perthe's disease. *Surg. Gynecol. Obstet.* 1929, *48*, 461.

[473] ZINN (W.M.). — *Idiopathic ischemic necrosis of the femoral head in adults. II. Clinical pictures and laboratory findings,* Stuttgart 1973. G. Thieme Publishers, p. 9.

INDEX